A Clinical Guide to Inherited Metabolic Diseases

Third Edition

Joe T. R. Clarke, MD, PhD, FRCPC

Division of Clinical & Metabolic Genetics, Hospital for Sick Children,
555 University Avenue, Toronto, Ontario M5G 1X8 CANADA

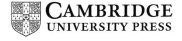
CAMBRIDGE
UNIVERSITY PRESS

CAMBRIDGE UNIVERSITY PRESS
Cambridge, New York, Melbourne, Madrid, Cape Town, Singapore, São Paulo

Cambridge University Press
The Edinburgh Building, Cambridge CB2 2RU, UK

Published in the United States of America by Cambridge University Press, New York

www.cambridge.org
Information on this title: www.cambridge.org/9780521614993

First published 1996
Second edition 2002
Third edition 2006

Printed in the United Kingdom at the University Press, Cambridge

A catalogue record for this publication is available from the British Library

ISBN-13 978-0-521-61499-3 paperback
ISBN-10 0-521-61499-6 paperback

A Clinical Guide to Inherited Metabolic Diseases

This user-friendly clinical handbook provides a clear and concise overview of how to go about recognizing and diagnosing inherited metabolic diseases. The reader is led through the diagnostic process from the identification of those features of an illness suggesting that it might be metabolic through the selection of appropriate laboratory investigation to a final diagnosis.

The book is organized into chapters according to the most prominent presenting problem of patients with inherited metabolic diseases: neurologic, hepatic, cardiac, metabolic acidosis, dysmorphism, and acute catastrophic illness in the newborn. It also includes chapters on general principles, laboratory investigation, neonatal screening, and the principles of treatment.

This new edition includes much greater depth on mitochondrial disease and congenital disorders of glycosylation. The chapters on neurological syndrome and newborn screening are greatly expanded, as are those on laboratory investigation and treatment, to take account of the very latest technological developments.

Dr J. T. R. Clarke is Professor of Paediatrics at the University of Toronto and a Senior Associate Scientist in the Research Institute of the Hospital for Sick Children, as well as continuing Head of the Genetic Metabolic Diseases Program of the Hospital. He is a Fellow of the Royal College of Physicians of Canada and the Canadian College of Medical Geneticists. He has won awards for postgraduate paediatric teaching and for excellence in paediatric medical care. He is consulted extensively by government and industry on matters relating to the management of inherited metabolic diseases and newborn screening. He is internationally respected for his expertise in the general area of metabolic genetics and is widely sought as a speaker and educator in this field. He has given over 100 invited lectures on inherited metabolic diseases in countries around the globe.

Contents

Reviews of first edition

'should be read thoroughly by any pediatric resident, genetic resident, or clinical fellow caring for patients with metabolic disorders'

American Journal of Medical Genetics

'In short, this is an excellent guide to metabolic disease; it represents good value for money and, I suspect, will be more likely found in the owner's pocket rather than on the shelf. It is recommended not only to the 'busy physician' and trainee, but to all those with an interest in metabolic disease.'

Journal of Inherited Metabolic Disease

'The writing is lucid, direct and salted with personal observations. Clarke's teaching skills shine forth from each page . . . It succeeds admirably, effectively demystifying the anxiety-provoking world of inherited biochemical illness.'

Canadian Medical Association Journal

'J. T. R. Clarke has performed the amazing feat of distilling practical knowledge about the diagnosis of metabolic diseases into a small, yet ultimately pragmatic 280-page clinical guide . . . On the whole, I found this to be an amazing book which contains a vast amount of information presented in a concise, logical and well-organized fashion . . . I would recommend this book wholeheartedly to anyone involved in the diagnosis of inherited metabolic diseases.'

Journal of Genetic Counseling

Reviews of second edition

'Dr Clarke's enthusiasm and erudition are evident on every page of this book.'

Archives of Diseases of Childhood

'An excellent book for physicians who find inherited metabolic diseases intimidating . . . The information is presented in such a clear and simple fashion that few people would find this book difficult to read . . . Clarke teaches a complex subject in a simple but complete manner.'

Canadian Medical Association Journal

'This book's strength lies in its simple straightforward clinical approach to this difficult area of medicine.'

Doctors.net.uk

'If your clinical work brings you into contact with patients who may be hiding an inherited metabolic disease, Clarke's *Guide* is clearly for you.'

Journal of the Royal Society of Medicine

'To guide the reader in this assessment, a compact volume such as has been written by Dr Clarke is invaluable. Dr Clarke has succeeded in providing the reader with a user-friendly, inexpensive book that is up to date, and provides directions for further reading.'

European Journal of Paediatric Neurology

List of tables

List of figures

Preface

In this enlarged third edition of *A Clinical Guide to Inherited Metabolic Diseases*, I have preserved the basic, clinical approach first developed in the first edition of the book. However, advances in many fields over the past 5 years have made it necessary to add significantly in some areas, such as mitochondrial disorders and the congenital disorders of glycosylation. The challenge continues to be to find ways to translate discoveries made in research laboratories, which understandably focus on biochemical and genetic principles, into a clinically relevant format organized in a way to facilitate the early recognition of the disorders by clinicians. For example, inherited defects in mitochondrial electron transport (ETC) may present as neurological syndromes (encephalopathy, myopathy, movement disorder), cardiac syndrome (cardiomyopathy), hepatic syndrome, metabolic acidosis, or catastrophic illness in the newborn. The challenge has been to develop and present a clinical approach to mitochondrial ETC defects without being unnecessarily repetitious. The chapter on 'Laboratory investigation' is important in this respect because it provides an approach to the transition in thinking between the recognition of various clinical signs and the biochemical and genetic investigation of possible causes of disease. By the very nature of laboratory investigation, it is also organized biochemically, which draws together the consideration of all those disorders presented in various different chapters as clinical problems. The book should, therefore, be viewed as a series of clinical chapters, which overlap in terms of biochemical and genetic organization and content in the chapter on 'Laboratory investigation'. It follows that reference to any topic presented in a clinical chapter ought to be considered also in the light of the appropriate section on the chapter on 'Laboratory investigation' – they go together.

I have added significantly to the chapter, 'Neurologic syndrome', as new mechanisms of disease are discovered, such as inherited disorders of neurotransmitter metabolism and the channelopathies. The chapter on 'Newborn screening' has also been expanded as this field grows, along with experience with the application of tandem mass spectrometry as a screening technology. The chapters on 'Laboratory investigation' and 'Treatment' have had to be modified significantly in the light of new technological developments in these areas. I have also added to and updated the bibliographies at the end of each chapter, though the number of publications cited is still a tiny fraction of the literature on the subjects discussed. In many cases, I have sacrificed some outstanding articles focusing on advances in basic research for articles I thought would be more relevant to clinicians dealing daily with patient problems.

For intellectual support and stimulation during the preparation of this edition of *A Clinical Guide*, I am again grateful to my colleagues, Annette Feigenbaum, Susan Blaser, Bill Hanley, Brian Robinson, John Callahan, and Eve Roberts, and to the people who slave away in the diagnostic labs, all at the Hospital for Sick Children. In addition, however, I owe a great deal to colleagues in other centers, scattered throughout the world, who read the second edition and suggested some changes which I am convinced will make this edition even better. I owe Charles Scriver special thanks for comments on the last edition of this book which have resulted in some important additions to the current edition. As usual, I am indebted to the large number of residents and fellows who rotated through the genetic metabolic service at the Hospital, stimulating me to think clearly about the clinical problems we tackled together. Gustavo Maegawa, from Brazil, Nouriya Al-Sannaa, now in Dhahran, Saudi Arabia, Aneal Khan, now at McMaster University in Hamilton, Pranesh Chakraborty, who is now at the Children's Hospital of Eastern Ontario, Nicola Poplawski, at the Adelaide Women's and Children's Hospital in Adelaide, and Julian Raiman, now at Guy's Hospital in London, merit special mention in this regard.

Many colleagues provided material for the figures in the book: Jim Phillips provided the electron micrographs of the liver, and Venita Jay supplied the electron micrographs of conjunctival epithelium and the photomicrograph of muscle. The photographs of patients with carbohydrate-deficient glycoprotein syndrome (now called congenital disorders of glycosylation) and mevalonic aciduria were provided by Jaak Jaiken and Georg Hoffmann, respectively. Jaak Jaiken also supplied the photograph of the isoelectric focusing of plasma transferrin shown in Chapter 6. Joe Alroy kindly provided the original electron micrographs showing the changes in skin in patients with lysosomal disorders appearing in Chapter 9. Margaret Nowaczyk and Chitra Prasad provided photographs of patients with Smith-Lemli-Opitz syndrome (Chapter 6), and Eric Shoubridge provided the photograph of the blue native PAGE in Chapter 9. I am again particularly grateful to Susan Blaser for the neuroimaging studies reproduced in Chapter 2 on 'Neurologic syndrome'.

Peter Silver, at Cambridge University Press, continued to provide moral and technical support during the preparation of the book. And once again, my wife, Cathy, encouraged and supported me throughout the project, often at great personal cost.

General principles

Introduction

In his 1908 address to the Royal College of Physicians of London, Sir Archibald Garrod (1857–1936) coined the expression inborn error of metabolism to describe a group of disorders – alkaptonuria, benign pentosuria, albinism, and cystinuria – which ". . . apparently result from failure of some step or other in the series of chemical changes which constitute metabolism".[1] He noted that each was present at birth, persisted throughout life, was relatively benign and not significantly affected by treatment; and that each was transmitted as a recessive trait within families in a way predictable by Mendel's laws of inheritance. In fact, alkaptonuria was the first example of Mendelian recessive inheritance to be recognized as such in humans. Garrod concluded, from the results of experiments on the effects of feeding phenylalanine and various putative intermediates of phenylalanine metabolism on homogentisic acid excretion by patients with the condition, that homogentisic acid is an intermediate in the normal metabolism of phenylalanine and tyrosine. Moreover, he observed that the specific defect was in the oxidation of homogentisic acid. La Du subsequently confirmed this 50 years later by demonstrating profound deficiency of homogentisic acid oxidase in a biopsy specimen of liver from a patient with alkaptonuria.[2]

Following Følling's discovery of phenylketonuria (PKU) in 1934, Garrod's concept underwent a major change, particularly with respect to its relationship with disease. Like alkaptonuria, PKU was shown to be caused by a recessively inherited point defect in metabolism, in the conversion of phenylalanine to tyrosine in the liver. However, unlike Garrod's original four inborn errors of metabolism, PKU was far from benign – it was associated with a particularly severe form of mental retardation. Moreover, although the underlying metabolic defect was 'inborn' and

[1] H. Harris, *Garrod's inborn errors of metabolism*, London: Oxford University Press, 1963, p. 13.
[2] La Du, B. N., Zannoni, V. G., Laster, L. & Seegmiller, J. E. (1958). The nature of the defect in tyrosine metabolism in alcaptonuria. *Journal of Biological Chemistry*, **230**, 251–60.

persisted throughout life, the associated mental retardation could be prevented by treatment with dietary phenylalanine restriction.

Harry Harris (1919–1994) applied the technique of starch gel electrophoresis, described originally by Smithies in 1955, to the demonstration of a large number of protein polymorphisms in humans, confirming the vast biochemical genetic diversity predicted by Garrod. He went on to show how the principle of one gene-one polypeptide chain applied to Garrod's inborn errors of metabolism, which he reviewed in some detail in his highly successful book, *The Principles of Human Biochemical Genetics*[3], published originally in 1970.

The discovery of PKU sparked the search for other clinically significant inborn errors of metabolism. The most recent edition of *The Metabolic and Molecular Bases of Inherited Disease*[4], edited by Charles Scriver and his colleagues, reports that the number of diseases in humans known to be attributable to inherited point defects in metabolism now exceeds 500. While the diseases are individually rare, they collectively account for a significant proportion of illness, particularly in children. They present clinically in a wide variety of ways, involving virtually any organ or tissue of the body, and accurate diagnosis is important both for treatment and for the prevention of disease in other family members.

While inborn errors of metabolism are a well-known cause of disease in children, their contribution to disease in adults is less well appreciated. This may be due in part to the lethal nature of many of the diseases, which often cause death before the patient reaches adulthood. However, owing primarily to advances in diagnostic technology, especially molecular genetics, a rapidly growing list of inherited metabolic diseases presenting in adulthood is emerging. Some of these, such as Scheie disease (MPS IS), are milder variants of diseases caused by the same enzyme deficiency that commonly causes death in childhood. Others, such as classical hemochromatosis, almost never present in childhood, though the disease in adults may be severe.

The purpose of this book is to provide a framework of principles to help clinicians recognize when an illness might be caused by an inborn error of metabolism. It presents a problem-oriented clinical approach to determining the type of metabolic defect involved and what investigation is needed to establish a specific diagnosis.

Some general metabolic concepts

Metabolism is the sum total of all the chemical reactions constituting the continuing process of breakdown and renewal of the tissues of the body. Enzymes play an

---

[3] H. Harris, *The Principles of Human Biochemical Genetics*, Amsterdam: North-Holland Publishing, 1970.
[4] Scriver, C. R., Beaudet, A. L., Sly, W. S. & Valle D. (eds). (2001). *The Metabolic and Molecular Bases of Inherited Disease*, 8th ed. New York: McGraw-Hill.

indispensable role in facilitating the process by serving as catalysts in the conversion of one chemical (metabolite) to another, often extracting the energy required for the reaction from a suitable high-energy source, such as ATP. All enzymes have at least two types of physico-chemical domains: one or more substrate-binding domains, and at least one catalytic domain. Mutations might affect enzyme activity by affecting the steady-state amount of enzyme protein because of a defect in enzyme production or as a result of abnormally rapid breakdown of the mutant protein. Deletions and insertions causing shifts in the reading frame, mutations to premature stop codons, and mutations affecting the processing of the primary RNA transcript all affect enzyme activity by decreasing the production of active enzyme protein. In contrast, studies on the turnover of mutant enzyme proteins have shown that many single amino acid substitutions resulting from single base substitutions cause deficiency of enzyme activity by causing abnormal folding of the nascent enzyme polypeptide which in turn causes aggregation and premature destruction of the polypeptide before it leaves the endoplasmic reticulum. This discovery is of signal importance to the development of new and specific treatments for diseases caused by inborn errors of metabolism because the stability of many mutant enzyme proteins, and therefore the activity of the enzymes, is enhanced by exposure to 'chemical chaperones'. These are relatively simple and inexpensive chemicals, in some cases substrate analogues, that bind to the mutant enzyme protein, preventing premature degradation. Mutations might also impair the activity of the enzyme without affecting the amount of enzyme protein by specifically impairing the catalytic properties of the protein. Of all the possible mechanisms of enzyme deficiency caused by mutation, this is the most uncommon.

The rapid transport of metabolites across cellular and subcellular membranes is facilitated in many cases by specific transport proteins that function like enzymes. This means that the process is susceptible to genetic mutations affecting the amount or function of the transporter in exactly the same way that mutation affects the activities of enzymes, and with similar consequences.

The coding sequences of most structural genes are comprised of at least a few thousand nucleotides, and the potential for mutation-generated variations in nucleotide sequence is vast. In the same way, the effects of mutation also vary tremendously. At one extreme, some mutations may totally disrupt the production of any gene product, resulting in severe disease. By contrast, other mutations might have no effect whatsoever apart from a functionally silent change in the nucleotide sequence of the gene. The relationship between genotype and disease phenotype is complex. Severe mutations, such as deletions or insertions, are generally associated with clinically severe disease, and the disease phenotype among different affected individuals tends to be similar. Structurally more subtle mutations, such

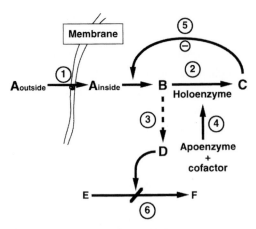

Figure 1.1   The primary consequences of inborn errors of metabolism.
The figure shows diagrammatically the various possible mutation-sensitive defects affecting the compartmentalization and metabolism of Compound A. **1**, transporter-mediated movement of A from one compartment to another; **2**, defect in the conversion of B to C; **3**, increased conversion of B to D caused by accumulation of B; **4**, defect in the interaction between an apoenzyme and an obligatory cofactor; **5**, decreased feedback inhibition of the conversion of A_{in} to B as a result of deficiency of C; and **6**, secondary inhibition of the conversion of E to F caused by accumulation of D.

as those resulting in single amino acid substitutions, are often associated with milder disease phenotypes. Moreover, the disease phenotype often varies markedly between different affected individuals, even within the same family, a reminder that the expression of any genetic information, including disease-causing mutations, is influenced by other genes (gene-gene interactions) and by environmental factors (gene-environment interactions).

Disease results from point defects in metabolism

The signs and symptoms of disease in patients with inborn errors of metabolism are the result of metabolic disturbances caused by deficiency of some catalytic or transport protein. Figure 1.1 shows schematically the relationship between various types of defects and their pathophysiologically and diagnostically important consequences.

Accumulation of substrate

Accumulation of the substrate of a mutant enzyme is an important cause of disease in many inborn errors of metabolism, particularly those involving strictly degradative processes. Some examples are shown in Table 1.1.

Table 1.1 Some examples of inborn errors of metabolism in which symptoms of disease are the result of substrate accumulation

Disease	Metabolic defect	Accumulating substrate	Main clinical findings
Tay-Sachs disease	β-Hexosaminidase A deficiency	GM2 ganglioside	Cerebral neurodegeneration
OTC deficiency	OTC deficiency	Ammonium	Acute encephalopathy
Methylmalonic acidemia	Methylmalonyl-CoA mutase deficiency	Methylmalonic acid	Metabolic acidosis
PKU	Phenylalanine hydroxylase deficiency	Phenylalanine	Progressive mental retardation
Hurler disease	α-L-iduronidase deficiency	Dermatan and heparan sulfates	Unusual facies, skeletal abnormalities, progressive mental retardation
Cystinuria	Dibasic amino acid transport defect in kidney	Cystine in urine	Recurrent obstructive uropathy
Hepatorenal tyrosinemia	Fumarylacetoacetase deficiency	Fumarylacetoacetate and maleylacetoacetate	Acute hepatocellular dysfunction, cirrhosis, rickets

Abbreviations: OTC, ornithine transcarbamoylase; PKU, phenylketonuria.

Accumulation of substrate is also diagnostically important. Specific diagnosis often follows quickly after identification of the accumulation of metabolites proximal to an enzyme defect, particularly among inborn errors of water-soluble substrates. This is generally true, for example, of the amino acidopathies and organic acidopathies, in which accumulation of substrate throughout the body is often massive, and is reflected by changes in plasma and urine.

In inborn errors of metabolism involving water-insoluble substrates, such as complex lipids, accumulation of the immediate substrate of the mutant enzyme is also important in the pathophysiology of disease. However, accumulation of the compounds is often limited to single tissues or organs, such as brain, which are relatively inaccessible. Moreover, chemical isolation and identification of the metabolites is often cumbersome, requiring laboratory expertise that is not routinely available.

In other disorders, such as the mucopolysaccharide storage diseases, the accumulation of substrate is a major factor in the pathophysiology of disease. However, because the metabolism of the substrate requires the participation of a number of different enzymes, any of which may be deficient as a result of mutation, the demonstration of accumulation is diagnostically important only to the extent that it indicates a class of disorders, not one specific disease. The demonstration of mucopolysaccharide accumulation is important as a screening test for inherited defects in mucopolysaccharide metabolism. However, the metabolism of the individual mucopolysaccharides involves 10 or more genetically distinct lysosomal enzymes, and accumulation of the same compound may occur as a consequence of deficiency of any one of the enzymes. Specific diagnosis in these disorders requires the demonstration of the specific enzyme deficiency in appropriate tissues, such as peripheral blood leukocytes or cultured skin fibroblasts (see Chapter 9).

Accumulation of a normally minor metabolite

In some disorders, the primary cause of disease is accumulation of a normally minor metabolite, produced in excess by a reaction that is usually of trivial metabolic importance. The cataracts in patients with untreated galactosemia occur as a result of accumulation the sugar alcohol, galactitol, a normally minor metabolite of galactose. In another example, accumulation of the normally minor complex lipid metabolite, psychosine, in the brain of infants with Krabbe globoid cell leukodystrophy excites a subacute inflammatory reaction, manifested by appearance in the brain of multinucleated giant cells, called globoid cells. It also causes rapid, severe demyelination, out of proportion to the accumulation of galactocerebroside, the immediate precursor of the defective enzyme, galactocerebrosidase.

Deficiency of product

Deficiency of the product of a specific reaction is another primary consequence of many inherited metabolic diseases. The extent to which it contributes to disease depends on the importance of the product. For example, most of the pathologic consequences of defects of biosynthesis are traceable to deficiency of the product of the relevant reaction – in these cases substrate accumulation plays little or no role in the development of disease. Table 1.2 shows a list of some conditions in which symptoms are the result of deficiency of the product of some enzymic reaction or transport process.

Among the inborn errors of amino acid biosynthesis, the signs of disease are often the combined result of substrate accumulation and product deficiency. For example, in the urea cycle disorder, argininosuccinic aciduria, the defect in the conversion of argininosuccinic acid to arginine causes arginine deficiency, and this, in turn, results in a deficiency of ornithine. Depletion of intramitochondrial ornithine causes accumulation of carbamoylphosphate and ammonia resulting in marked hyperammonemic encephalopathy. The importance of arginine deficiency in the pathophysiology of the encephalopathy is shown by the dramatic response to administration of a single large dose of arginine (4 mmoles/kg given intravenously).

Deficiency of products of reactions is important in two other situations that are common among the inborn errors of metabolism. One of these could be regarded as the result of a 'metabolic steal', a term used to explain the occurrence of myopathy in some patients with glycogen storage disease due to debrancher enzyme deficiency. It was postulated that increased gluconeogenesis in patients with the disease causes accelerated muscle protein breakdown as free amino acids are diverted from protein biosynthesis to gluconeogenesis in an effort to maintain the blood glucose in the face of impaired glycogen breakdown. Another example of the consequences of a metabolic steal is the occurrence of hypoglycemia in patients with hereditary defects in fatty acid oxidation. The over-utilization of glucose and resulting hypoglycemia are a consequence of the inability to meet energy requirements by fatty acid oxidation because of deficiency of one of the enzymes involved in the process.

Another mechanism by which a metabolic defect causes symptoms because of deficiency or inaccessibility of a product might be called 'metabolic sequestration'. Transport defects caused by mutations affecting proteins involved in carrier-mediated transport often produce disease through a failure of the transfer of a metabolite from one subcellular compartment to another. The HHH syndrome, named for the associated hyperammonemia, hyperornithinemia, and homocitrullinemia, is caused by a defect in the transport of the amino acid, ornithine, into the

Table 1.2 Some examples of inborn errors of metabolism in which symptoms of disease are the result of product deficiency

Disease	Metabolic defect	Product deficiency	Main clinical findings
Vitamin D dependency	25-Hydroxycholecalciferol-1α-hydroxylase deficiency	1α, 25-Dihydroxycholecalciferol	Rickets
Hartnup disease	Neutral amino acid transport defect	Niacinamide	Pellagra-like condition
Lysinuric protein intolerance	Dibasic amino acid transport defect	Ornithine	Recurrent hyperammonemia
Hereditary thrombophilia	Protein C defect	Protein C (physiologic anticoagulant)	Recurrent phlebothrombosis
Transcobalamin II deficiency	Transcobalamin II defect	Vitamin B_{12}	Megaloblastic anemia
Congenital hypothyroidism	Various defects in thyroid hormone biosynthesis	Thyroid hormone	Cretinism, goitre
X-linked hypophosphatemic rickets	Renal phosphate transport defect	Phosphate	Rickets

mitochondria. The resulting intramitochondrial ornithine deficiency causes accumulation of carbamoylphosphate and ammonia, ultimately causing hyperammonemic encephalopathy, in a manner similar to that causing the hyperammonemia in argininosuccinic aciduria described above.

Secondary metabolic phenomena

Because of the close relationship between the various processes comprising intermediary metabolism, enzyme deficiencies or transport defects inevitably have effects beyond the immediate changes in the concentrations of substrate and product of any particular reaction. These secondary metabolic phenomena often cause diagnostic confusion. For example, ketotic hyperglycinemia was initially thought to be a primary disorder of glycine metabolism. However, subsequent studies showed that glycine accumulation was actually a secondary metabolic phenomenon in patients with a primary defect of propionic acid metabolism. Furthermore, the acute forms of other organic acidopathies, such as methylmalonic acidemia (see Chapter 3), were also found to be associated with marked accumulation of glycine, severe ketoacidosis, and hyperammonemia, all the result of secondary metabolic effects of organic acid or organic acyl-CoA accumulation. Table 1.3 lists some examples of potentially confusing secondary metabolic responses to point defects in metabolism.

Inborn errors of metabolism are inherited

Determination of the pattern of inheritance of a condition is often helpful in making a diagnosis of genetic disease, and it provides the foundation for genetic counselling. The most important information required for establishing the pattern of inheritance is a family history covering at least three generations of relations.

Autosomal recessive disorders

Most of the inherited metabolic diseases recognized today are inherited in the same manner as Garrod's original inborn errors of metabolism: they are Mendelian, single-gene defects, transmitted in an autosomal recessive manner. Disease expression requires that an individual be homozygous for significant, though not necessarily the same, mutations in the same gene. In the overwhelming majority of cases, homozygosity occurs as a result of inheritance of a mutant gene from each parent, who are both heterozygous for the defect. Although it is theoretically possible for one, or even both, of the mutations to arise in the patient as a result of *de novo* mutation, this is so unlikely that for practical purposes it is ignored. Inheritance of two copies of a mutation from one heterozygous parent may occur as a result of uniparental isodisomy. However, this phenomenon is very rare.

Table 1.3 Some examples of inborn errors of metabolism in which secondary metabolic defects play a prominent role in the production of symptoms of disease

Disease	Metabolic defect	Secondary metabolic abnormalities	Main clinical findings
CAH	21-Hydroxylase deficiency	Androgen accumulation and deficiencies of aldosterone and cortisol	Addisonian crisis; virilization of females
GSD type I	Glucose-6-phosphatase deficiency	Lactic acidosis; hyperuricemia; hypertriglyceridemia	Massive hepatomegaly; hypoglycemia; failure to thrive
HFI	Fructose-1-phosphate aldolase deficiency	Lactic acidosis; hypoglycemia; hyperuricemia; hypophosphatemia	Severe metabolic acidosis; hypoglycemia
Methylmalonic acidemia	Methylmalonyl-CoA mutase deficiency	Hyperammonemia; hyperglycinemia	Acute encephalopathy; metabolic acidosis
HHH syndrome	Ornithine transport defect	Homocitrullinemia	Hyperammonemic encephalopathy
OTC deficiency	OTC deficiency	Orotic aciduria	Hyperammonemic encephalopathy
Abetalipoproteinemia	Apolipoprotein B deficiency	Malabsorption of vitamin E	Spinocerebellar degeneration

Abbreviations: CAH, congenital adrenal hyperplasia; GSD, glycogen storage disease; HFI, hereditary fructose intolerance; OTC, ornithine transcarbamoylase; HHH, hyperammonemia-hyperornithinemia-homocitrullinemia.

Most individuals with autosomal recessive inherited metabolic diseases have no family history of the disorder. However, the occurrence of a similar disorder in a sibling or in a cousin raises the possibility that the condition is not only hereditary, but that it is transmitted as an autosomal recessive disorder. Obtaining the information may be difficult because the occurrence of serious disease in children, particularly if it is associated with mental retardation, early infant death, or physical deformities, may be concealed by the family out of shame, or simply forgotten.

Consanguinity increases the likelihood that an inherited disorder is autosomal recessive because it increases the probability that both parents of a child are carriers of a rare recessive mutation. As a rule, the more rare it is, the more likely the occurrence of an autosomal recessive condition will be affected by inbreeding. For some very rare disorders, the frequency of consanguinity of the parents of affected individuals is as high as 30–40%. Geographic or socio-cultural isolation of relatively small and demographically stable communities increases the risk of inadvertent inbreeding, no doubt contributing to the high incidence of certain diseases in specific ethnic groups. When considering the possibility that the disease in an individual may be the result of an autosomal recessive mutation, the family history should include specific questions to assess the possibility of parental consanguinity. Simply asking the parents if they are related will often reveal the fact. The origins of the parents are also important. The possibility of consanguinity is increased, for example, if the parents of a patient both come from a small village with a history of population stability and isolation, and if relatives on both sides of the family share the same surname.

The increased incidence of a specific genetic defect in a demographically isolated population as a result of the introduction of the mutation by a founding member is called a 'founder effect'. The high incidences of certain rare inherited metabolic disorders in specific ethnic groups or communities are well known examples of a putative founder effect, though the role of an element of environmental selection favoring heterozygotes has not been eliminated in some cases. Some examples of inborn errors of metabolism occurring in particularly high frequency in specific ethnic groups are shown in Table 1.4.

X-linked recessive disorders

In males, it only takes one mutation of a gene on the X-chromosome to produce disease. Unlike autosomal recessive disorders, in which the contribution of new mutations to the occurrence of disease in individuals is negligible, about a third of males with X-linked recessive diseases are born to mothers who are not carriers of the mutation: the boys are affected as a result of new mutations. For the purposes of genetic counselling, once the medical diagnosis has been confirmed and the

Table 1.4 Some examples of inborn errors of metabolism occurring in high frequency among specific ethnic groups

Disease	Ethnic group	Estimated incidence (per 100,000 births)
Tay-Sachs disease	Ashkenazi Jews	33[*]
Gaucher disease	Ashkenazi Jews	100
Hepatorenal tyrosinemia	French-Canadians (Saguenay-Lac Saint-Jean region)	54
Porphyria variegata	South African (white)	300
Congenital adrenal hyperplasia	Yupik Eskimos	200
Phenylketonuria (PKU)	Turkish	38.5
	Yemenite Jews	19
	Ashkenazi Jews	5
Glutaric aciduria, type I	Ojibway Indians (Canada)	>50[†]
Maple syrup urine disease	Mennonites (Pennsylvania)	3.3
Salla disease	Finnish	568

Note: [*]Before the introduction of screening and prenatal diagnosis to prevent the condition.
[†]Estimated.
Source: Data derived in part from Weatherall, D. J. (1991) and Scriver et al. (1995).

possibilities of autosomal recessive and non-genetic phenocopies have been eliminated, it is critical to determine whether the disease caused by an X-linked mutation developed as a result of inheritance of the mutation, or as a result of a new mutation. The family history is particularly important in this situation. The likelihood that the mother of a boy with an X-linked recessive disease inherited the mutation from her own mother can be estimated from the number of healthy male relatives she has related to her through her mother and sisters. For example, the mother of a boy with Hunter disease (MPS II), an X-linked recessive mucopolysaccharide storage disease, is unlikely to have inherited the mutation from her own mother if she has a large number of healthy brothers and nephews (i.e., sons of her sisters). The larger the number of healthy male relatives, the more likely the affected boy has the disease as a result of a new mutation, either in the boy himself or in his mother during gametogenesis in each case. In the first situation, the risk of recurrence of the disease in subsequent offspring is negligible. However if the boy's mother is a carrier as a result of a new mutation, the risk of recurrence is the same as if the mother had inherited the mutation from her mother.

It is a mistake to assume automatically that a woman is a carrier of an X-linked disease if she has a son affected with it. But, if a woman has two affected sons, or she has an affected brother as well as an affected son, she is regarded as an obligate

Table 1.5 Some mechanisms of autosomal dominance

Mechanisms	Gene product	Disease example
Abnormal assembly of the subunits of a multimeric protein	Fibrillin	Marfan syndrome
Abnormal interaction between the subunits of multimeric protein	Hemoglobin	Hemoglobin M disease
Derepression of rate-limiting enzyme activity	Porphobilinogen deaminase	Acute intermittent porphyria (derepression of δ-aminolevulinic acid dehydratase)
Cell receptor defects	LDL-receptor	Familial hypercholesterolemia (derepression of HMG-CoA reductase)
Cell membrane defects	Spectrin	Hereditary spherocytosis
Deposition of an abnormal structural protein	Transthyretin	Hereditary amyloidosis
Somatic cell mutation coupled with inheritance of a recessive gene	pp110^{RB}	Retinoblastoma

Abbreviations: LDL, low-density lipoprotein; HMG-CoA, 3-hydroxy-3-methylglutaryl-CoA.

carrier of the disease-causing mutation. It also follows that all the female offspring of a man affected with an X-linked disorder are obligate carriers of the disease; in contrast, none of his sons would be affected because male-to-male transmission of X-linked conditions does not occur.

Autosomal dominant disorders

Although autosomal dominant mutations are common causes of genetic disease in humans, they contribute relatively little to the sum total of inherited metabolic disorders. This is probably because, with a few exceptions, most inherited metabolic diseases are caused by abnormalities in enzymes or transport proteins that are not involved in the types of interactions or processes required to produce dominance (Table 1.5).

Autosomal dominant inheritance is characterized by:

- every affected individual has an affected parent (unless the individual has the disease as a result of a new mutation, or the mutation is non-penetrant);
- on average half of the offspring of an affected individual will themselves have only unaffected children (assuming penetrance is complete);
- males and females are equally represented among affected members of the kindred;
- transmission of the condition occurs vertically through successive generations, unless the condition impairs reproduction.

Because only one mutation is required to cause disease, new mutations contribute significantly to the incidence of autosomal dominant disorders. The rate of spontaneous mutation, and hence the likelihood in any particular situation that disease is due to spontaneous mutation, varies from one disease to another. In some noteworthy cases, the autosomal dominant inheritance of a condition may be overlooked because disease in a particular patient may be the result of a new mutation. Many of the diseases, such as acute intermittent porphyria and dopa-responsive dystonia (Segawa syndrome), are also characterized by incomplete penetrance[5] and marked variability in expressivity[6], even among members of the same family, further obscuring the dominant mode of inheritance. A careful family history is invaluable in recognizing the familial nature of these disorders.

Mitochondrial inheritance

Each mitochondrion in every cell contains several copies of a small, circular, double-stranded DNA molecule (mtDNA) containing genes coding for the production of ribosomal RNA and various tRNAs necessary for mitochondrial protein biosynthesis, and for the production of some of the proteins involved in mitochondrial electron transport (Figure 1.2). The mitochondrial genome consists of 16,569 basepairs, comprising 5523 codons, coding for the production of 37 gene products.

The vast majority of mitochondrial proteins, including most of the proteins of subunits involved in electron transport (see Table 9.13), are encoded by nuclear genes. Mutations of these genes cause diseases transmitted as autosomal recessive disorders. As in the case of other autosomal recessive conditions, the disease phenotype of various affected individuals in the same family tends to be very similar.

The situation is quite different with regard to the pattern of inheritance and clinical expression of disease caused by mtDNA mutations. The mitochondria in the cells of each individual are derived at the time of conception from the mitochondria in the cytoplasm of the ovum; the mitochondria and mtDNA of the sperm are lost during the process of fertilization. It follows that mtDNA mutations are also inherited only from the mother. When multiple members of a family are affected with a condition because of inheritance of an mtDNA mutation, the pattern of inheritance is quite specific:

---

[5] Penetrance is the *probability* that an individual with a specific disease-associated genotype will exhibit clinical manifestations of the disease. It is a statistical concept generally derived from pedigree analysis. Incomplete penetrance refers to the observation that some individuals with a specfic disease-causing mutation may exhibit no clinical manifestations of the disease at all – the disease appears to skip generations in families with multiple affected members.

[6] Expressivity is the *extent* to which individuals with a specific disease-associated genotype, all of whom have disease, exhibit manifestations of the disease. Variable expressivity refers to the observation that several individuals with the same genotype may have disease manifestations varying from very mild to very severe. It is not to be confused with penetrance.

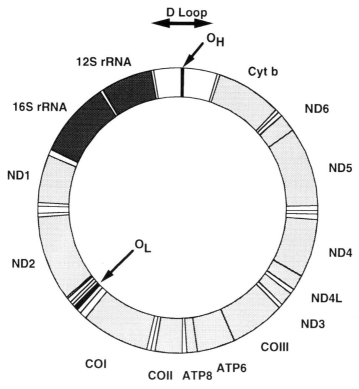

Figure 1.2   The human mitochondrial genome.
The human mitochondrial genome is encoded in a double-stranded, circular mtDNA molecule. The figure show in a simplified way the identity and relative locations of various mitochondrial genes.

- all the offspring of a woman carrying a mtDNA mutation can generally be shown to have inherited the mutation, whether they are clinically affected with disease or not;
- the phenotypic expression of disease in different individuals who have inherited mtDNA mutations is often highly variable, both in terms of the systems involved and the severity of clinical disease;
- transmission of the condition from father to offspring does not occur.

Each cell contains at least hundreds of mitochondria, and any mtDNA may affect all (homoplasmy) or only a fraction (heteroplasmy) of the total mitochondria in each cell. The phenotypic effect of any particular mutation depends on the severity of the mtDNA mutation, the proportion of mitochondria affected, and the susceptibility of various tissues to impaired mitochondrial energy metabolism. This makes the relationship between the proportion of mutant mtDNA and clinical phenotype very complex. Owing to different thresholds for susceptibility to mitochondrial

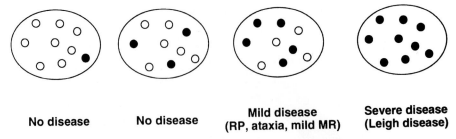

| No disease | No disease | **Mild disease**
(RP, ataxia, mild MR) | **Severe disease**
(Leigh disease) |

Figure 1.3   The effect of heteroplasmy on the clinical expression of mtDNA mutations.
The figure represents four cells, each containing nine mitochondria. Mitochondria bearing normal mtDNA are shown as open circles; those with a mtDNA mutation are shown as filled circles. As the proportion of mutant mitochondria in the cells of various tissues increases, different thresholds are reached for the production of disease-causing cell damage. While lower proportions of mutant mitochondria are well tolerated, severe disease results when the proportion is very high.

energy defects, the tissues and organs involved in the clinical phenotype may vary markedly from one affected individual to another with the same mtDNA mutation, depending on the degree of heteroplasmy in each individual. Increasingly, families are being identified in which variations in the extent of the heteroplasmy in the offspring of a clinically healthy woman carrying a specific mtDNA mutation may result in some being clinically completely normal, some, for example, dying in early infancy with severe Leigh disease, and some being affected with clinically intermediate disease variants (mental retardation, retinitis pigmentosa, and ataxia). Figure 1.3 gives some idea of what heteroplasmy is and how it relates to phenotype. Obtaining a family history appropriate to the recognition of this type of inheritance of a specific mtDNA mutation is particularly challenging. No clinical abnormality in a relative, no matter how apparently trivial or how different it may seem from the disease phenotype in the proband, can be dismissed.

The mutation rate for mtDNA is much higher than that for nuclear DNA, and the relative contribution of *de novo* mtDNA mutations especially deletions, to disease is much greater than the contribution of new mutations to disease due to nuclear DNA mutations. Conditions, like Kearns-Sayre syndrome, which is usually the result of mtDNA deletions or duplications, are almost always sporadic, and the risk of recurrence of the condition in the family is low.

Inherited metabolic diseases may present at any age

Historically and traditionally, inherited metabolic diseases have been thought of as primarily pediatric problems, even though three of Garrod's four original inborn errors of metabolism are generally more commonly identified for the first time in adults rather than in children affected with the disorders. The strong association with pediatrics seems to have grown out of experience with PKU and the possibility that other serious conditions presenting in infancy might be caused by point defects in metabolism. Moreover, as the contribution of infectious diseases and malnutrition to pediatric mortality declined over the middle years of the 20th century, the proportion of mortality caused by inborn errors of metabolism increased rapidly. One thing is certain, reports of the identification and characterization of specific inherited metabolic diseases began to appear in exponentially growing numbers in the pediatric literature long before comparable articles appeared in significant numbers in the general medical literature.

As a result of advances in diagnostic technology, particularly as it relates to lysosomal and mitochondrial disorders, the number of inherited metabolic diseases recognized to present in adulthood has increased enormously. Many, if not most, inborn errors of metabolism originally described in infants and children are now known to occur as adult-onset variants. In most cases, the late-onset variants are clinically milder than variants that are often rapidly fatal in infancy. The clinical presentation and course are often significantly different from those of the pediatric variants (Table 1.6). In some cases, such as milder variants of ornithine transcarbamoylase (OTC) deficiency, the presentation in adults, with severe hyperammonemic encephalopathy, often precipitated by severe physiological stress, may resemble that in infants with a similarly lethal outcome. An increasing number of examples are being found of inborn errors of metabolism that seem never to present in childhood. Some are familiar, such as many of the hereditary hyperlipidemias. In others, recognition of the diseases is more recent, such as with Leber hereditary optic neuropathy (LHON) and gyrate atrophy. This is an area that is bound to expand over the coming years.

Three sources of diagnostic confusion

The commonest error in the management of inherited metabolic disorders is probably delayed or wrong diagnosis. There are three common sources of potential confusion in the diagnosis of inherited metabolic disease.

Confusion with common acquired conditions

Some inborn errors are often misdiagnosed as acquired disease, particularly some infections, intoxications, or nutritional deficiencies (Table 1.7). Failure to consider both classes of disorders simultaneously in the differential diagnosis of an acutely ill child may result in the loss of an opportunity to carry out critical diagnostic investigations, and may result in unnecessary morbidity, or even death.

Table 1.6 Some examples of inborn errors of metabolism presenting in adulthood in which the clinical phenotype differs significantly from that in childhood

Disease	Enzyme defect	Pediatric phenotype	Adult-onset phenotype
GM2 gangliosidosis (Tay-Sachs disease and Sandhoff disease)	β-hexosaminidase	Rapid cognitive (developmental) deterioration, with seizures, blindness, progressing to early death	Slowly progressive movement disorder, ataxia, psychiatric problems, with little or no intellectual impairment until late in the course of the disease
Gaucher disease	Glucocerebrosidase	Marked hepatosplenomegaly with early and severe neurological impairment, progressing rapidly to death (type 2); or hepatosplenomegaly and progressive movement disorder, seizures, intellectual deterioration, progressing to death within a few years (type 3)	Hepatosplenomegaly, which is often asymptomatic, though frequently associated with hypersplenism, bone pain, fractures, avascular necrosis of large joints, but no CNS involvement (type 1)
Niemann-Pick disease	Acid sphingomyelinase	Marked hepatosplenomegaly with early and severe neurological impairment, progressing rapidly to death (type A)	Hepatosplenomegaly, bone pain, cirrhosis, chronic infiltrative lung disease, but no CNS involvement (type B)
MPS I	α-L-iduronidase	Dysmorphic facial features, corneal clouding, dysostosis multiplex, hepatosplenomegaly, valvular heart disease, obstructive pulmonary disease, marked growth retardation, with severe (Hurler disease), or little or no (Hurler-Scheie disease) CNS involvement	Little or no facial dysmorphism, corneal clouding, marked restriction of joint movement, with early-onset osteoarthritis, but no primary CNS involvement (Scheie disease)
MLD	Arylsulfatase A	Ataxia, developmental delay, cognitive regression, progressing rapidly to severe neurological impairment and death	Psychiatric problems primarily affecting executive function, late slowly progressive motor impairment and dementia

GSD type 2	Acid maltase (acid α-glucosidase)	Severe, rapidly progressive muscle weakness and cardiomyopathy	Very slowly progressive skeletal muscle weakness with minimal myocardial involvement
OTC deficiency	OTC	Severe, often lethal, neonatal hyperammonemic encephalopathy in affected males; failure to thrive, recurrent hyperammonemic encephalopathy in affected females	Recurrent headaches; rarely presents as severe hyperammonemic encephalopathy
LHON	mtDNA mutations	None	Progressive blindness
Gyrate atrophy	OAT	None	Progressive blindness
NARP	mtDNA mutations	Leigh disease: failure to thrive, persistent lactic acidosis, irregularly progressive neurological deterioration with episodes of acute encephalopathy	Peripheral neuropathy, retinitis pigmentosa, intellectual impairment, ataxia, with episodes of acute deterioration associated with lactic acidosis
Adult-onset type II citrullinemia (CTLN2)	citrin	Neonatal hepatitis with intrahepatic cholestasis, generalized amino acidemia (including methionine, tyrosine, citrulline, lysine, threonine and arginine), and galactosemia	Hyperammonemia, disorientation, delirium, delusions, stupor progressing to coma, associated with marked hypercitrullinemia

Abbreviations: CNS, central nervous system; MPS, mucopolysaccharidosis; MLD, metachromatic leukodystrophy; OTC, ornithine transcarbamoylase; LHON, Leber hereditary optic neuropathy; OAT, ornithine aminotransferase; NARP, neuropathy-ataxia-retinitis pigmentosa

Table 1.7 Some common non-metabolic conditions that are often confused with inherited metabolic diseases

Inherited metabolic 'syndrome'	Common non-metabolic disease phenocopy
Syndrome (Chapter)	*Infections*
Hepatic syndrome (4)	Hepatitis, enterovirus infection, infectious mononucleosis
Cardiomyopathy (5)	Enterovirus infection
Storage syndrome (6)	Congenital CMV infection, congenital toxoplasmosis
Encephalopathy (2)	Arbovirus infections, enterovirus infections, herpes infections (especially newborn), postinfectious encephalopathy (e.g., chicken pox)
	Intoxications
Neurologic syndrome (2)	CNS depressants, antihistaminics, anticonvulsants
Lactic acidosis (3)	Ethanol, methanol, ethylene glycol, salicylism
Hepatic syndrome (4)	Valproic acid intoxication, amiodarone reaction
Cardiac syndrome (5)	ACTH reaction (cardiomyopathy)
	Nutritional deficiencies
Lactic acidosis (3)	Thiamine deficiency
Methylmalonic acidemia (3)	Vitamin B_{12} deficiency
	Hematopoietic disorders
Storage syndrome (6)	FEL, hemoglobinopathies, lymphoma, malignant histiocytosis
Hepatic syndrome (4)	

Abbreviations: CMV, cytomegalovirus; CNS, central nervous system; FEL, familial erythrophago-cytic lymphohistiocytosis.

Confusion caused by association with intercurrent illness

Metabolic decompensation in a child with a marginally compensated inherited metabolic disorder commonly occurs as a result of the physiological stress of inter-current illness. Preoccupation with the intercurrent illness often delays diagnosis of the underlying genetic disorder. Owing to an impaired ability to compensate adequately for the metabolic pressures caused by intercurrent illness, particularly infection, children with inherited metabolic diseases often decompensate when they contract relatively trivial infections. The child with intermittent MSUD (maple syrup urine disease) or a fatty acid oxidation defect, or the girl with OTC (ornithine transcarbamylase) deficiency, is often the one in the family who is described as 'sickly'. They get sicker and take longer to recover from trivial viral infections than their healthy siblings.

However, some inherited metabolic diseases significantly increase the risk of intercurrent illness. For example, recurrent, treatment-resistant, otitis media is a common problem in children of all ages with mucopolysaccharide storage diseases in which distortion of the Eustachian tubes and the production of particularly tenacious mucus combine to create a favorable environment for bacterial colonization of the middle ear. The neutropenia that is a prominent feature of glycogen disease (GSD), type Ib, and some of the organic acidopathies, predisposes to pyogenic infections. Classical galactosemia predisposes infants to neonatal *Escherichia coli* sepsis by a mechanism that is not yet understood.

Confusion arising from genetic heterogeneity

Among the inherited metabolic diseases, two or more clinically similar disorders may be caused by mutations in completely different genes. This follows from the fact that the net result of a defect in any one of a number of steps in a complex metabolic process may be functionally the same. A prominent example of this is the mucopolysaccharide storage disease, Sanfilippo disease, a group of clinical indistinguishable diseases caused by defects in different enzymes involved in the breakdown of the glycosaminoglycan, heparan sulfate. This has important implications for carrier testing and for prenatal diagnosis, situations in which major decisions are made on the strength of the results of a single laboratory test. Doing the wrong test has a high probability of producing the wrong results, sometimes with tragic consequences.

Congenital malformations and inborn errors of metabolism

On the one hand, major congenital malformations, such as meningomyelocele, complex congenital heart disease, and major congenital limb deformities, are not generally considered signs of an underlying inherited metabolic disease. On the other hand, the recent discovery of a specific defect in cholesterol biosynthesis in patients with Smith-Lemli-Opitz syndrome has forced some modification of this view. There are some inherited metabolic conditions in which dysmorphism is so characteristic that a strong presumptive diagnosis can be made on physical examination alone. This is discussed in detail in Chapter 6.

The internet is particularly important

The internet has revolutionized the management of inherited metabolic diseases by making vast amounts of information readily available – not only to physicians, but to patients, as well. The number of newly recognized disorders, new developments

Table 1.8 A list of a selection of Internet websites related to inherited metabolic disorders, either for health professionals or patients and their families

Website	Organization maintaining the site	Comments
Websites with extensive resource directories		
www.ncbi.nlm.nih.gov/entrez/query.fcgi	National Library of Medicine	Excellent search engine for articles and abstracts in vast array of journals dating back over 50 years
www.genetests.org	University of Washington	Resource for information on clinics and laboratories providing genetic diagnostic services
www3.ncbi.nlm.nih.gov/Omim	National Center for Biotechnology Information	The 'gold standard' for information on the genetics of hereditary single gene disorders
www.slh.wisc.edu/newborn/guide	Wisconsin State Laboratory of Hygiene	Health professionals' guide to newborn screening
www.ninds.nih.gov/health_and_medical/disorders	National Institute of Neurological Disorders and Stroke	Information and links related to several inherited metabolic diseases
www.umm.edu/glossary/	University of Maryland Medicine	Information and links related to several inherited metabolic diseases
archive.uwcm.ac.uk/uwcm/mg/docs/oth_mut.html	Cardiff Human Gene Mutation Database	Index of locus-specific mutation databases with many links
www.ulf.org	United Leukodystrophy Foundation	Information and links related to several inherited metabolic neurodegenerative diseases
www.rarediseases.org	National Organization for Rare Disorders (NORD)	Information and links related to several inherited diseases
www.ntsad.org	National Tay-Sachs and Allied Diseases Association	Information and links related to several inherited metabolic neurodegenerative diseases
www.nfjgd.org	National Foundation of Jewish Genetic Diseases	Information and links related to several inherited metabolic diseases prevalent among Ashkenazi Jews
mcrcr2.med.nyu.edu/murphp01/frame.htm	New York University Medical Center	International directory to many genetic diseases and support groups
Disease-specific websites		
www.oaanews.org	Organic Acidemia Association, Inc.	Information on several inherited disorders of organic acid metabolism
www.pkunews.org	National PKU News	Information on PKU for patients, parents and professionals

Organization	Website	Description
National Urea Cycle Disorders Foundation	www.nucdf.org	Information on urea cycle disorders for patients, parents and professionals
Maple Syrup Urine Disease Family Support Group	www.msud-support.org	Information on MSUD for patients, parents and professionals
Parents of Galactosemic Children, Inc.	www.galactosemia.org	Information on galactosemia primarily for patients and parents
Association for Glycogen Storage Disease (UK)	www.agsd.uk/home/	Information on glycogen storage diseases for patients, parents and professionals
Lysosomal Storage Disease Network	www.lsdn.com	Information and links related to many lysosomal storage diseases
Lysosomal Diseases Australia	www.lda.org.au	Information and links related to many lysosomal storage diseases
New Zealand LSD Support Group	www.ldnz.org.nz	Information and links related to many lysosomal storage diseases
United Mitochondrial Disease Foundation	www.umdf.org	Information and links related to various mitochondrial diseases
Wilson's Disease Association International	www.wilsonsdisease.org	Information and links related to many Wilson diseases
National MPS Society, Inc.	www.mpssociety.org	Information on mucopolysaccharide storage diseases for patients, parents and professionals
National Niemann-Pick Disease Foundation, Inc.	www.nnpdf.org	Information on Niemann-Pick disease for patients, parents and professionals
Mead Johnson Nutritionals	www.meadjohnson.com/metabolics/metabolichandbook.html	Information and links related to several inherited metabolic diseases treatable by dietary manipulation
Batten Disease Support and Research Association	www.bdsra.org	Information and links related to neuronal ceroid lipofuscinosis (Batten disease)
Fabry Support and Information Group	www.fabry.org	Information and links related to Fabry disease
National Gaucher Foundation	www.gaucherdisease.org	Information and links related to Gaucher disease
Canavan Foundation	www.canavanfoundation.org	Information and links related to Canavan disease
Canavan Research Foundation	www.canavan.org	
Fatty Oxidation Disorder Communication Network	www.fodsupport.org	Information and links related to various fatty acid oxidation disorders
International Pompe Association	www.worldpompe.org/index.html	A federation of patients' groups with information and links related to Pompe disease

Table 1.9 A selection of locus-specific mutation databases

Disease	Gene	Website	Institution maintaining the site
X-linked adrenoleukodystrophy	*ABCD1*	www.x-ald.nl and	Academic Medical Center, Amsterdam, Netherlands
		www.peroxisome.org	Kennedy Krieger Institute, Baltimore, MD
Hereditary fructose intolerance	*ALDH9*	www.bu.edu/aldolase	Boston University, Boston, MA
Congenital disorders of glycosylation	*ALG6, DPM1, GCS1, MGAT2, not561, PMM2*	www.kuleuven.ac.be/med/cdg	Leuven University, Leuven, Belgium
Hypophosphatasia	*ALPL*	www.sesep.uvsq.fr/Database.html	University of Versailles-Saint Quentin en Yvelines, France
Wilson disease	*ATP7B*	www.medgen.med.ualberta.ca/database.html and	University of Alberta, Edmonton, Canada
		life2.tau.ac.il/GeneDis/Tables/Wilson/Wilson.html	Tel-Aviv University, Tel-Aviv, Israel
Homocystinuria	*CBS*	www.uchsc.edu/sm/cbs/cbsdata/cbsmain.html	University of Colorado Health Sciences Center, Denver, CO
Albinism	*CHS1, TYR, TYRP1*	www.cbc.umn.edu/tad/tyasemut.html	University of Minnesota, Minneapolis, MN
		www.cbc.umn.edu/tad/tyr1mut.html	
		www.retina-international.com/sci-news/tyrmut.htm	Retina International
Chediak-Higashi syndrome	*CHS1*	www.cbc.umn.edu/tad/chsmut.html and	University of Minnesota, Minneapolis, MN
		www.retina-international.com/Sci-news/chsmut.htm	Retina International
Neuronal ceroid lipofuscinosis (Batten disease)	*CLN2, CLN3, CLN5, CLN8, PPT1 (CLN1)*	www.ucl.ac.uk/ncl and	University College London, UK
		www.retina-international.com/Sci-news/cln3mut.htm	Retina International
G6PD deficiency	*G6PD*	rialto.com/favism/mutat.htm	Scripps Research Institute, La Jolla, CA
Pompe disease (GSD II)	*GAA*	www.eur.nl/FGG/CH1/pompe	Erasmus University, Rotterdam, Netherlands
Krabbe globoid cell leukodystrophy	*GALC*	life2.tau.ac.il/GeneDis/Tables/Krabbe/krabbe.html	Tel-Aviv University, Tel-Aviv, Israel
Galactosemia	*GALT*	www.ich.bris.ac.uk/galtdb and	Institute of Child Health, Bristol, UK
		www.emory.edu/PEDIATRICS/medgen/research/galt.htm	Emory University, Altanta, GA
Gaucher disease	*GBA*	www.tau.ac.il/~racheli/genedis/gaucher/gaucher.html	Tel-Aviv University, Tel-Aviv, Israel

Disease	Gene	URL	Institution
Phenylketonuria (PKU)	*PAH*	ww2.mcgill.ca/pahdb	McGill University, Montreal, Canada
Dihydropteridine reductase deficiency	*QDPR*	www.bh4.org	University Children's Hospital, Zurich, Switzerland
Pterin-4a-carbinolamine dehydratase deficiency	*PCBD*	www.bh4.org	University Children's Hospital, Zurich, Switzerland
GTP cyclohydrolase I deficiency	*GCH1*	www.bh4.org	University Children's Hospital, Zurich, Switzerland
6-Pyruvoyloo-tetrahydropterin synthase deficiency	*PTS*	www.bh4.org	University Children's Hospital, Zurich, Switzerland
GM2 gangliosidosis	*GMA*	data.mch.mcgill.ca/gm2adb	McGill University, Montreal, Canada
Tay-Sachs disease	*HEXA*	data.mch.mcgill.ca/hexadb and life2.tau.ac.il/GeneDis/Tables/Tay_Sachs/tay_sachs.html	McGill University, Montreal, Canada Tel-Aviv University, Tel-Aviv, Israel
Sandhoff disease	*HEXB*	data.mch.mcgill.ca/hexbdb	McGill University, Montreal, Canada
Lesch-Nyhan disease	*HPRT1*	www.ibilio.org/dnam/mainpage.html	University of North Carolina, NC
Congenital adrenal hyperplasia	*HSD3B2*	life2.tau.ac.il/GeneDis/Tables/CAH/cah.html	Tel-Aviv University, Tel-Aviv, Israel
Familial hypercholesterolemia	*LDLR*	www.ucl.ac.uk/fh and www.umd.necker.fr	University College London, UK Hôpital Necker-Enfantrs Malades, Paris, France
Sanfilippo disease, type B	*NAGLU*	www.peds.umn.edu/gene/mutation	University of Minnesota, Minneapolis, MN
Lowe syndrome	*OCRL*	www.nhgri.nih.gov/DIR/GDRB/Lowe	The National Human Genome Research Institute, Bethesda, MD
Ornithine transcarbamoylase deficiency	*OTC*	63.75.201.100/otc	University of Minnesota, Minneapolis, MN
X-linked hypophosphatemia	*PHEX*	data.mch.mcgill.ca/phexdb	McGill University, Montreal, Canada
Cystinuria	*SLC3A1*	data.mch.mcgill.ca/cysdb	McGill University, Montreal, Canada
Mitochondrial cytopathies	Various	www.gen.emory.edu/mitomap.html	Emory University, Atlanta, GA

in diagnostic technology, and advances in treatment are growing at such a rapid rate that staying abreast of the field is a daunting task. Information available through the internet includes:

- peer-reviewed journal articles. Various search engines are available which allow the reader to find in a matter of moments specific articles on a subject, by searching on keyword, author, or journal. A particularly useful site is that maintained by the National Library of Medicine of the U.S. (www.ncbi.nlm.nih.gov/entrez/query.fcgi). A vast array of journals is accessible by this technique, covering over 50 years of publications. Access to abstracts is generally free. Some journals also provide full text versions of the articles free of charge, though most require the reader to have an individual or institutional subscription, or to pay for access. This is a particularly valuable resource for physicians.
- Disease-specific foundation sites. These sites can generally be found by conducting a general search on the name of the disease or class of diseases of interest. A partial list is provided in Table 1.8. The material provided by these sites generally includes a wide range of information, from very basic descriptions and explanations in layman terms to references to the medical-scientific literature for physicians. Most also provide the opportunity for readers, including patients, to ask questions about the disease of interest. Some provide 'bulletin boards' for the exchange of information, opinions, and experiences between readers. These are particularly valuable sites, for patients, as well as for treating physicians.
- Medical-scientific databases. A number of sites has been developed to gather and collate technical information of relevance to specific technical aspects of inherited metabolic diseases. These include databases reporting the current status of the identification and characterization of mutations associated with specific diseases. Mutation analysis has become particularly important for carrier detection and prenatal diagnosis of inherited metabolic diseases for which specific mutations have been described. A partial list of these sites is provided in Table 1.9.
- Diagnostic services sites. GeneTests (www.genetests.org/) is a website funded by the National Institutes of Health of the U.S. providing information on a range of services provided by clinics and laboratories for the diagnosis of genetic diseases. Of specific interest is the international laboratory directory of genetic testing laboratories offering accredited laboratory testing for specific diseases, including mutation analyses.
- Metabolic list-serve. This is an extraordinarily useful electronic forum providing physicians around the world with the opportunity to exchange questions and viewpoints, including unpublished experience, related to inherited metabolic diseases. It is accessed by application to the administrator at metab-l-admin@franken.de.

SUGGESTED READING

Blau, N., Duran, M., Blaskovics, M. E. & Gibson, K. M. (eds). (2003). *Physician's Guide to the Laboratory Diagnosis of Metabolic Diseases*, 2nd ed, Heidelberg: Springer-Verlag.

DiMauro, S. & Schon, E. A. (2003). Mitochondrial respiratory-chain diseases. *New England Journal of Medicine*, **348**, 2656–68.

Fernandes, J. Saudubray, J. M. & Van den Berghe, G. (eds). (2000). *Inborn Metabolic Diseases*, 3rd ed, Heidelberg: Springer-Verlag.

Gilbert-Barness, E. & Barness, L. A. (2000). *Metabolic Diseases: Foundations of Clinical Management, Genetics, and Pathology*. Natick, MA: Eaton Publishing Co.

Guttmacher, A. E., Collins, F. S. & Carmona, R. H. (2004). The family history – more important than ever. *New England Journal of Medicine*, **351**, 2333–6.

Hoffmann, G. F., Nyhan, W. L., Zschocke, J., Kahler, S. G. & Mayatepek, E. (2001) *Inherited Metabolic Diseases*, Philadelphia: Lippincott Williams & Wilkins.

Korf, B. R. (2000). *Human Genetics. A Problem-Based Approach*, 2nd ed, Malden, Massachusetts: Blackwell Science Inc.

Nyhan, W. L. & Ozand, P. T. (1998). *Atlas of Metabolic Diseases*. London: Chapman & Hall Medical.

Saudubray, J. M., Ogier, H. & Charpentier, C. Clinical approach to inherited metabolic diseases. In: Fernandes, J., Saudubray, J. M. & Van den Berghe, G. (eds). (1996). *Inborn Metabolic Diseases: Diagnosis and Treatment*, 2nd ed. Berlin: Springer-Verlag, pp 3–39.

Scriver, C. R., Beaudet, A. L., Sly, W. S. & Valle D. (eds). (2001). *The Metabolic and Molecular Bases of Inherited Disease*, 8th ed, New York: McGraw-Hill.

Thorburn, D. R. (2004). Mitochondrial disorders: prevalence, myths and advances. *Journal of Inherited Metabolic Diseases*, **27**, 349–62.

Vogel, F. & Motulsky, A. G. (1996). *Human Genetics*, 3rd ed, Berlin: Springer-Verlag.

Zschocke, J. & Hoffmann, G. F. (2004). *Vademecum metabolicum: manual of metabolic paediatrics*, 2nd ed, Stuttgart: Schattauer.

2

Neurologic syndrome

Neurologic symptoms are the presenting and most prominent clinical problems associated with many inherited metabolic disorders. However, neurologic problems in general are common, especially psychomotor retardation, and deciding whom to investigate, and the type of testing to be done, is often difficult. The age of onset and clinical course often provide important clues to the metabolic nature of the disorder. This is also one situation in which delineation of the extent of the pathology is often invaluable. Besides determining the range of pathology within the nervous system, it is important to establish the extent to which other organs and tissues are involved in order to make a rapid diagnosis of inherited metabolic disease.

Careful and comprehensive clinical assessment, along with imaging studies, electrophysiologic investigation, and histopathologic and ultrastructural information from selected biopsies help to establish the distribution and type of abnormalities within the nervous system. Some patterns of abnormalities are so typical of certain disorders that metabolic studies are required only to confirm the diagnosis. Similarly, the pattern and degree of involvement of other organs and tissues is sometimes sufficiently characteristic to suggest a specific course of metabolic investigation. On one hand, for example, the presence of retinitis pigmentosa, hepatocellular dysfunction, and renal tubular dysfunction, in a child with psychomotor retardation, muscle weakness and seizures, strongly suggest the possibility of a mitochondrial defect. On the other hand, the presence of hepatosplenomegaly without significant hepatocellular dysfunction in a child with slowly progressive psychomotor retardation and ataxia without seizures suggests that the pursuit of a diagnosis of a lysosomal storage disease is likely to be more productive.

Among the inherited metabolic diseases, there are six particularly common neurologic presentations:
• Chronic encephalopathy
• Acute encephalopathy
• Stroke

- Movement disorder
- Myopathy
- Psychiatric or behavioral abnormalities

Chronic encephalopathy – without non-neural involvement

Whether the signs of disease are primarily signs of gray matter or white matter involvement, or both, is a useful guide to diagnostic investigation.

Gray matter disease (poliodystrophy)

Psychomotor retardation or dementia, seizures, impairment of special senses, such as blindness, and extrapyramidal disturbances generally occur early in the course of gray matter diseases.

Psychomotor retardation or dementia

Of all the neurologic problems that occur in patients with inherited metabolic diseases, developmental delay or psychomotor retardation is the commonest. The diagnosis of psychomotor retardation involves assessment of age appropriateness in a number of developmental spheres, including IQ in older patients, and gross motor, fine motor, socio-adaptive, and linguistic milestones in young children and infants. In young children, the Denver Developmental Screening Test is relatively easy to master and apply on a routine basis. Other screening tests are more sophisticated and require special training or access to special supplies or equipment. The periodic reports provided by teachers on the social and academic progress of a child in class provide invaluable information on development, particularly on any deterioration over a period of several months.

In adults, chronic encephalopathy may take the form of progressive dementia. Early recognition and assessment of the progression of the disorder is facilitated by use of any one of a number of mini-mental state examinations, such as the Folstein Mini Mental State Examination (MMSE). They are short, easy to execute and score, and require no special equipment to administer. They are useful as screening instruments; however, in order for any clinical test of higher integrative functioning to be reliably interpretable, the afferent and efferent components of any task must be intact. In other words, the application of tests requiring the patient to be able to see are worthless in patients who are blind. Similarly, the performance of complex actions requiring coordination, such as drawing shapes, are uninterpretable in patients with severe motor disturbances, whether higher integrative functions are intact or not.

Screening tests of mental state are unreliable in individuals who are not fluently comfortable speaking English, or in individuals with little formal education. They are also relatively insensitive to defects in executive functioning, which often emerge before other signs of dementia, but require the use of more sophisticated testing, such as Raven's Progressive Matrices, to identify. The clock-drawing test is more sensitive than the MMSE as a screening test for executive dysfunction, and it is easy to administer in the clinic or at the bedside. However, it does take some practice to learn how to score it.

Psychomotor retardation is a prominent feature of many inherited metabolic diseases presenting in childhood, but only a fraction of the mental retardation encountered in practice will turn out to be caused by inborn errors of metabolism. Who, then, should be investigated, and what type of investigation is most appropriate in each case?

Some general characteristics of the psychomotor retardation caused by inborn errors of metabolism in children

There are some characteristics of the cognitive disabilities caused by inherited metabolic disease which, when present, should alert the clinician to the possibility of an underlying inborn error of metabolism.

First, it tends to be *global*, affecting all spheres of development to some extent. Although a mild developmental problem may present as speech delay, in most cases, a careful history and developmental examination show that the defect extends to other developmental spheres. Older children with mental retardation caused by inborn errors of metabolism commonly show discrepancies in performance on tests of general intelligence, such as the Wechsler Intelligence Scale for Children (revised) (WISC-R): they often perform better on tests of verbal skills compared with motor skills. On the other hand, conditions characterized by progressive myopathy may present as developmental delay characterized by deficits limited to gross motor activities. The nature of the underlying disability usually becomes obvious on physical examination.

Secondly, *severe irritability, impulsivity, aggressiveness, and hyperactivity are also more common* among infants with mental retardation caused by inborn errors of metabolism than among infants with nonmetabolic diseases. Infants with Krabbe globoid cell leukodystrophy are often implacable. Patients with Sanfilippo disease (MPS III) and boys with Hunter disease (MPS II) exhibit particularly disruptive behavior, which in the case of Sanfilippo disease may be the presenting complaint. Motor automatisms and stereotypic behavior are also common in these disorders. Compulsive chewing of the thumb and fingers often results in maceration of the skin and chronic paronychia. The self-mutilatory behavior of boys with Lesch-Nyhan syndrome (X-linked HPRT deficiency) is particularly prominent, sometimes resulting in traumatic amputation of fingers or severe laceration of the lips. Nocturnal restlessness is a common problem in both children and adults with inherited metabolic diseases affecting the brain.

Thirdly, the psychomotor retardation is *usually progressive.* There is generally a history of a period of apparently normal development, followed by loss of developmental milestones or progressive deterioration in school performance. Initially, the progression may be subtle, amounting to an apparent arrest of development during which the gap between the developmental level of the patient and normal children of the same age grows wider with time, without any obvious loss of developmental milestones. Ultimately, loss of previously acquired skills makes the progressive nature of the problem obvious.

On the one hand, earlier onset signals a more rapidly progressive course of the mental handicap. The developmental deficit in a six-year-old with a history of mild mental retardation dating from early infancy, and associated with no regression or other neurologic problems, is unlikely to be attributable to any known inherited metabolic disease. On the other hand, the progression of the intellectual deficit in late-onset GM2 gangliosidosis is usually very slow, tending to be obscured by the prominence of the movement disorder or psychiatric problems associated with the disease. The course of the deterioration in some inherited metabolic diseases, such as metachromatic leukodystrophy, is sigmoidal: a period of relatively slow progression is followed by rapid deterioration, which is then followed by a long period in a relatively stable near-vegetative state.

It is important to distinguish primary developmental regression, occurring as a result of progression of the disease, from pseudo-regression due to environmental or other secondary effects on the nervous system (Table 2.1).

Fourthly, the psychomotor retardation is *usually associated with other objective evidence of neurologic dysfunction,* such as disorders of tone, impairment of special senses, seizures, pyramidal tract signs, evidence of extrapyramidal deficits, or cranial nerve deficits. Moreover, the likelihood that the mental retardation is due to an inborn error of metabolism is increased if the associated neurologic deficits involve more than one part of the nervous system, such as evidence of central nervous system (CNS) disease, along with signs of a peripheral neuropathy.

A general approach to the investigation of inherited metabolic causes of chronic encephalopathy is presented in Figure 2.1. It is based on the early determination of the extent of involvement of non-neural tissues and the degree of involvement of different components of the nervous system. Those disorders in which metabolic acidosis is a prominent aspect of the presentation are discussed in Chapter 3. Similarly, conditions in which hepatic involvement dominates the clinical presentation are considered in Chapter 4, and conditions typically associated with unusual physical features of dysmorphism are discussed in Chapter 6.

This approach serves well when the clinical manifestations of disease are well established, but many of the signs that are particularly characteristic of inherited metabolic diseases only emerge with observation over a period of time.

Table 2.1 Causes of developmental pseudo-regression

Emotional problems, such as depression
The apparent developmental regression of emotionally disturbed infants is well-recognized. This is not a common cause of pseudo-regression in very young children, but must be considered in patients who are mature and lucid enough to be aware of their advancing disease.

Poorly controlled seizure activity
Apparent developmental regression is a common consequence of poor seizure control. The problem is particularly difficult to unravel when the seizures themselves are clinically subtle, but frequent enough to impair consciousness for significant periods of time.

Over-medication with anticonvulsants
The relationship between apparent regression and the introduction of new drugs or changes in drug dosages is usually obvious. An understanding of the usual course of the response to anticonvulsant therapy and possible drug interactions (e.g., erythromycin and carbamazepine), helps to identify this common cause of pseudo-regression.

Intercurrent systemic illness
Children with severe static brain lesions, such as cerebral palsy, often show developmental regression during intercurrent systemic illnesses. This is generally recognized to be reversible in time. However, the recovery of skills is sometimes so slow it raises the question of possible neurological regression that may prompt needless investigation. The relationship to intercurrent illness is usually obvious.

Secondary neurological problems
Secondary neurological problems arising as part of the natural history of some static brain lesions may result in the loss of some previously acquired skills. One example is the loss of mobility arising from skeletal and joint deformities caused by spasticity. A previously ambulatory child with cerebral palsy may stop walking as a result of shortening of the Achilles tendons. The resulting discrepancy between gross motor and other developmental spheres is a clue to the mechanism of the regression in these patients.

Initial investigation

A strategy for the initial investigation of young patients presenting with what might be regarded as undifferentiated chronic encephalopathy or psychomotor retardation without evidence of non-neurologic involvement is shown in Table 2.2. It includes studies:
- to determine the extent and degree of neurologic damage,
- to ensure that the early stages of some treatable metabolic disorder are not missed, and
- studies to establish a baseline for monitoring the natural history of the condition.
   Any metabolic abnormality would be an indication for further investigation. Primary disorders of amino acid metabolism would be unlikely to be missed through this approach. Similarly, most primary defects of organic acid metabolism would

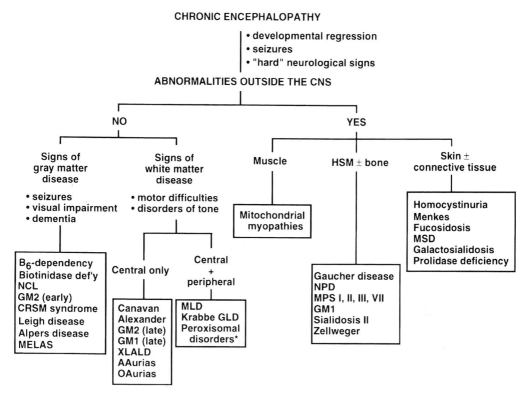

Figure 2.1   An approach to inherited metabolic diseases with chronic encephalopathy.
Abbreviations: NCL, neuronal ceroid-lipofuscinosis; CRSM, cherry-red spot-myoclonus syndrome; MELAS, mitochondrial encephalomyopathy-lactic acidosis and stroke-like episodes syndrome; XLALD, X-linked adrenoleukodystrophy; AAurias, amino acidurias; OAurias, organic acidurias; MLD, metachromatic leukodystrophy; GLD, globoid cell leukodystrophy; NPD, Niemann-Pick disease; MPS, mucopolysaccharidosis; MSD, multiple sulfatase deficiency; HSM, hepatosplenomegaly.

be detected, particularly those in which the psychomotor retardation is severe. It is impossible to exaggerate the importance of imaging techniques, especially MRI with spectroscopy, in the diagnosis of inherited metabolic diseases presenting as neurological syndrome. Many of these conditions are associated with imaging abnormalities that are so characteristic they are virtually diagnostic. Marked reduction in the size of the creatine peak on magnetic resonance spectroscopy of the brain may be the only significant laboratory finding in patients with defects of creatine biosynthesis or in boys with X-linked creatine transporter defects causing severe developmental delay and hypotonia.

The schedule and protocol for reassessment would depend primarily on the age of the patient, the severity of the psychomotor disability, the findings at the initial investigation, and the reproductive plans of the parents. One must be alert to the

Table 2.2 Initial investigation of chronic encephalopathy

Thorough developmental assessment and neurologic examination

Brain imaging: CT or MRI scan

Electrophysiologic studies: auditory brain stem responses, visual evoked potentials, somatosensory evoked potentials, nerve conduction studies, EMG

Radiographs of the hands, chest, and lateral of the spine: for evidence of dysostosis multiplex (see Chapter 6)

Plasma amino acid analysis: screening by thin-layer chromatography will meet most needs; quantitative amino acid analysis, if abnormalities are found (see Chapter 9)

Urinary amino acid thin-layer or paper chromatography

Urinary organic acid analysis, even in the absence of overt metabolic acidosis

Plasma ammonium, preferably two hours after a normal meal of protein-containing food

Plasma lactate

Urinary MPS screening test (see Chapter 9)

Urinary oligosaccharide screening test (see Chapter 9)

Abbreviations: MPS, mucopolysaccharide; EMG, electromyography.

emergence of new clinical signs and be prepared to depart from a protocol that might have been generated in the first place by the feeling that the problem was not the result of an inborn error of metabolism. Often the clinical signs of disease at presentation in early childhood may suggest an inherited metabolic disorder, but intensive metabolic investigation fails to demonstrate any diagnostically specific abnormality, and the subsequent clinical course of the disease turns out to be more consistent with a static neurological lesion.

In other cases, like Rett syndrome, the subsequent clinical course of the condition is sufficiently typical to indicate the diagnosis. In other situations, new information may emerge that redirects the metabolic investigation, leading to the identification of a specific primary metabolic abnormality or a new disease.

Seizures

Recurrent seizures by themselves, in the absence of other evidence of brain disease or systemic metabolic abnormalities, such as hypoglycemia, are unusual as the first manifestation of inherited metabolic diseases. The specific characteristics of seizures that might suggest they are in fact the result of a primary disorder of brain metabolism include:

- onset early in life.
- association with other neurologic signs, such as psychomotor retardation, disorders of tone, movement disorders, or visual impairment.
- complex partial or myoclonic seizures.
- resistance to conventional anticonvulsant therapy.

Intractable seizures in the newborn are considered in detail in Chapter 7. Beyond the newborn period, there is a small number of inherited metabolic diseases in which presentation primarily as a seizure disorder is common (Table 2.3), perhaps with little or no evidence of other problems. In these, the seizure phenotype often resembles West syndrome, with a mixture of partial complex seizures, absence attacks, and frequent massive myoclonic jerks.

One of the most difficult of this category is the group of patients with atypical pyridoxine-dependent seizures. Pyridoxine-dependent seizures typically present in the newborn period (Chapter 7) as generalized tonic-clonic seizures, which are dramatically responsive to administration of large intravenous doses (100 mg) of pyridoxine (vitamin B_6). The diagnosis of atypical pyridoxine dependency is also based on the response to treatment with pyridoxine; however, the response is slower and more variable. Rapid response to therapy seems to be the exception, and exclusion of the diagnosis may require a trial of up to 50 mg of vitamin B_6 per kilogram of body weight, given daily for at least three weeks.

Biotinidase deficiency, a form of multiple carboxylase deficiency, commonly presents between three and six months of life with failure to thrive, metabolic acidosis, a skin rash resembling seborrheic dermatitis, and alopecia, in addition to seizures (see Chapter 3). However, any of the usual features of the disorder may be absent. Some infants have been reported presenting as early as one month of age with infantile spasms. The skin rash, hair changes, and acidosis may only develop some weeks or months later. Presumptive diagnosis is by urinary organic acid analysis, though in some infants the typical abnormalities are sometimes absent. Confirmation of the diagnosis is by enzyme assay on as little as a few drops of blood. The response to treatment with biotin is dramatic. If the diagnosis is considered, treatment with 20 mg per day should be begun without delay while awaiting the results of laboratory studies.

Seizures are generally the only early sign of inherited defects in glucose transport across the blood-brain barrier, caused by mutations in the *GLUT1* gene. Infants with this disorder characteristically present a few months after birth with a history of complex partial, myoclonic, or absence seizures that are typically resistant to conventional anticonvulsant medication. Routine biochemical studies of blood and urine are normal. The EEG and imaging studies are also often normal. However, simultaneous measurement of plasma and CSF shows hypoglycorrhachia: the ratio of CSF to plasma glucose, which is normally >0.65, is decreased to < 0.35. This condition generally responds well to treatment with a ketogenic diet.

Seizures may be the presenting sign of early-onset variants of neuronal ceroid-lipofuscinosis (NCL). They are invariably a major problem in the later stages of the disease, regardless of the age of onset. Developmental delay, psychomotor regression, or dementia are almost always present, usually preceding the onset of myoclonus, which may be interpreted as seizures. Visual impairment progressing

Table 2.3 Inherited metabolic disease in which seizures are particularly prominent in the absence of obvious non-neural involvement

Disease	Other clinical features	Diagnosis
Pyridoxine dependency	Neonatal or early infantile onset of intractable tonic–clonic seizures	Absence of metabolic acidosis or specific abnormalities of intermediary metabolism; rapid EEG and clinical response to pyridoxine.
Atypical pyridoxine dependency	Early infantile onset of intractable tonic-clonic seizures	Absence of metabolic acidosis or specific abnormalities of intermediary metabolism; delayed clinical response to pyridoxine without significant EEG changes.
Tay-Sachs disease	Developmental arrest, hypotonia, visual inattentiveness, markedly exaggerated startle reflex, and macrocephaly	Deficiency of β-hexosaminidase A in serum, leukocytes, or fibroblasts.
Sandhoff disease	Developmental arrest, hypotonia, visual inattentiveness, markedly exaggerated startle reflex, and macrocephaly	Deficiency of total β-hexosaminidase in serum, leukocytes, or fibroblasts.
Multiple carboxylase deficiency	Early infantile onset of intractable tonic-clonic seizures, often with skin rash, alopecia, and lactic acidosis	Urinary organic acids generally, though not always, show presence of 3-methylcrotonate, 3-methylcrotonylglycine, 3-hydroxyisovalerate, and other metabolites (see Chapter 3)
Infantile NCL (Santavuori-Hagberg syndrome)	Early infantile-onset psychomotor retardation, myoclonic seizures, blindness, early flattening of the EEG	Typical lysosomal inclusions seen on electron microscopic examination of skin, leukocytes, or conjunctival epithelium; mutation analysis
Late-infantile NCL (Jansky-Bielschowsky syndrome)	Onset of partial complex and myoclonic seizures at 2–4 years of age, progressive visual impairment, developmental regression, ataxia and tremor	Typical lysosomal inclusions seen on electron microscopic examination of skin, leukocytes, or conjunctival epithelium; mutation analysis
Juvenile NCL (Spielmeyer-Vogt syndrome)	Tonic-clonic seizures, usually preceded by visual failure, and later onset of intellectual regression	Typical lysosomal inclusions seen on electron microscopic examination of skin, leukocytes, or conjunctival epithelium; mutation analysis
MELAS	Lactic acidosis, small stature, seizures, stroke, cortical blindness, psychomotor retardation	Defects in mitochondrial ETC in fibroblasts or skeletal muscle; mitochondrial mutation analysis (see Chapter 9)

Disorder	Clinical features	Laboratory findings
Late-onset galactosialidosis	Myoclonus, seizures, corneal clouding, cherry-red spots, mental retardation	Deficiency of β-galactosidase and α-neuraminidase in fibroblasts
Krabbe GLD	Marked irritability, generalized hypertonia, feeding difficulties, partial complex seizures	Deficiency of galactocerebrosidase in leukocytes or fibroblasts
3-Phosphoglycerate dehydrogenase deficiency	Microcephaly, early-onset severe psychomotor retardation, mixed-type seizures, i.e., tonic, clonic, absence, myoclonic	Abnormally low concentrations of glycine and serine in plasma and CSF; low CSF 5-methylTHF; deficiency of enzyme in cultured fibroblasts
Peroxisomal disorders	Early-onset, marked failure to thrive, severe developmental delay, partial complex seizures	Elevated VLCFA in plasma
GAMT deficiency	Early-onset developmental delay, hypotonia, dystonia, choreiform movements	Marked elevation of GAA levels in plasma, urine and CSF; decreased plasma arginine and urinary creatinine; marked attenuation of creatine peak on MRS; deficiency of GAMT in fibroblasts
CDG syndrome	Marked psychomotor retardation, generalized hypotonia, dysmorphic features (see Chapter 6)	Abnormal isoelectric focusing of plasma transferrin reflecting under-glycosylation
BFNC	Neonatal-onset seizures, with normal neurological and cognitive outcome	Mutations in neuronal potassium channel genes (*KCNQ2* or *KCNQ3*)
GEFS+	Febrile seizures occurring over age 6 years	Mutations in neuronal sodium channel gene (*SCNB1*)

Abbreviations: ETC, electron transport chain; NCL, neuronal ceroid-lipofuscinosis; PDH, pyruvate dehydrogenase; MMA, methylmalonic acidemia; THF, tetrahydrofolate; MELAS, mitochondrial encephalomyopathy with lactic acidosis and stroke-like episodes; GLD, globoid cell leukodystrophy; VLCFA, very long-chain fatty acids; GAMT, guanidinoacetate methyltransferase; GAA, guanidinoacetic acid; MRS, magnetic resonance spectroscopy; CDG, congenital disorder of glycosylation; BFNC, benign familial neonatal convulsions; GEFS+, generalized epilepsy with febrile seizures plus syndrome.

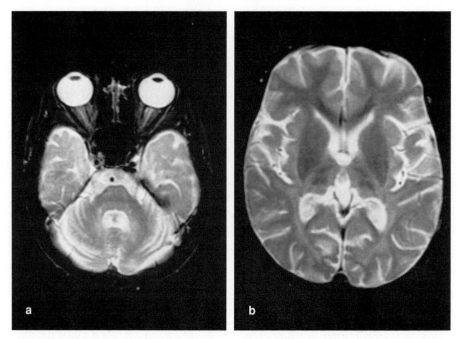

Figure 2.2   MRI scans of the brain of a patient with juvenile neuronal ceroid-lipofuscinosis.
T2-weighted axial MRI scans [TR2800/TE90] through the posterior fossa (**a**) and basal ganglia (**b**) of a 4-year-old child with juvenile neuronal ceroid-lipofuscinosis showing volume
loss of both supra- and infra-tentorial structures, most marked in the cerebellum. Abnormal
signal is also seen in the internal capsules and internal medullary lamina of the thalamus
bilaterally.

to blindness is a prominent and early feature of most of the variants of this group
of disorders. It is more likely to be the presenting problem in children over the age
of three years, but it is not a feature of adult-onset variants of the disease. Macular degeneration, marked attenuation of retinal blood vessels, peripheral 'bone
spicule' pigment deposits, and optic atrophy are typical ocular findings in the
early-onset variants. Early extinction of the electroretinogram (ERG) is a classical
feature of most early-onset variants of NCL. Figure 2.2 shows MRI findings in
juvenile NCL. Electron microscopic examination of conjunctival epithelium, skin,
peripheral blood leukocytes, or rectal mucosa, shows the presence of typical amor-
phous or membranous inclusions (Figure 2.3). The various subtypes of NCL are
summarized in Table 2.4.

Cherry-red spot-myoclonus syndrome (sialidosis, type I) may present with
seizure-like polymyoclonia in later childhood or adolescence with little or no evidence of dementia. However, vision is usually impaired, and ophthalmoscopic
examination reveals the presence of a prominent cherry-red spot in the macula.
The urinary oligosaccharide pattern is abnormal, and demonstrating deficiency of
α-neuraminidase in cultured fibroblasts confirms the diagnosis.

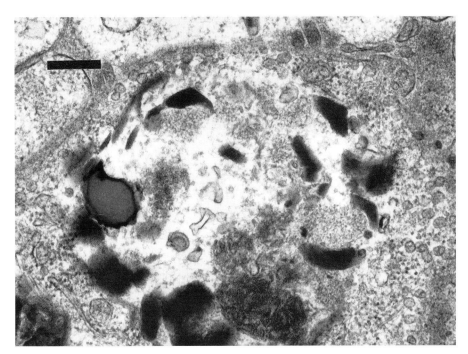

Figure 2.3   Electron micrograph of conjunctival epithelium showing curvilinear and fingerprint inclusions in a patient with neuronal ceroid-lipofuscinosis.
The bar represents 1 μm. (Courtesy of Dr. Venita Jay, Toronto, Canada.)

Seizures with persistent lactic acidosis may be the first indication of an inherited metabolic disorder of mitochondrial energy metabolism, such as pyruvate dehydrogenase (PDH) deficiency or mitochondrial electron transport chain (ETC) defects. The most aggressive clinical variant of this group of disorders is Leigh disease (subacute necrotizing encephalomyelopathy). It is characterized by onset of feeding difficulties and failure to thrive, usually in the first or second year of life. Seizures generally occur on a background of psychomotor retardation then regression, hypotonia, oculomotor abnormalities, recurrent episodes of apnea, ataxic breathing, and tachypnea. The course of the disease is variable. The neurologic deterioration is often punctuated by periods of partial recovery, then acute deterioration. In some infants, progression of the disease appears to arrest for periods of up to several months. There is no effective treatment for the disease, and death generally occurs within weeks to a few years after the onset of symptoms.

Persistent lactic acidosis is typical of most patients with Leigh disease, regardless of the underlying biochemical lesion. However, sometimes it is difficult to determine whether lactate accumulation is the result of a primary defect in lactic acid metabolism, or simply the normal response to uncontrolled seizure activity. In a small proportion of patients, plasma lactate levels may be normal much of the time. Measurement of cerebrospinal fluid (CSF) lactate levels is helpful in these

Table 2.4 Classification of neuronal ceroid lipofuscinoses

Clinical variant	Clinical features	Anatomic abnormalities	Biochemical abnormality	Gene
INCL (Santavuori-Haltia disease)	Onset in the first year of life of developmental delay, hypotonia, exaggerated startle, followed by psychomotor regression, visual failure, ataxia, dystonia, spasticity, myoclonic seizures; retinal dystrophy; extinction of ERG; cerebral atrophy on MRI	GROD	Palmitoyl protein thioesterase (PPT)	_**CLN1**_
LINCL (Jansky-Bielschowsky disease)	Onset at 2–4 years of seizures, myoclonus, psychomotor retardation, ataxia, progressive visual impairment, early extinction of ERG	Lysosomal curvilinear bodies	Tripeptidyl peptidase 1 (TPP1); neuronal accumulation of SCMAS	CLN1, _**CLN2**_
JNCL (Batten disease or Spielmeyer-Vogt-Sjögren disease)	Onset at 4–7 years of progressive visual impairment, followed sometimes years later by dysarthria, intellectual deterioration, seizures, behavioral and other psychiatric disturbances, myoclonia, ataxia	Vacuolated lymphocytic inclusions on peripheral smear; intralysosomal finger-print bodies	Lysosomal membrane glycoprotein of uncertain function	CLN1, CLN2, _**CLN3**_[1]
ANCL (Kufs disease)	Onset in third decade of progressive intractable myoclonic epilepsy with dementia, ataxia and pyramidal and extrapyramidal signs, or behavior disturbances and dementia, ataxia, pyramidal and extrapyramidal signs, suprabulbar deficits. Eyes unaffected.	Mixed intralysosomal inclusions of finger-print, curvilinear, and granular osmiophilic inclusions	Unknown	Unknown

Finnish vLINCL	Onset at 4–7 years of age of motor clumsiness, then progressive visual failure, psychomotor deterioration, and later by ataxia, myoclonia and seizures.	Mixed finger-print, curvilinear, and rectilinear[2] inclusions	Soluble lysosomal glycoprotein of uncertain function; immunoreactive staining for SCMAS	CLN5
Gypsy/Indian vLINCL (Lake-Cavanagh disease; early juvenile NCL)	Onset at 18 mons–5 years of speech delay, then seizures, ataxia, myoclonus, and rapidly progressive psychomotor regression, late progressive visual impairment.	Cytosomal finger-print and rectilinear inclusions in brain; finger-print bodies in neurones of myenteric plexus	Endoplasmic reticulum membrane protein of uncertain function	CLN6
Turkish vLICNL	Onset at 3–7 years of progressive visual impairment, delayed speech, seizures, cognitive deterioration, myoclonia, ataxia.	Cytosomal finger-print, rectilinear and curvilinear inclusions; immunoreactive staining for SCMAS	Endoplasmic reticulum membrane protein of uncertain function	CLN8
Northern EPMR (rare)	Onset at 5–10 years of generalized tonic-clonic seizures, then slowly progressive psychomotor deterioration.			CLN8

Note: For updated catalogue of mutations, see www.ucl.ac.uk/ncl

Abbreviations: GROD, granular osmiophilic deposits; ERG, electroretinogram; SCMAS, subunit c of mitochondrial ATP synthase; EPMR, epilepsy and progressive mental retardation; INCL, infantile neuronal ceroid lipofuscinosis; LINCL, late-infantile neuronal ceroid lipofuscinosis; JNCL, juvenile neuronal lipofuscinosis; vLINCL, variant LINCL; ANCL, adult neuronal ceroid lipofuscinosis.

[1] A large deletion involving two exons of *CLN3* accounts for over 70% of the mutant alleles associated with this disease.

[2] Stacks of short, straight, oligolamellar structures.

Source: Table is adapted from Goebel & Wisniewski (2004).

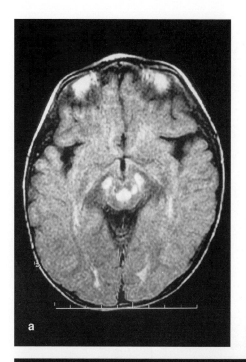

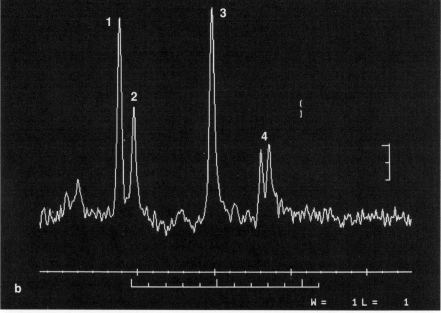

Figure 2.4   Axial MRI scan and MRS of the brain of a patient with Leigh disease.
Panels **a**, Axial FLAIR MRI scan [TR9000/TE160, TI2200] of a 17-month-old child showing increased signal in periaqueductal gray matter and cerebral peduncles; **b**, MRS showing prominent lactic acid doublet. 1, choline; 2, creatine; 3, N-acetylaspartate; 4, lactate.

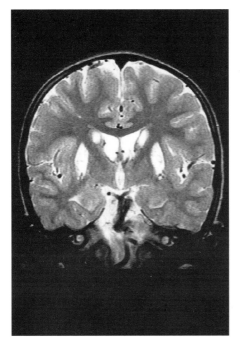

Figure 2.5   Coronal MRI scan of the brain of a child with Leigh disease.
Coronal fast spin echo, T2-weighted MRI scan [TR4000/TE63] of the brain of a $4\frac{1}{2}$-year-old
child showing typical increased signal in the putamina and caudate heads.

situations. CSF lactate levels are not as likely to be spuriously elevated as plasma lactate levels, and they are often elevated in patients with primary disorders of lactic acid metabolism even when plasma levels are normal. Rarely, both plasma and CSF lactates are normal. Imaging studies often show destructive lesions in the brainstem (Figure 2.4) and basal ganglia and thalamus (Figure 2.5). Confirmation of the diagnosis requires biochemical studies on fibroblasts or skeletal muscle (see Chapter 9).

Alper's disease (progressive infantile poliodystrophy) is a clinical syndrome, similar to Leigh disease, characterized by onset in early childhood of psychomotor retardation, then regression, disturbances of tone, myoclonic or tonic-clonic seizures, ataxia, and episodic tachypnea. The principal differences are the prominence in Alpers disease of seizures and cortical blindness, a reflection of the greater involvement of the cerebral cortex, and evidence of hepatocellular dysfunction. This syndrome has been reported in infants with various inborn errors of energy metabolism, particularly PDH deficiency and mitochondrial ETC defects. Persistent lactic acidosis is common, often becoming severe during intercurrent infections. The approach to diagnosis is the same as for Leigh disease.

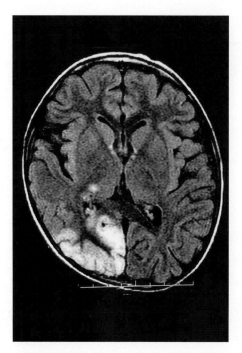

Figure 2.6   Axial MRI scan of the brain of a child with MELAS.
Axial FLAIR MRI scan [TR9002/TE165] through the basal ganglia of an 8-year-old child showing stroke-like lesion in the occipital lobe and junction of the thalamus and internal capsule.

Patients with mitochondrial encephalomyopathy, lactic acidosis, and stroke-like episodes (MELAS) generally present in middle-to-late childhood with a history of psychomotor delay, growth failure, headaches, vomiting, and seizures. Alternating hemiparesis and visual field defects or blindness, exercise intolerance, and muscle weakness, are also common and prominent features of the disease. During episodes of acute encephalopathy, lactate levels may rise to 10–20 mmol/L. Despite the name given to the disease, plasma lactate levels between episodes of metabolic decompensation are not always elevated. However, CSF lactate levels are generally two to three times above normal. CSF protein concentrations are also increased. Imaging studies typically show patchy cortical abnormalities indicative of ischemic damage (Figure 2.6). These do not always conform to the distribution of major cerebral arteries. Histochemical studies on skeletal muscle biopsies show ragged-red fibers. Biochemical studies on muscle often show deficiency of Complex I or Complexes I and IV of the mitochondrial ETC. A particularly common defect in patients with this disease is a point mutation in mitochondrial tRNA$^{Leu(UUR)}$. Endocrinopathies, especially type I diabetes mellitus, are common in patients with MELAS. In fact, diabetes may be the first, and sometimes the only, manifestation of the disease, predating the onset of neurological disturbances by several months or even years.

Measurement of the ratio of lactate to pyruvate (L/P) in plasma or CSF in patients with chronic progressive encephalopathy and lactic acidosis establishes whether lactate accumulation is the result of pyruvate accumulation or accumulation of NADH (see Chapter 3). If the L/P ratio is normal, the accumulation of lactate is the result of a defect in pyruvate metabolism, either pyruvate carboxylase (PC) deficiency, type A, or PDH deficiency. Measurement of the enzyme activities in leukocytes or fibroblasts will confirm the diagnosis. If the L/P ratio is increased and the 3-hydroxybutyrate-to-acetoacetate ratio is decreased, a diagnosis of PC deficiency, type B, should be considered, though this condition always presents in the newborn period and is associated with the presence of other abnormalities (hyperammonemia and increased plasma levels of citrulline, lysine and proline) which should suggest the diagnosis. Again, measurement of PC activity in leukocytes or fibroblasts confirms the diagnosis. Although mitochondrial ETC defects are sometimes identifiable from studies on cultured skin fibroblasts, confirmation of a diagnosis often requires muscle biopsy with histochemical studies, electron microscopy, and biochemical studies on mitochondrial electron transport in mitochondria isolated fresh from the tissue (see Chapter 9).

Leigh disease presenting in early infancy with seizures, severe lactic acidosis, renal tubular dysfunction, and cardiomyopathy has been reported in some infants with muscle coenzyme Q_{10} (ubiquinone, CoQ_{10}) deficiency. Although treatment of infants with the disease with CoQ_{10} may improve the lactic acidosis, the long-term outcome is uniformly poor. By contrast, adults with encephalopathic CoQ_{10} deficiency, presenting as a similar Leigh-like, acute-on-chronic, encephalopathy, appear to improve on treatment with high-dose coenzyme Q_{10}.

Infants with the classical infantile variants of GM2 gangliosidosis – Tay-Sachs disease and Sandhoff disease – usually present at 6–12 months of age with a history of developmental arrest, hypotonia, visual inattentiveness, markedly exaggerated startle reflex, and macrocephaly. Visual failure and seizures occur early and are difficult to control. Fundoscopic examination reveals macular cherry-red spots, which are, in this clinical context, virtually pathognomonic of the disease. CT scans of the brain often show typical abnormalities in the thalamus (Figure 2.7). Although Tay-Sachs mutations are common among Ashkenazi Jews, the incidence of the disease in the Jewish community has dropped dramatically over the past 30 years as a result of carrier screening, genetic counselling, and prenatal diagnosis. In our own experience, the majority of affected infants seen over the past 20 years have not been Jewish. Tay-Sachs disease is caused by deficiency of β-hexosaminidase A. The diagnosis is confirmed by measurement of the enzyme in plasma, leukocytes, or fibroblasts.

Sandhoff disease is a panethnic disease that is much more rare than Tay-Sachs disease, though clinically almost indistinguishable from it. Infants with Sandhoff disease often show mild hepatomegaly, some thickening of alveolar ridges, and radiographic evidence of very mild dysostosis multiplex in addition to all the features of

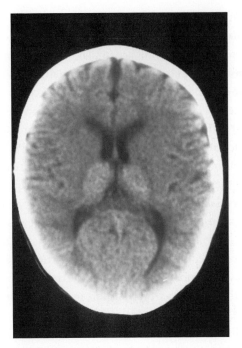

Figure 2.7   Axial CT scan of the brain of an infant with Tay-Sachs disease.
Axial CT scan of the brain of a 16-month-old child showing 'bright thalami', typical of classical Tay-Sachs disease.

Tay-Sachs disease, including macrocephaly and typical macular cherry-red spots. The disease is caused by deficiency of both β-hexosaminidase A and B, which is easily demonstrated in plasma, leukocytes, or fibroblasts.

In children with peroxisomal disorders, such as Zellweger syndrome, pseudo-Zellweger syndrome, neonatal adrenoleukodystrophy, infantile Refsum disease, and rhizomelic chondrodysplasia punctata, cerebral cortical disorganization is often prominent, and seizures are a common early manifestation of the disorders. Dysmorphism, severe psychomotor retardation, sensorineural deafness, peripheral neuropathy, pigmentary retinopathy, failure to thrive, and evidence of hepatocellular dysfunction, may be absent or subtle compared with the prominence of the seizures, particularly early in the course of the later-onset variants. These conditions are discussed in more detail in Chapter 6. Analysis of very long-chain fatty acids, pipecolic acid, and bile acid intermediates in plasma and plasmalogen concentrations in erythrocytes is usually sufficient to establish the diagnosis (see Chapter 9).

Early-onset, severe psychomotor retardation, profound generalized hypotonia, variable facial dysmorphism, and intractable seizures are also characteristic of most of the variants of congenital disorders of glycosylation (CDG) syndrome. These, too, are discussed in more detail in Chapter 6.

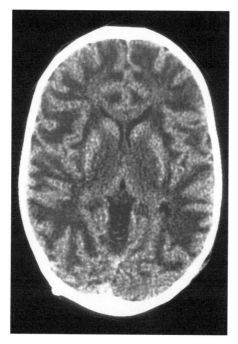

Figure 2.8   CT scan of the brain of an infant with Canavan disease.
Axial CT scan of the brain of a $2\frac{1}{2}$-year-old child showing diffuse abnormal attenuation of white matter and subcortical gray structures.

White matter disease (leukodystrophy)

In diseases predominantly affecting cerebral white matter, the clinical presentation tends to be dominated by motor difficulties, including gross motor delay, weakness, and incoordination. White matter disease (leukodystrophy) is a common feature of many inherited metabolic disorders presenting with chronic encephalopathy, including many 'small molecule' diseases. Therefore, the investigation of any patient presenting with signs of leukodystrophy should routinely include analysis of plasma amino acids and urinary organic acids.

The leukodystrophy in patients with Canavan disease is particularly aggressive and typically associated with rapidly developing megalencephaly. Affected infants present in the first few months of life with a history of developmental arrest, irritability, hypotonia, and failure to thrive, followed by spasticity and seizures. Imaging studies show severe, diffuse white matter attenuation (Figure 2.8). The disease is caused by deficiency of aspartoacylase, which is associated with accumulation of N-acetylaspartate (NAA) in the CSF, blood, and urine. Diagnosis is suggested by finding increased NAA levels in urine by GC-mass spectrometry, or in the brain by magnetic resonance spectroscopy, and it is confirmed by direct demonstration of the enzyme deficiency in fibroblasts. The incidence of this disease is high among Ashkenazi Jews in whom a single mutation (E285A) accounts for 80–85% of the mutant alleles, with only two other mutations accounting for the bulk of the remainder.

Classical Alexander disease is a phenocopy of Canavan disease with early onset of developmental arrest, hypotonia, seizures, and marked megalencephaly. Imaging studies show severe white matter disease. The diagnosis is usually made by demonstration of Rosenthal fibers in the brain at autopsy. The disease has recently been shown to be associated with autosomal dominant mutations in the GFAP gene, coding for glial fibrillary acidic protein. Late-onset variants of Alexander disease are not associated with megalencephaly. Pseudobulbar and bulbar signs dominate the onset of the juvenile-onset variant; patients with adult-onset disease show signs of pyramidal tract and cerebellar dysfunction, mimicking multiple sclerosis, with palatal myoclonus in at least some. Imaging studies show atrophy of the cerebellum, medulla, and spinal cord.

Boys with X-linked adrenoleukodystrophy (XL-ALD) generally present in middle childhood with a history of behavior problems (irritability, withdrawal, obsessiveness) or school failure, followed by the development of gait disturbances, increased muscle tone progressing to spasticity, visual failure, and deafness. Deterioration to a neuro-vegetative state occurs rapidly, though death may be delayed for several years. Some boys present with overt clinical evidence of adrenal insufficiency, such as a history of fatiguability and deep tanning of the skin. All boys with the condition show at least biochemical evidence of adrenal failure sometime in the course of the disease. The CT and MRI changes are so typical that they immediately suggest the diagnosis (Figure 2.9), which is confirmed by measurement of very long-chain fatty acids in plasma.

The onset of disease in males who have inherited an ALDP mutation causing XL-ALD may be delayed for several years. Late-onset variants of the disease, called adrenomyeloneuropathy (AMN), are often clinically difficult to distinguish from progressive multiple sclerosis. Progressive spastic paraplegia occurs in a small but significant number of female carriers of XL-ALD. Dementia is late and only very slowly progressive. However, the biochemical abnormalities are the same as in classical juvenile-onset XL-ALD. Curiously, many different clinical variants of the disease may occur in male members of the same family. This makes genetic counselling and the evaluation of any treatment for this disorder particularly difficult.

Many patients with late-onset variants of GM2 gangliosidosis present with motor difficulties, such as ataxia, dysarthria, and dystonia, caused by generalized white matter involvement with the disease. Imaging studies show generalized brain atrophy, but posterior fossa structures are usually particularly severely affected (Figure 2.10). Unlike the common infantile-onset variants of the disease (Tay-Sachs disease and Sandhoff disease), macular cherry-red spots are not seen in patients

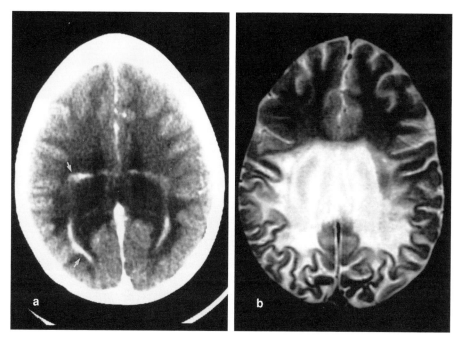

Figure 2.9   CT and MRI scans of the brain in X-linked adrenoleukodystrophy.
Panel **a**, shows a CT scan of the brain with enhancement done early in the course of the
disease in a nine-year-old boy. It shows diffuse white matter attenuation in the peritrigonal
area and corpus callosum. The arrows indicate the rim of active demyelination characteristic
of the disease. Panel **b**, shows a T2-weighted MRI scan [TR2800/TE90] done 10 years later.
It shows extensive demyelination of the peritrigonal area and corpus callosum extending
into subcortical white matter with incomplete sparing of U-fibers.

with late-onset forms of the disease. The diagnosis is confirmed by measurement
of β-hexosaminidase A and B in plasma, leukocytes, or fibroblasts.

The presence of *peripheral neuropathy* may not be clinically obvious, but it is
an important feature of inherited disorders of myelin lipid metabolism, such as
metachromatic leukodystrophy and Krabbe globoid cell leukodystrophy. Metachromatic leukodystrophy (MLD) is caused by deficiency of arylsulfatase A and is characterized by accumulation of the myelin lipid, sulfatide, in the brain and peripheral
nerve. The clinical presentation in early onset variants of MLD is usually dominated by signs of motor difficulties, such as weakness, clumsiness, and stumbling,
resembling ataxia. Nerve conduction studies show slowing, and the CSF protein
concentration is characteristically elevated. Cognitive functioning is only minimally affected at first. The diagnosis is confirmed by measurement of arylsulfatase
A in leukocytes or fibroblasts. Later in the course of the disease, and early in the
course of late-onset variants of MLD, cognitive dysfunction is more prominent.

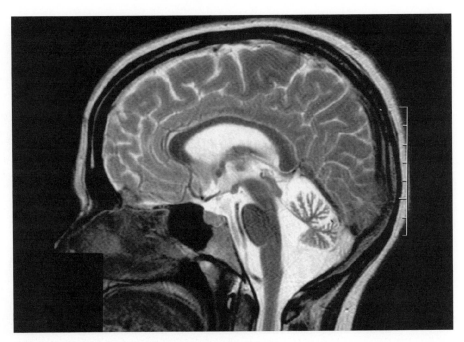

Figure 2.10 MRI scan of the brain in late-onset GM2 gangliosidosis.
Sagittal fast spin echo T2-weighted MRI [TR4000/TE63] of the brain of a 31-year-old woman showing severe volume loss of the cerebellum.

Children with juvenile-onset MLD generally come to attention as a result of deteriorating school performance, though the presence of motor difficulties and some dysarthria can usually be demonstrated on careful physical examination. In patients with adult-onset MLD, cognitive impairment is commonly accompanied by psychiatric disturbances. General physical and routine neurological examinations are often normal, though careful mental state examination will usually show deficits, which in the early stages may be limited to higher cognitive abnormalities, especially executive dysfunction.

Chronic encephalopathy – with non-neural tissue involvement

The pattern of non-neural tissue involvement in patients presenting with chronic encephalopathy is an important clinical clue to the underlying defect. Many of the diseases exhibiting significant non-neurologic involvement are caused by defects in organelle metabolism. Those in which myopathy is particularly prominent are considered in the section on 'Myopathy'.

Hepatosplenomegaly is a prominent feature of many of the lysosomal storage diseases presenting as chronic encephalopathy. In some, such as Hurler disease

(MPS IH), Hunter disease (MPS II), and Sly disease (MPS VII), the non-neurologic manifestations of disease dominate the clinical presentation, and they are discussed in Chapter 6. In contrast, the hepatosplenomegaly in patients with Sanfilippo disease (MPS III) is rarely very impressive and the radiographic evidence of dysostosis multiplex may be very subtle. Patients with Sanfilippo disease usually present in the second or third year of life with a history of developmental delay, particularly affecting speech, and characteristically horrendous behavior problems characterized by marked impulsivity, aggressiveness, hyperactivity, stereotypic motor automatisms, and nocturnal restlessness. The behavior problems are sufficiently characteristic to suggest the diagnosis. The four biochemically and genetically distinct variants of Sanfilippo disease (MPS IIIA, B, A, and D) are clinically indistinguishable from each other. Urinary MPS screening tests are sometimes falsely negative. Thin-layer chromatography of urinary MPS typically shows increased excretion of heparan sulfate. The diagnosis is confirmed by analysis in fibroblasts of each of the four enzymes found deficient in different variants of the disease (see Chapter 9).

Infants with acute neuronopathic Gaucher disease (type 2) present in the first few months of life with developmental arrest, hypertonia, neck retraction, strabismus, visual impairment, and major feeding difficulties as a result of inability to swallow. The liver and especially the spleen are typically huge, but bone changes, which are so prominent in many patients with non-neuronopathic Gaucher disease (type 1), do not occur. Storage cells are not seen in the peripheral circulation. However, bone marrow aspirates contain typical Gaucher cells, which are indistinguishable from those seen in non-neuronopathic variants of the disease. The diagnosis is confirmed by demonstrating deficiency of lysosomal β-glucosidase (or glucocerebrosidase) in leukocytes or fibroblasts. Most infants with acute neuronopathic Gaucher disease carry at least one L444P mutation. This is a rapidly progressive disease, generally ending in death before age two years.

Children with subacute neuronopathic Gaucher disease (type 3) usually present in early or middle childhood with a history of slowly progressive ataxia, dysarthria, and cognitive deterioration, similar is many respects to juvenile MLD. However, unlike children with MLD, children with type 3 Gaucher disease almost always have significant hepatosplenomegaly. Some children with type 3 disease present in early childhood with aggressive visceral disease, with little or no clinical evidence of neurologic involvement for some years. Superficially, the disease in these children resembles a very severe form of type 1 Gaucher disease. In fact, some patients with type 3 disease die of hepatic failure before they develop significant neurologic problems. Survivors invariably develop an unusual oculomotor abnormality, characterized by vertical looping movements of the eyes on lateral gaze, the first clinical clue to the true nature of the condition, sometimes long before the appearance of other neurologic abnormalities. Biochemically, patients with this disease are indistinguishable from patients with severe non-neuronopathic Gaucher disease (see Chapter 6). Mutation analysis is of some help: most patients with type 3 Gaucher disease, like those with type 2 disease have at least one L444P allele. In contrast, the presence of the common N370S allele is virtually unknown in patients with neuronopathic Gaucher disease, either type 2 or type 3.

Infants with Niemann-Pick disease (NPD), especially type A, also present in the first few months of life with typically massive enlargement of the liver and spleen causing marked protuberance of the abdomen. However, neurologic involvement with the disease occurs later and is more slowly progressive that in the acute neuronopathic variant of Gaucher disease. Feeding problems commonly cause severe failure to thrive, and pulmonary involvement often causes chronic respiratory problems. Liver function tests may be mildly abnormal. Skeletal radiographs are usually normal. However, radiographs of the chest commonly show diffuse reticular infiltrations of the lungs. Bone marrow smears usually show the presence of foamy storage histiocytes, which are typical though not specific for the disease. The disease is caused by deficiency of lysosomal acid sphingomyelinase. The diagnosis of the disease is confirmed by measuring the enzyme in leukocytes or fibroblasts.

NPD type C (NPD-C) may present in infancy or early childhood as hepatic syndrome (see Chapter 4), or as a progressive neurodegenerative condition with relatively little evidence of visceral involvement. Presentation as neurologic disease is usually in early to middle childhood with progressive gait disturbance, dysarthria, emotional lability, and developmental arrest, then regression. The liver and spleen are usually enlarged, and liver function test is often mildly abnormal. One of the characteristic features of the condition is early-onset supranuclear gaze palsy, manifested as impaired vertical saccadic eye movements. Bone marrow aspirates usually show the presence of foamy histiocytes and 'sea-blue' histiocytes. The basic biochemical defect in NPD-C is incompletely understood. It appears to involve some disturbance in the intracellular processing of cholesterol. The esterification of cholesterol by cultured skin fibroblasts is typically impaired. The cells also show strong staining with filipin as a result of cholesterol accumulation in the cells. Confirming the diagnosis of NPD-C by laboratory studies is often difficult because the diagnostic abnormalities are secondary manifestations of the primary metabolic defect. Mutation analysis is particularly important in this group of diseases because it is the only reliable method for the identification of carriers of the disease, and it greatly facilitates prenatal diagnosis. Most cases of NPD-C are caused by mutations in the *NPC1* gene; some are caused by *NPC2* mutations.

GM1 gangliosidosis and sialidosis, along with other glycoproteinoses, are reviewed in Chapter 6. Both conditions may present in early infancy with severe, rapidly progressive, neurovisceral storage disease associated with dysmorphic facial features resembling Hurler disease, but without corneal clouding, often with cherry-red macular spots, and radiographic evidence of bone involvement. Patients with later-onset variants have little or no evidence of non-neurologic disease. As a rule, they present with gait disturbances, dysarthria, and psychomotor retardation. Spasticity and seizures follow. Analysis of urinary oligosaccharides is abnormal in both conditions. Definitive diagnosis requires demonstration of deficiency of β-galactosidase in plasma, leukocytes, or fibroblasts in the case of GM1 gangliosidosis. Confirmation of the diagnosis of sialidosis requires the demonstration of α-neuraminidase deficiency in cultured fibroblasts.

Fucosidosis and mannosidosis commonly present as chronic encephalopathy with developmental delay. Although both, especially fucosidosis, are associated with the development of 'storage facies' as they grow older, psychomotor retardation is often the only clinical complaint at initial presentation. Radiographic evidence of mild dysostosis multiplex is usually present, though subtle and often overlooked. Vacuolated mononuclear cells are often found in peripheral blood smears. Patients with mannosidosis characteristically develop sensorineural hearing loss early in the course of their disease. Angiokeratomata, indistinguishable from those seen in patients with Fabry disease, are a typical feature of fucosidosis.

The non-neurologic features of homocystinuria and Menkes disease clearly set them apart from other inherited metabolic diseases in which chronic encephalopathy is a prominent aspect of the clinical presentation. They are discussed in Chapter 6.

Acute encephalopathy

Acute encephalopathy, regardless of the cause, is a medical emergency. In addition to being a common manifestation of a variety of acquired medical or surgical conditions, it is a presenting feature of a number of inherited metabolic diseases, particularly in young children (Figure 2.11). Deterioration of consciousness occurring as a result of inherited metabolic disease:

• often occurs with little warning in a previously healthy infant or child;
• may be missed because the early signs may be mistaken as a behavior disorders;
• often progresses rapidly, may fluctuate markedly;
• usually shows no focal neurologic deficits.

The earliest signs of encephalopathy may be no more obvious than excessive drowsiness, unusual behavior, or some unsteadiness of gait. Acute or intermittent

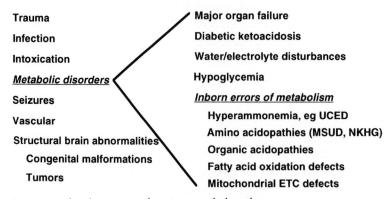

Figure 2.11 Summary of major causes of acute encephalopathy.
Abbreviations: UCED, urea cycle enzyme defects; MSUD, maple syrup urine disease; NKHG, nonketotic hyperglycinemia; ETC, electron transport chain.

Table 2.5 Causes of metabolic acute encephalopathy to be considered at various ages

Condition	Age		
	Newborn	Early childhood	Later childhood
Urea cycle defects	++++	+ (girls with OTC)	(+)
NKHG	++++	0	0
Organic acidopathies	++++	+	(+)
MSUD	++++	++	++
FAOD	+	++++	?
Reye syndrome	0	++	+++
Drug ingestion	+ (maternal)	+++	+++

Abbreviations: NKHG, nonketotic hyperglycinemia; MSUD, maple syrup urine disease; FAOD, fatty acid oxidation defects; OTC, ornithine transcarbamoylase deficiency.

ataxia is a common sign of acute encephalopathy in older children with inborn errors of metabolism. A history of recurrent attacks of unsteadiness of gait or ataxia, especially when associated with vomiting or deterioration of consciousness, should be considered a strong indication for investigation of a possible inherited metabolic disease.

The progression to stupor and coma is often irregular, with periods of apparent lucidity alternating with periods of obtundation. Failure to recognize the inherent instability of the situation, and to monitor clinical neurologic vital signs closely, may end in disaster. The likely causes of acute metabolic encephalopathy are age-dependent (Table 2.5).

Table 2.6 Initial investigation of acute encephalopathy

Blood gases and electrolytes (calculate anion gap), blood glucose
Urinalysis, including tests for ketones and reducing substances
Liver function tests
Blood ammonium
Plasma lactate
Urinary organic acids (15 ml urine, no preservative, stored frozen)
Plasma amino acid analysis, quantitative
Plasma carnitine and acylcarnitines, including tandem MSMS

Table 2.7 Differential diagnosis of inherited metabolic diseases presenting as acute encephalopathy

	UCED	MSUD	OAuria	FAOD	ETC defects
Metabolic acidosis	0	±	+++	±	++
Plasma glucose	N	N or ↓	↓↓	↓↓↓	N
Urinary ketones	N	↑↑	↑↑	0	0
Plasma ammonium	↑↑↑	N	↑↑	↑	N
Plasma lactate	N	N	↑	±	↑↑↑
Liver function	N	N	N	↑↑	N
Plasma carnitine	N	N	↓↓↓	↓↓	N
Plasma amino acids	Abnormal	↑ BCAA	↑ glycine		↑ alanine
Urinary organic acids	N	Abnormal	Abnormal	Abnormal	N

Abbreviations: UCED, urea cycle enzyme defect; MSUD, maple syrup urine disease; OAuria, organic aciduria; FAOD, fatty acid oxidation defect; ETC, mitochondrial electron transport chain; BCAA, branched-chain amino acids; ↑ elevated; ↓ decreased; +, present; ±, variably present; N, normal; 0, not present.

Initial investigation

Because of the importance of identifying treatable inherited metabolic diseases early, initial investigation of any patient presenting stuporous or obtunded must not be delayed (Table 2.6).

A summary of the results of initial laboratory studies in various inborn errors of metabolism presenting as acute encephalopathy is shown in Table 2.7.

Hyperammonemia

The plasma or blood ammonium should be measured immediately, along with the plasma glucose and electrolytes, in any child presenting with acute or sub-acute encephalopathy of obscure etiology. However, the interpretation of the results requires additional information. Plasma ammonium levels are often elevated in patients with severe hepatocellular dysfunction, regardless of the cause, including viral infections, intoxications, or some inborn errors of metabolism. Inherited metabolic diseases presenting with hyperammonemia due to liver failure are discussed in Chapter 4. Apart from marked elevation of plasma ammonium levels, liver function tests in patients with primary disorders of urea biosynthesis are usually near normal. Ornithine transcarbamoylase (OTC) deficiency is an exception to this generalization. Transaminases in patients with the disease are often mildly to moderately elevated, but the hyperammonemia is generally much more severe than can be explained by the degree of hepatocellular dysfunction, as reflected by the transaminases and other tests of liver cell damage.

The investigation and diagnosis of possible urea cycle enzyme defects (UCED) is facilitated by reference to a simplified diagram showing the main elements of ammonium metabolism (Figure 2.12).

The key features of the metabolism of waste nitrogen are:
- The process is divided between two sets of reactions, one set in the cytosol, the other inside mitochondria.
- The first reaction, the carbamoylphosphate synthase I (CPS I)-catalyzed condensation of ammonium with bicarbonate to form carbamoylphosphate, requires the presence of N-acetylglutamate (NAG), an obligatory effector, not a substrate, for the reaction.
- One of the two waste nitrogen atoms that become part of urea is derived from the non-essential amino acid, aspartate. Aspartate is produced by transamination of oxaloacetate in a reaction catalyzed by liver and muscle aspartate aminotransferase (AST).
- The entire process is highly dependent on an adequate supply of intramitochondrial ornithine.

Ornithine is a five-carbon amino acid analogue of the essential amino acid, lysine. It is formed from arginine by a reaction catalyzed by arginase. The concentration of the amino acid is directly related to the availability and metabolism of arginine. Ornithine is not incorporated into body protein. Transport into mitochondria is facilitated by a specific carrier system. Ornithine is a precursor in the biosynthesis of spermine and putrescine, as well as the amino acids, glutamate and proline.

Intramitochondrial ornithine condenses with carbamoylphosphate in a reaction catalyzed by OTC, which is coded by a gene on the short arm of the X chromosome. The product, citrulline, diffuses out of the mitochondrion into the cytosol where it condenses with aspartate to form argininosuccinic acid (ASA) in a reaction catalyzed by ASA synthetase. ASA is cleaved to produce arginine and fumarate in a reaction catalyzed by ASA lyase. The renal clearance of ASA is extremely high.

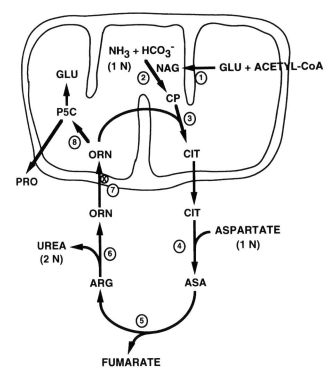

Figure 2.12 Summary of normal ammonium metabolism.
The various enzyme of transport systems involved are: **1**, N-acetylglutamate synthetase (NAGS); **2**, carbamoylphosphate synthetase I (CPS I); **3**, ornithine transcarbamoylase (OTC); **4**, argininosuccinic acid synthetase (ASA synthetase); **5**, argininosuccinic acid lyase (ASA lyase); **6**, arginase; **7**, mitochondrial ornithine transport system; **8**, ornithine aminotransferase. Other abbreviations: GLU, glutamate; CIT, citrulline; ARG, arginine; ORN, ornithine; P5C, Δ^1-pyrroline-5-carboxylic acid; PRO, proline. The figure shows how one of the waste nitrogen atoms excreted as urea is derived from ammonia (NH_3); the other comes from the amino acid, aspartate.

A widely used algorithmic approach to the differential diagnosis of hyperammonemic encephalopathy is presented in Figure 2.13. The presence of moderate to severe metabolic acidosis indicates that the hyperammonemia is a manifestation of an inherited disturbance of organic acid metabolism, which is discussed in Chapter 3.

Urea cycle enzyme defects presenting as acute hyperammonemic encephalopathy, whether in early infancy or later in childhood, are clinically indistinguishable from each other. The most important diagnostic information, after ammonium determination, liver function tests, and analysis of blood gases and plasma glucose

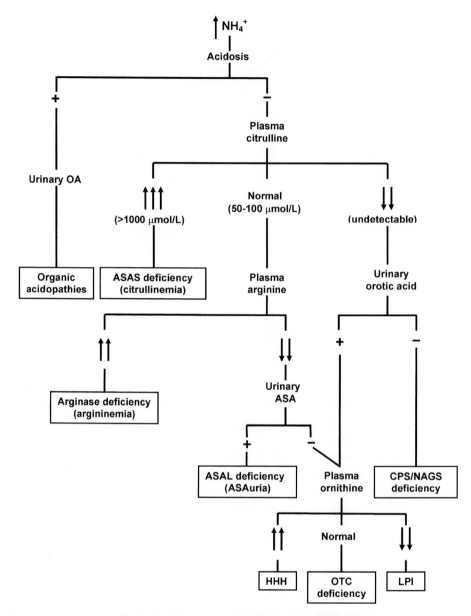

Figure 2.13 An approach to the diagnosis of hyperammonemia in older children.
Abbreviations: OA, organic acids; ASAS, argininosuccinic acid synthetase; ASAL, argininosuccinic acid lyase; CPS/NAGS, carbamoylphosphate synthetase I or N-acetylglutamate synthetase; HHH, hyperammonemia-hyperornithinemia-homocitrullinemia syndrome; OTC, ornithine transcarbamoylase; LPI, lysinuric protein intolerance.

and electrolytes, is *quantitative* analysis of plasma amino acids. The reliance on semi-quantitative or screening tests to measure amino acid levels is a common error in the investigation of inherited metabolic diseases. In the investigation of a patient with hyperammonemia, these are particularly inappropriate. Low concentrations of certain amino acids are as important as excesses in the differential diagnosis of hyperammonemia, and subnormal amino acid levels cannot be detected by any of the qualitative or semi-quantitative amino acid screening tests (see Chapter 9). The analytical chemist should be alerted to the need to identify low levels of amino acids, as well as excesses.

The concentration of citrulline is central to the interpretation of the results of amino acid analyses. If the citrulline concentration is markedly elevated, the child has citrullinemia as a result of ASA synthetase deficiency. Citrulline levels that are extremely low suggest the presence of a defect in citrulline biosynthesis, the result of deficiency of OTC, CPS I, or NAG synthetase (NAGS).

OTC deficiency is transmitted as an X-linked recessive condition. Affected boys usually present in the newborn period with severe, usually life-threatening, hyperammonemia (see Chapter 7). Symptomatic carrier girls generally present later in childhood with an antecedent history of feeding problems, failure to thrive, intermittent ataxia, or intermittent encephalopathy. Unfortunately, the diagnosis in symptomatic girls is often missed until the patients present with acute encephalopathy, commonly resulting in irreparable brain damage. Recently, we have encountered a small number of adults with variants of OTC deficiency which presented in the third or fourth decades of life as sudden onset of progressive hyperammonemic encephalopathy, often progressing rapidly to coma and death, in previously completely healthy individuals. Decompensation in some cases was clearly associated with some intercurrent infection or major surgery; in others, no cause could be identified.

Deficiency of OTC causes accumulation of carbamoylphosphate and ammonium; diffusion of the excess carbamoylphosphate into the cytosol results in overproduction of pyrimidines and the pyrimidine intermediates-orotic acid and orotidine. OTC is differentiated from CPS I and NAGS deficiencies by the demonstration of increased concentrations of orotic acid and orotidine in the urine.

Citrulline levels that are normal or only moderately elevated are generally an indication of argininosuccinic aciduria, the result of argininosuccinic acid lyase deficiency, or argininemia, caused by arginase deficiency. However, argininemia almost never presents as acute encephalopathy. Instead, patients with this disorder tend to have only mild to moderate elevations of plasma ammonium, and they present clinically later in infancy and early childhood with 'cerebral palsy'. The elevation of plasma arginine is generally sufficiently specific to make the diagnosis.

Argininosuccinic aciduria is characterized by subnormal arginine levels in plasma and the presence of markedly increased amounts of the amino acid, argininosuccinate, in plasma and urine. The renal clearance of this amino acid is very high, and the concentrations in urine are generally very high compared with the levels in plasma. However the demonstration of the presence of increased concentrations of argininosuccinate in plasma requires no more analysis than has already been done for the usual quantitative analysis of plasma amino acids.

Lysinuric protein intolerance (LPI) may also present in later infancy or early childhood as hyperammonemic encephalopathy. This is a protean metabolic disorder, which may present as growth retardation and hepatomegaly, hematologic abnormalities, pulmonary disease, or renal disease. It is caused by a generalized hereditary defect in dibasic amino acid transport. Plasma arginine, ornithine, and lysine levels are typically markedly subnormal. At the same time, quantitative analysis of urinary amino acids shows marked increases in the excretion of the same compounds. Intracellular ornithine deficiency causes accumulation of carbamoylphosphate and ammonium resulting in increased urinary orotic acid and orotidine excretion.

Hyperammonemia-hyperornithinemia-homocitrullinemia (HHH) syndrome is another disorder of ammonium metabolism caused by a defect in amino acid transport. In this case, the transport of ornithine into mitochondria is defective, resulting in intramitochondrial ornithine deficiency. Paradoxically, plasma ornithine levels are markedly elevated in this condition. However, intramitochondrial ornithine deficiency causes accumulation of carbamoylphosphate and ammonium, and in the same manner as in LPI, this causes carbamoylphosphate accumulation resulting in increased urinary orotic acid and orotidine concentrations.

Citrin deficiency, or adult-onset type II citrullinemia (CTLN2), is an autosomal recessive disease characterized by the sudden onset, often precipitated by drug or alcohol ingestion or infection, of hyperammonemia and acute organic brain syndrome – disorientation, delirium, delusions, stupor – often progressing rapidly to death. The disease is caused by mutations of the *SLC25A13* gene, a mitochondrial aspartate-glutamate carrier protein. The hyperammonemia appears to be the result of cytosolic aspartate deficiency, caused by the defect in aspartate transport from inside mitochondria into the cytosol. Plasma citrulline levels are characteristically elevated, and plasma aspartate concentrations are typically low. Argininosuccinic acid synthase activity is impaired, partly because of the deficiency of aspartate, along with an absolute deficiency of the enzyme activity in liver by some currently unknown mechanism. The importance of cytosolic aspartate in urea biosynthesis is shown in Figure 2.12.

Unlike patients with other urea cycle enzyme defects, who have an aversion to high protein foods and do better on high-carbohydrate diets, patients with CTLN2 report a preference for high-protein foods and dislike carbohydrates. Most are very thin. The prognosis is generally poor, though the response to liver transplantation is excellent. Almost all known cases have been Japanese.

Leucine encephalopathy (maple syrup urine disease – MSUD)

This usually presents in the newborn period as an acute encephalopathy, initially without metabolic acidosis (Chapter 7). Milder variants of the disease may present at any age during childhood. Acute encephalopathy without hyperammonemia or significant metabolic acidosis, on a background of chronic failure to thrive and mild to moderate psychomotor retardation, is typical of MSUD. Decompensation is usually heralded by drowsiness, anorexia, and vomiting. The odor widely described as resembling the aroma of maple syrup is more like the smell of burnt sugar. The urine typically tests positive for ketones. Testing the urine for the presence of α-ketoacids by addition of DNPH (dinitrophenylhydrazine) reagent produces a strongly positive reaction. Plasma ammonium levels are characteristically normal. The course of subsequent deterioration is often highly irregular with periods of lucidity alternating with stupor, progressing to coma. Signs of intracranial hypertension (posturing, dilated and sluggish pupils, periodic breathing) are an indication that the situation is grave and the chances of recovery, even with aggressive treatment, are seriously compromised. Quantitative analysis of plasma amino acids is the most rapid and reliable method to confirm the diagnosis, and it should be done without delay. Marked elevations of leucine, isoleucine, and valine, and the presence of alloisoleucine, are diagnostic of MSUD. Modest increases in the branched-chain amino acids are common in children during short-term starvation and should not be confused with mild variants of MSUD.

Analysis of urinary organic acids as oxime derivatives shows the presence of a number of branched-chain α-ketoacids. However, this generally takes longer than plasma amino acid analysis and does not add much to the diagnosis of MSUD.

Reye-like acute encephalopathy (fatty acid oxidation defects)

Acute encephalopathy resembling Reye syndrome is a common presenting feature of the primary inherited disorders of fatty acid oxidation. The commonest of these is medium-chain acyl-CoA dehydrogenase (MCAD) deficiency. Affected children are usually completely well until they present, usually in the first year or two of life, with what may appear initially to be nothing more sinister than 'stomach flu', with anorexia, vomiting, drowsiness, and lethargy. The fact that metabolic decompensation is usually precipitated by intercurrent illness, generally associated with poor feeding, often obscures the nature of the underlying metabolic disorder. Drowsiness and lethargy progress rapidly to stupor and coma, hepatomegaly with evidence of hepatocellular dysfunction, hypotonia, hypoketotic hypoglycemia (see

Chapter 4), and mild to moderate hyperammonemia. Hypoglycemic seizures may be the first serious sign of the disease. Although it is often clinically indistinguishable from Reye syndrome, onset in the first two years of life, a positive family history, and recurrence of acute metabolic decompensation during trivial intercurrent illnesses or fasting, are features peculiar to MCAD deficiency and other fatty acid oxidation defects.

Acute encephalopathy may also occur in the absence of hypoglycemia or significant hepatocellular dysfunction, suggesting that accumulation of fatty acid oxidation intermediates plays some role in its pathogenesis. Sudden unexpected death is tragically common in infants with unrecognized MCAD deficiency, perhaps as a result of cardiac arrhythmias caused by accumulated fatty acid oxidation intermediates (see Chapter 5). Successful management of this condition rests on a high index of suspicion coupled with early treatment with glucose while awaiting the results of definitive laboratory tests.

Analysis of urinary organic acids during acute metabolic decompensation characteristically shows the presence of large amounts of C-6 to C-10 dicarboxylic acids (adipic, suberic, and sebacic acids), the (ω-1)-hydroxy derivatives of hexanoic and octanoic acids, but little or no ketones (see Chapter 4). Urinary organic acid analysis when the child is clinically well may be completely normal. However, analysis of acylcarnitines and acylglycines generally shows the presence of octanoylcarnitine, and hexanoylglycine and phenylpropionylglycine, respectively, in urine. Analysis of acylcarnitines in plasma or dried blood spots by tandem MSMS shows accumulation of octanoylcarnitine, even when the child is clinically well. Tandem MSMS is being employed by several centers as a method for screening newborns for fatty acid oxidations defects (see Chapter 8).

MCAD deficiency is an inherited metabolic disorder in which specific mutation analysis is particularly useful for making a diagnosis: one mutation, K329E, accounts for over 90% of all MCAD deficiency-associated alleles discovered to date. Testing for the presence of this mutation provides helpful confirmatory evidence for this disease.

Other inborn errors of fatty acid oxidation are rare compared with MCAD deficiency. Systemic carnitine deficiency and long-chain acyl-CoA dehydrogenase (LCAD) deficiency may present with a Reye-like acute encephalopathy, but the evidence of skeletal muscle involvement is usually more obvious, and cardiomyopathy, which is never seen in MCAD deficiency, is generally prominent. Similarly, short-chain acyl-CoA dehydrogenase (SCAD) deficiency is very rare, and may present as encephalopathy with metabolic acidosis in the newborn period (see Chapter 7). Rarely, carnitine palmitoyltransferase II (CPT II) deficiency, which is usually associated with a myopathy presenting in later childhood, may present in infancy with recurrent Reye-like acute encephalopathy clinically indistinguishable from MCAD deficiency. A summary of the urinary organic acid abnormalities in these conditions is shown in Table 2.8.

Acute encephalopathy with metabolic acidosis

The inherited organic acidopathies commonly present as acute encephalopathy, the presence of severe metabolic acidosis is usually recognized early in the management of the problem. Detailed treatment of this particular group of disorders is presented in Chapter 3 and Chapter 7.

Hypoglycemia

Although conditions like glycogen storage disease, type I (GSD I), often present in infancy with alteration of consciousness, sometimes progressing rapidly to coma and to seizures, the presence of hypoglycemia generally directs the investigation (see Chapter 4).

Stroke

Stroke is a well-recognized result of some inherited metabolic diseases, such as familial hypercholesterolemia and homocystinuria. Over the past few years, an increasing number of inborn errors of metabolism has been reported to be associated with stroke or stroke-like episodes (Table 2.9). Stroke in infancy and childhood is more likely to be the result of inherited defects in metabolism than that occurring in adults. It is generally, though not always, associated with other abnormalities, such as metabolic acidosis, psychomotor retardation, or failure to thrive. In some cases, it is may be the presenting problem.

Episodic unilateral migraine headache associated with hemiplegia, aphasia, hemianopia, or facial paresthesia, lasting from hours to days, suggests the possibility of familial hemiplegic migraine (FHM) caused by mutations in one of the calcium channel genes (*CACNA1A*).

Movement disorder

Extrapyramidal movement disorders in patients with inborn errors of metabolism are almost always associated with neurologic signs referable to other parts of the nervous system (Table 2.10). Unsteadiness of gait, particularly in children, which may be a manifestation of immaturity or muscle weakness, is a particularly common finding in inherited metabolic diseases.

Ataxia

One productive approach to the diagnosis in patients in whom ataxia is a prominent is to determine early on whether the problem is static or progressive, and if it is

Table 2.8 Organic acid abnormalities in the hereditary fatty acid oxidation defects

MCAD deficiency	SCAD deficiency	LCAD deficiency	LCHAD deficiency	ETF/ETF-DH deficiency
5-hydroxyhexanoate	**ethylmalonate**	adipate	adipate	3-hydroxybutyrate
adipate	**methylsuccinate**	suberate	3-hydroxyadipate	**glutarate**
suberate		octenedioate	suberate	**ethylmalonate**
octenedioate	**n-butyrylglycine**	decenedioate	octenedioate	**methylsuccinate**
7-hydroxyoctanoate		**dodecanedioate**	**3-hydroxysuberate**	
sebacate		**tetradecanedioate**	sebacate	**n-butyrylglycine**
decenedioate			decenedioate	isobutyrylglycine
3-hydroxysebacate			**3-hydroxysebacate**	2-methylbutyrylglycine
			dodecanedioate	**isovalerylglycine**
hexanoylglycine			**3-hydroxydodecanedioate**	**hexanoylglycine**
suberylglycine			**3-hydroxydodecenedioate**	
phenylpropionylglycine			**3-hydroxytetradecanedioate**	
			3-hydroxytetradecenedioate	
octanoylcarnitine				

Abbreviations: MCAD, medium-chain acyl-CoA dehydrogenase; SCAD, short-chain acyl-CoA dehydrogenase; LCAD, long-chain acyl-CoA dehydrogenase; LCHAD, long-chain 3-hydroxyacyl-CoA dehydrogenase; ETF/ETF-DH, electron transfer flavoprotein/electron transfer flavoprotein dehydrogenase. Bold type indicates the presence of the compound is particularly characteristic of the disease.

Table 2.9 Inherited metabolic diseases associated with strokes or stroke-like episodes

Disease	Diagnosis
Homocystinuria, including cystathionine β-synthase deficiency, MTHFR deficiency and cobalamin defects	Elevated plasma homocysteine and demonstration of specific enzyme defect
Fabry disease	Deficiency of plasma or leukocyte α-galactosidase A activity (males) or demonstration of disease-causing mutation in *GLA* gene (males or females)

Organic acidopathies
  Methylmalonic acidemia
  Propionic acidemia
  Isovaleric acidemia
  Glutaric aciduria, types I and II
	Abnormalities of urinary organic acids or plasma acylcarnitines and demonstration of specific enzyme defect

Ornithine transcarbamoylase (OTC) deficiency	Hyperammonemia, elevated urinary orotic acid, demonstration of mutations in *OTC* gene
MELAS	Persistent lactic acidosis, typical changes on MRI of the brain, demonstration of disease-associated mtDNA mutations (see Table 9.14)
CDG type Ia	Abnormal isoelectric focusing pattern of plasma transferrin
Familial hemiplegic migraine	Demonstration of mutations in P/Q-type calcium channel gene (*CACNA1A*)

Abbreviations: MTHFR, methylene tetrahydrofolate reductase; MELAS, mitochondrial encephalomyopathy, lactic acidosis, and stroke-like episodes; CDG, congenital disorder of glycosylation.

progressive, whether the course is a relentless one, or if it is intermittent. Early-onset, static ataxia is almost never caused by an inherited metabolic disease. It is more likely to be traceable to a congenital malformation of the brain or brain injury sustained early in life. In childhood, generalized muscle weakness may present as unsteadiness during walking or running, resembling ataxia caused by a primary extrapyramidal disorder.

In any child presenting with a history of ***recurrent acute ataxia*** separated by periods free of neurologic abnormalities, the possibility of an inherited metabolic disease should be considered. Recurrent episodes of ataxia are a common manifestation of metabolic decompensation in patients with 'small molecule' disorders, such as urea cycle enzyme defects, organic acidopathies, and the mild or intermittent variants of MSUD. It may be the only clinical manifestation of various 'channelopathies' or of mild pyruvate dehydrogenase deficiency (PDH) deficiency. Mild

Table 2.10 Inherited metabolic disease in which movement disorders are prominent

Disease	Other clinical features	Diagnosis
Intermittent ataxia		
UCED (e.g., OTC deficiency, CPS I deficiency, ASAuria, etc.)	Encephalopathy, dietary protein intolerance, hyperammonemia	Plasma amino acid abnormalities and deficiency of specific urea cycle enzymes
Organic acidopathies (e.g., MMA, PA, IVA)	Metabolic acidosis, hyperammonemia	Marked excretion of organic acid intermediates in the urine
PDH deficiency (mild)	Lactic acidosis	Deficiency of PDH in leukocytes and fibroblasts
Episodic ataxia, type 1 (EA1)	Brief attacks of cerebellar ataxia, with later development of myokymia of facial, arm and hand muscles, precipitated by sudden changes in posture or stress	Mutations in potassium channel gene, *KCNA1*.
Episodic ataxia type 2 (EA2)	Attacks of headache and ataxia, vertigo, dysarthria, and nystagmus	Mutations in P/Q-type calcium channel genes (*CACNA1A*)
Progressive ataxia		
Friedreich ataxia	Progressive gait ataxia, pes cavus, kyphoscoliosis, sensory neuropathy, dysarthria, nystagmus, sensorineural deafness, absent deep tendon reflexes, extensor plantar reflexes, cardiomyopathy, diabetes mellitus in some	Expansion of GAA repeats in frataxin gene (*FRDA*)
AVED	Onset in first or second decade of progressive ataxia, visual impairment with retinitis pigmentosa (in some), head titubation, flexor plantar reflexes	Marked decrease of plasma α-tocopherol levels
Abetalipoproteinemia	Steatorrhea, anemia, acanthocytosis, psychomotor retardation, retinitis pigmentosa	Marked deficiency of apolipoprotein B in plasma
Infantile NCL (Santavuori-Haltia syndrome)	Psychomotor retardation, myoclonic seizures, blindness, early flattening of the EEG	Typical lysosomal inclusions seen on electron microscopic examination of skin, leukocytes, or conjunctival epithelium

Mitochondrial ETC defects (e.g., KSS, MERRF)	Lactic acidosis, small stature, retinal degeneration, psychomotor retardation, seizures, myopathy, sensorineural deafness	Defects in mitochondrial ETC in fibroblasts or skeletal muscle; mitochondrial mutation analysis (see Chapter 9)
Late-onset galactosialidosis	Myoclonus, seizures, corneal clouding, cherry-red spots, mental retardation	Deficiency of β-galactosidase and α-neuraminidase in fibroblasts
Late-onset GM2 gangliosidosis	Muscle wasting, dysarthria, exaggerated deep tendon reflexes, psychosis	Deficiency of β-hexosaminidase in serum, leukocytes or fibroblasts
Late-onset MLD	Muscle wasting, dysarthria, peripheral neuropathy	Deficiency of arylsulfatase A in leukocytes or fibroblasts
Late-onset Krabbe GLD	Spasticity, visual failure	Deficiency of galactocerebrosidase in leukocytes or fibroblasts
Refsum disease	Retinitis pigmentosa, peripheral neuropathy, sensorineural deafness, cataracts, ichthyosis	Elevated phytanic acid levels in plasma; defect in phytanic acid oxidation in fibroblasts
Niemann-Pick disease, type C	Hepatosplenomegaly, supranuclear vertical gaze palsy, sea-blue histiocytes in bone marrow	Defect in cholesterol esterification in fibroblasts; NPC1 mutation analysis
Hartnup disease	Pellagra-like skin rash	Massive neutral, monoamino-monocarboxylic aminoaciduria
L-2-Hydroxyglutaric aciduria	Psychomotor retardation, choreoathetosis ± seizures	Marked increase in levels of L-2-hydroxyglutaric acid in urine
Mevalonic aciduria	Psychomotor retardation, facial dysmorphism, failure to thrive, recurrent fever, diarrhea, arthralgia, edema, skin rash	Increased mevalonic acid in urine on organic acid analysis
Spinocerebellar ataxia type 6	Late-onset, slowly progressive cerebellar ataxia	Demonstration of mutations in P/Q-type calcium channel genes (CACNA1A)
Dystonia/choreoathetosis		
Glutaric aciduria, type I	Psychomotor retardation, episodes of acute encephalopathy with metabolic acidosis	Marked increase in excretion of glutaric and 3-hydroxyglutaric acids in urine; deficiency of glutaryl-CoA dehydrogenase in fibroblasts
Lesch-Nyhan disease	Psychomotor retardation, self-mutilatory behavior	Increased uric acid levels in plasma and urine; HPRT deficiency in leukocytes or fibroblasts

(*cont.*)

Table 2.10 (cont.)

Disease	Other clinical features	Diagnosis
TPI deficiency	Chronic hemolytic anemia, susceptibility to infection, cardiomyopathy, death in early childhood	Deficiency of TPI in erythrocytes
4-Hydroxybutyric aciduria	Psychomotor retardation, oculomotor abnormalities, choreoathetosis	Massive excretion of 4-hydroxybutyric acid in urine, decreasing with age
Segawa syndrome	Dystonia of extremities growing worse during the course of the day, normal intellect	Dramatic response to treatment with L-dopa; GTP-cyclohydrolase assay in fibroblasts
Parkinsonism		
Wilson disease	Dementia, psychiatric problems, hepatocellular dysfunction (Chapter 4). Kayser-Fleischer rings	Marked decrease of plasma ceruloplasmin and copper levels and increased urinary excretion of copper
Tyrosine hydroxylase deficiency	Onset in infancy or generalized rigidity, ptosis, drooling, truncal hypotonia, marked tremor in upper extremities, occasional myoclonic jerks. Reduced deep tendon reflexes. Normal MRI and CT scans	CSF neurotransmitter analysis: ↓HVA, normal 5HIAA, ↓MHPG, normal 3OMD, normal BH4, normal BH2, normal Neopterin
Aromatic amino acid decarboxylase deficiency	Early-onset bradycardia, temperature instability, irritability and poor feeding. Generalized hypotonia with paroxysmal extension of arms and legs accompanied by eye-rolling, evolving into an extrapyramidal movement disorder with oculogyric crises and convergence spasm.	CSF neurotransmitter analysis: ↓HVA, ↓5HIAA, ↓MHPG, ↑3OMD, normal BH4, normal BH2, normal Neopterin

Abbreviations: MLD, metachromatic leukodystrophy; ETC, electron transport chain; KSS, Kearns–Sayre syndrome; MERRF, myoclonic epilepsy and ragged-red fiber disease; AVED, ataxia with vitamin E deficiency; NCL, neuronal ceroid-lipofuscinosis; UCED, urea cycle enzyme defects; CPS I, carbamoylphosphate synthetase 1; ASAuria, argininosuccinic aciduria; PDH, pyruvate dehydrogenase; MMA, methylmalonic aciduria; PA, propionic acidemia; IVA, isovaleric acidemia; HPRT, hypoxanthine phosphoribosyltransferase; TPI, triose phosphate isomerase; GLD, globoid cell leukodystrophy; HVA, homovanillic acid; 5HIAA, 5-hydroxyindoleacetic acid; MHPG, 3-methoxy-4-hydroxyphenylglycol; 3OMD, 3-O-methyldopa; BH4, tetrahydrobiopterin; BH2, 7,8-dihydrobiopterin.

PDH deficiency, presenting as recurrent ataxia, occurs almost exclusively in young boys, and the episodes of unsteadiness are usually, though not always, associated with lactic acidosis.

Intermittent ataxia may be the presenting clinical problem in young children with acute intermittent muscle weakness, such as occurs in the early-onset ion channelopathies (see below).

Progressive ataxia is often the presenting problem in many of the late-infantile or juvenile-onset variants of organelle diseases, such as late-infantile metachromatic leukodystrophy (often called classical MLD), or the juvenile-onset variants of Niemann-Pick disease, type C, the GM2 gangliosidoses (juvenile Tay-Sachs disease and juvenile Sandhoff disease), or GM1 gangliosidosis. Differentiation from nonmetabolic hereditary ataxias is usually possible on the basis of the presence of other neurologic signs, such as psychomotor retardation or regression, spasticity, or peripheral neuropathy, and evidence of non-neurologic involvement with the disease. The diagnosis in each case is confirmed by demonstrating deficiency of the relevant enzyme activity in plasma, peripheral blood leukocytes, or cultured skin fibroblasts (see Chapter 9).

Coenzyme Q_{10} (CoQ_{10}) deficiency may also present in young children as a very slowly progressive cerebellar ataxia with muscle weakness and pyramidal tract signs, associated in some cases with seizures and mental retardation. Imaging of the CNS typically shows cerebellar atrophy. Routine biochemical studies levels, are generally normal, though some patients have persistent mild lactic acidosis. Measurements of mitochondrial electron transport chain (ETC) activity often show deficiencies of one or more complexes of the ETC; however, the pattern of the abnormalities varies from patient to patient. When ataxia is the dominant cause of disability, muscle histology and histochemistry is normal. CoQ_{10} concentrations in muscle are decreased, and treatment with high doses of the cofactor, up to 3000 mg per day, produces dramatic improvements in muscle strength, ataxia, and seizure control.

Choreoathetosis and dystonia

Choreoathetosis is a prominent feature of Lesch-Nyhan syndrome, caused by X-linked hypoxanthine phosphoribosyltransferase (HPRT) deficiency. Many, though not all, patients with the disease show psychomotor retardation. Self-mutilation, another feature of the condition in many affected boys, may not be present. The diagnosis is suggested by finding increased uric acid levels in blood and urine, and it is confirmed by specific enzyme assay on leukocytes or fibroblasts.

Choreoathetosis and dystonia are characteristic of glutaric aciduria, type I. This disorder, caused by deficiency of glutaryl-CoA dehydrogenase, is characterized by

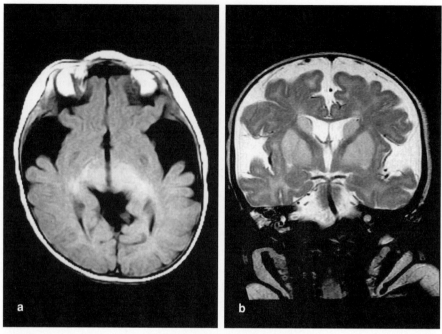

Figure 2.14 MRI scans of the brain of an infant with glutaric aciduria, type I.
Panel **a**, Axial T1-weighted MRI scan [TR550/TE11] of a 10-month-old infant showing marked prominence of the Sylvian fissures with hypoplasia of the temporal lobes and generalized delayed myelination. Panel **b**, Coronal fast spin echo T2-weighted MRI scan [TR4000/TE65] through the enlarged Sylvian fissures showing increased signal intensity of the heads of the caudate nuclei and putamen bilaterally.

the acute onset in early infancy of intermittent episodes of encephalopathy with ketoacidosis, hypotonia, seizures, posturing (arching, grimacing, tongue-thrusting, rigidity), and evidence of hepatocellular dysfunction. Recovery is usually incomplete, with the extrapyramidal movement disorder tending to persist. The MRI of the brain typically shows cerebral atrophy particularly prominent in the temporal lobes, producing changes that are virtually diagnostic of the disease (Figure 2.14). The urine usually contains large amounts of glutaric acid and smaller amounts of 3-hydroxyglutaric acid, though sometimes the organic acid pattern is not abnormal; the presence of 3-hydroxyglutaric acid is more specific and is particularly important in establishing the diagnosis.

Dystonia is a prominent feature of disorders of neurotransmitter metabolism (Table 2.10). In many cases, the disturbance is intermittent and may be associated with choreoathetosis or parkinsonism. Dopa-responsive dystonia (Segawa syndrome) is characterized by the onset in middle childhood of dystonia, spasticity, and parkinsonian rigidity and tremor, that grows progressively more pronounced as the day progresses and the patient becomes tired. The response to treatment with L-dopa is dramatic and virtually diagnostic. The condition is most often transmitted as an autosomal dominant disorder with decreased penetrance and marked variability in clinical expression of the disease, even among members of the same family. It is caused by mutations in *GCH1* resulting in GTP cyclohydrolase deficiency. It is associated with typical abnormalities of CSF neurotransmitter metabolites (see Table 9.7). The diagnosis is confirmed by demonstrating deficiency of the enzyme in cultured skin fibroblasts or phytohemagglutinin-stimulated peripheral blood lymphocytes, or by specific mutation analysis. An autosomal recessive form of the same syndrome is caused by deficiency of tyrosine hydroxylase. The onset of symptoms is earlier, and the course is more rapidly progressive in this variant of Segawa syndrome. It is often associated with intellectual impairment. Nevertheless, the response to treatment with L-dopa is just as dramatic as in patients with the autosomal dominant variant of the disease.

Involuntary choreiform movements, progressive hypotonia, developmental delay, dystonia, and intractable seizures presenting in early infancy are prominent features of cerebral creatine deficiency caused by deficiency of guanidinoacetate methyltransferase (GAMT), an autosomal recessive disorder of creatine biosynthesis. The plasma and urinary creatinine concentrations may be abnormally low. However, confirmation of the diagnosis requires the demonstration of increased concentrations of guanidinoacetate in plasma, urine, or CSF. MRS of the brain typically shows marked reduction in the size of the creatine peak. Treatment with creatine monohydrate, together with dietary arginine restriction and ornithine supplementation, is reported to produce a significant improvement in seizure control.

Parkinsonism

Parkinsonism, dystonia, and cerebellar dysfunction are prominent symptoms in many patients with Wilson disease. Most patients with the disease come to medical attention in later childhood with evidence of severe hepatocellular dysfunction (see Chapter 4). However, many present somewhat later, in adolescence or early adulthood, with neuropsychiatric problems, usually dominated by extrapyramidal or cerebellar dysfunction, or psychiatric disturbances. Cerebellar ataxia is often associated with tremors, titubation, dysmetria, and scanning speech. In other patients, other signs of extrapyramidal disease dominate, with dystonia, cog-wheel rigidity, facial grimacing, drooling, dysphagia, and stereotypic gestures. In spite of profound disturbances of motor function, intelligence usually remains normal. On the other hand, psychiatric problems are often prominent. They may even be the first indication of disease (see Table 2.18).

Myopathy

Inherited metabolic disorders presenting as myopathy are commonly the result of defects in energy metabolism. These can be divided into five categories on the basis of the clinical characteristics of the muscle disease and associated findings:
- Acute intermittent muscle weakness
- Progressive muscle weakness.
- Exercise intolerance with cramps and myoglobinuria (myophosphorylase deficiency phenotype).
- Exercise intolerance with cramps and myoglobinuria (CPT II deficiency phenotype).
- Myopathy as a manifestation of multisystem disease (mitochondrial myopathies).

Acute intermittent muscle weakness

Episodes of acute onset of marked muscle weakness, hypotonia and unsteadiness of gait lasting from a few hours to a few days is a feature of hyperkalemic and hypokalemic periodic paralysis. These present a particularly challenging diagnostic problem. Onset is generally in later childhood, with episodes of flaccid muscle weakness associated with hyperkalemia or hypokalemia, lasting some hours. Attacks typically occur during rest following intensive exercise. In patients with hyperkalemic periodic paralysis (HyperPP), attacks may also be precipitated by ingestion of potassium. Between attacks, patients with HyperPP often exhibit myotonia of the facial muscles and extremities. The disease is caused by mutations in the sodium channel gene, *SCN4A*, in skeletal muscle.

Paramyotonia congenita (PMC), which is also caused by *SCN4A* mutations, is characterized by attacks of muscle stiffening (myotonia) precipitated by exercise or exposure to cold. The stiffness typically evolves into flaccid muscle weakness lasting for some hours before resolving spontaneously. Between attacks, patients show myotonia of the muscles of the face and throat, with delayed eye-opening and percussion myotonia of the tongue.

The attacks of weakness in hypokalemic periodic paralysis (HypoPP) are associated with low plasma potassium concentrations. They are typically precipitated by ingestion of a high-carbohydrate meal. Myotonia is not a feature of this disorder, and patients apparently do not develop progressive myopathy later in life. The condition is caused by mutations in the calcium channel gene, *CACNL1A3*, in skeletal muscle.

What is remarkable about patients with these disorders is the absence of any evidence of acute encephalopathy, systemic illness, or underlying neurological deficits or psychomotor retardation. In some, the diagnosis is suggested by the presence of typical electrolyte disturbances (i.e., hypokalemia or hyperkalemia) during episodes of weakness. Electrolyte analyses done when the patient is well are almost always normal. Most of these disorders are transmitted as autosomal dominant conditions, and the family history may reveal that one or other of the parents will have had similar transient episodes of marked weakness during later childhood, or has developed a slowly progressive myopathy. A predominance of affected males is a characteristic of HypoPP.

Progressive muscle weakness

One of the most striking examples of inherited metabolic diseases presenting with progressive myopathy is Pompe disease (GSD II), caused by deficiency of the lysosomal enzyme, α-glucosidase (acid maltase). It is characterized by the onset, at three to five months, of rapidly progressive weakness and hypotonia. Affected infants are remarkable for the marked paucity of spontaneous movement and their frog-leg posture, but who have normal social interaction. The face is myopathic, and the tongue is characteristically enlarged; however, extraocular movements are spared. Despite marked muscle weakness and hypotonia, muscle bulk is initially not significantly decreased, and the muscles have a peculiar woody texture on palpation. Deep tendon reflexes, which may initially be preserved, are soon lost. The liver is not significantly enlarged unless the infant is in heart failure. Cardiac muscle involvement is prominent and severe (see Chapter 5). The course of the disease is relentlessly progressive, culminating in death within a few months. The excess glycogen in the muscles of infants with Pompe disease accumulates in lysosomes, and lysosomal glycogen contributes next to nothing to meeting the energy needs of the tissue. Why the muscle weakness in the disease is so severe is not understood. Treatment by enzyme replacement therapy is currently in clinical trials and offers some hope for the families of infants with this otherwise uniformly lethal disease.

In late-onset variants of acid maltase deficiency, the onset of the myopathy is more insidious and the progression more gradual. Muscle biopsy typically shows the presence of large accumulations of intra-lysosomal glycogen. Cardiomyopathy is much less prominent in late-onset disease; death is invariably the result of respiratory failure caused by respiratory muscle weakness.

Progressive skeletal myopathy, sometimes involving the heart, may be a major problem in patients with glycogen storage disease, type III (GSD III). This disease is caused by deficiency of glycogen debrancher enzyme, usually in liver and muscle, but sometimes only in liver. While the consequences of liver involvement usually improve with age (see Chapter 4), the myopathy gradually becomes worse, often only becoming clinically significant after age 20 or 30 years. The creatine phosphokinase (CPK) is often, though not always, elevated in patients with muscle involvement. The mechanism of the myopathy in GSD III is uncertain. Some feel that it is the result of local glycogen accumulation; others think, on the basis of apparent improvement using high protein dietary treatment, that increased muscle protein breakdown to fuel gluconeogenesis is responsible.

Muscle weakness and exercise-induced myoglobinuria, associated with seizures, ataxia, pyramidal tract signs, and developmental retardation, are particularly prominent in some cases of CoQ_{10} deficiency (Table 2.10). Muscle biopsies in patients with this variant of the disorder show the presence of ragged-red fibres, and measurement of mitochondrial electron transport chain (ETC) activity in muscle or cultured skin fibroblasts typically shows deficiencies of CoQ_{10}-dependent complexes I+II and I+III. The diagnosis is confirmed by showing marked deficiency of CoQ_{10} in muscle or cultured skin fibroblasts. Treatment with large doses of CoQ_{10} results in significant improvement in muscle power in most and the ataxia in some patients with CoQ_{10} deficiency.

Myoglobinuria (myophosphorylase deficiency phenotype)

The clinical course of myophosphorylase deficiency (McArdle disease or GSD V) is typical of a number of inherited defects of glycolysis presenting as exercise intolerance. It is characterized by the onset in early adulthood of severe muscle cramps shortly after the initiation of intense exercise; mild, sustained exercise, such as level walking, is well-tolerated. Typically, if the patient rests briefly, moderate levels of activity can be resumed without discomfort. This is the so-called 'second-wind' phenomenon. Presumably as the muscle switches to fatty acid oxidation in order to meet its energy needs, the requirement for glucose is decreased, and the cramps disappear. Episodes of cramping are often followed within hours by the development of wine-colored pigmentation of the urine (myoglobinuria) as a result of rhabdomyolysis. CPK levels are typically markedly elevated and rise further during exercise. Rhabdomyolysis and resulting myoglobinuria occur in all myopathies occurring as a result of defects in skeletal muscle energy metabolism. Rarely, it is severe enough to cause acute renal failure.

The normal accumulation of lactic acid in the course of an ischemic forearm exercise test does not occur, and the normal increase in plasma ammonium is exaggerated. The test (Table 2.11) involves the measurement of lactate and ammonium in blood collected from the antecubital vein before and after a defined period of vigorous exercise during which the circulation to the forearm is temporarily interrupted by application of a partially inflated blood pressure cuff. In many patients, discomfort associated with the task forces interruption of the test before completion of the two minutes of vigorous exercise. In that case, blood samples for measurement of lactate and ammonium should continue to be collected as scheduled.

Table 2.11 Protocol for the ischemic forearm exercise test

1. An intravenous is established in one arm with an ample needle in the antecubital vein kept open with a slow infusion of 0.9% NaCl.
2. The patient is given a rolled-up, partially-inflated, blood pressure cuff attached to a sphygmomanometer to squeeze.
3. A second cuff is applied to the arm, above the elbow, but it is not inflated.
4. Blood is taken for analysis of lactate, ammonium, and CPK (baseline).
5. The cuff on the arm is inflated to 120–140 mm of mercury, and the patient is instructed to squeeze the cuff in her hand rapidly (30–60 times per minute), trying as hard as possible to produce a pressure ≥ 100 mm of mercury. After 2 minutes, the cuff on the arm is deflated and the patient is instructed to relax.
6. Blood samples are obtained from the intravenous line for measurement of lactate, ammonium, and CPK at 2, 5, 10, and 15 minutes after termination of the 2 minutes of ischemic exercise and deflation of the cuff on the arm.

Abbreviations: CPK, creatine phosphokinase.

Muscle phosphofructokinase (PFK) deficiency (GSD VI) shares many features in common with myophosphorylase deficiency, including severe muscle cramping during short-term exercise, a 'second-wind' phenomenon, abnormal ischemic forearm exercise test, and myoglobinuria. However, onset in childhood is more common, the attacks of muscle cramps are generally more severe, and they are aggravated by ingestion of high-carbohydrate meals. Like patients with other inborn errors of glycolysis, patients with PFK deficiency generally show evidence of a compensated hemolytic anemia, and it may be associated with marked hyperuricemia. The disorder is more prevalent among Ashkenazi Jews and Japanese than in people of other ethnic groups.

Exercise intolerance of the 'myophosphorylase deficiency phenotype' occurs in patients with other glycolytic defects (Table 2.12), but these are rare. Myoadenylate deaminase deficiency is often clinically indistinguishable from myophosphorylase deficiency. However, the average age of onset is somewhat later, and the attacks of exercise-induced cramping tend to be less severe. CPK levels are increased in half the patients, and the electromyogram (EMG) is often normal. The ischemic forearm exercise test produces a normal increase in plasma lactate, but the normal increase in plasma ammonium does not occur. The diagnosis is confirmed by enzyme analysis, specific histochemical staining of the muscle, or mutation analysis. In about half the patients with adenylate deaminase deficiency, the symptoms are due to secondary or acquired enzyme deficiency associated with other chronic neuromuscular problems or with collagen vascular disease.

Table 2.12 Inherited metabolic diseases presenting as muscle cramping or myoglobinuria

Disease	Clinical features	Diagnosis
Myophosphorylase deficiency phenotype		
Muscle phosphorylase deficiency (McArdle disease)	Muscle cramps during exercise, 'second-wind' phenomenon, normal pre-test lactate and no increase on ischemic forearm exercise test, elevated CPK, myoglobinuria	Deficiency of phosphorylase in muscle
PFK deficiency	Muscle cramps during exercise, myoglobinuria, hyperuricemia (and gout), excessive increase of ammonium on ischemic forearm exercise test, compensated hemolytic anemia, elevated CPK, more common in Ashkenazi Jews and Japanese	Marked deficiency of PFK activity in muscle; half normal activities in erythrocytes
PGK deficiency	X-linked recessive, chronic hemolytic anemia, mental retardation, psychiatric problems	Deficiency of PGK in erythrocytes
PGAM deficiency	May be clinically indistinguishable from PFK deficiency	Deficiency of PGAM in muscle
LDH deficiency	May be clinically indistinguishable from PFK deficiency. No lactic acidosis, but marked hyperpyruvic acidemia during ischemic forearm exercise test	Deficiency of LDH-M subunit in erythrocytes
CPT II deficiency phenotype		
CPT II deficiency	Post-exercise cramps or myalgia, cold-induced muscle cramps and stiffness, increased CPK during fasting, normal lactate and ammonium responses but increased CPK on ischemic forearm exercise test, myoglobinuria	Deficiency of CPT II in fibroblasts
Myoadenylate deaminase deficiency	Post-exercise muscle cramps or myalgia, normal lactate response, but no increase in ammonium on ischemic forearm exercise test, elevated CPK in about 50%	Deficiency of adenylate kinase on histochemical or biochemical analysis of skeletal muscle
LCAD deficiency	Similar to CPT II deficiency, episodes of Reye-like encephalopathy, decreased plasma carnitine	Deficiency of LCAD in fibroblasts
SCHAD deficiency	Extremely rare, chronic muscle weakness with episodic acute deterioration and myoglobinuria, prominent myocardial involvement	Deficiency of SCHAD in muscle. Enzyme activity in fibroblasts is normal.

Abbreviations: CPT II, carnitine palmitoyltransferase II; LCAD, long-chain acyl-CoA dehydrogenase; LDH, lactate dehydrogenase; PFK, phosphofructokinase; PGK, phosphoglycerate kinase; PGAM, phosphoglycerate mutase; CPK, creatine phosphokinase; SCHAD, short-chain 3-hydroxyacyl-CoA dehydrogenase.

Table 2.13 Differences between myophosphorylase deficiency and CPT II deficiency phenotypes

	Phenotype	
	Myophosphorylase	CPT II
Short-term intense exercise	Not tolerated	Well tolerated
Prolonged mild-moderate exercise	Well tolerated	Not tolerated
Second wind phenomenon	Present	Absent
Effect of fasting	Beneficial	Detrimental
High carbohydrate-low fat diet	No benefit*	Beneficial

Note: *Although high carbohydrate dietary treatment is not beneficial in patients with myophosphorylase deficiency, a high-protein diet appears to be beneficial in some, and ingestion of glucose immediately before exercising often enhances exercise tolerance.
Abbreviations: CPT II, carnitine palmitoyltransferase II.
Source: Adapted from Di Mauro, Bresolin & Papadimitriou (1984).

Myoglobinuria (CPT II deficiency phenotype)

In patients with myopathy resulting from defects in fatty acid oxidation, the muscle cramps and tenderness characteristically develop after periods of exercise, when the patient is actually at rest, and the muscle is drawing heavily on fatty acid oxidation to meet its energy requirements.

The main difference between the myophosphorylase deficiency and CPT II deficiency phenotypes are shown in Table 2.13. Most patients with CPT II (carnitine palmitoyltransferase II) deficiency present as young adults with a history of episodic muscle stiffness, pain, tenderness, weakness, and myoglobinuria precipitated by prolonged exercise, exposure to cold, fasting, or intercurrent infection. Patients do not experience a 'second-wind' phenomenon. Between attacks, they may be completely asymptomatic, though some experience residual muscle weakness and fatiguability. The CPK is elevated during attacks, but it is generally normal at other times. Muscle biopsy typically shows lipid accumulation in many, though not all, affected individuals. The myoglobinuria is severe enough in many patients to precipitate renal failure. The normal ketotic response to fasting (see Chapter 4) is blunted, though acute metabolic decompensation in older patients is rare. The diagnosis is confirmed by demonstrating deficiency of CPT II activity in fibroblasts.

Myopathy as a manifestation of multisystem disease (mitochondrial myopathies)

Progressive myopathy is often the principal manifestation of the multisystem involvement of diseases caused by defects in the mitochondrial ETC, though other systems are invariably involved. The extent and degree of involvement of various tissues and organs inpatients with different mitochondrial ETC defects varies enormously, not only between unrelated patients, but also between patients within the same family. In some disorders, such as Leigh subacute necrotizing encephalomyelopathy and Alpers disease (see section on 'Chronic encephalopathy'), the myopathy is clinically mild compared with the effects of the disease on the CNS. In others, hepatocellular dysfunction or other gastrointestinal disturbances, such as pseudo-obstruction, dominate the presentation. However, in others, muscle weakness may be the presenting symptom and the multisystem nature of the condition is only appreciated after careful examination and laboratory studies. In most, the course of the disease is relentlessly progressive; in some, it is marked by episodes of acute deterioration superimposed on a background of chronic deterioration; and in a few, mostly young infants, spontaneous recovery occurs over a period of a few months. Most are associated with persistent lactic acidosis, though lactate levels are generally not >10 mmol/L except during acute metabolic decompensation. The mode of inheritance may be autosomal recessive, autosomal dominant, X-linked, or mitochondrial (matrilineal). Among patients with disease due to mitochondrial mutations, a large proportion of them is *de novo* mutations, rather than inherited. However, the clinical symptomatology associated with mitochondrial mutations is often highly variable owing to the phenomenon of heteroplasmy (see Chapter 1), and other family members should be studied in detail before the mutation in a particular patient is concluded to be new. Characteristics that suggest the myopathy is due to a mitochondrial ETC defect are shown in Table 2.14.

In spite of the enormous variability between patients with mitochondrial ETC defects, many patients exhibit patterns of clinical findings that have made it possible to identify some relatively distinct syndromes. Many of these are attributable to mtDNA mutations (Table 2.15). However, some conditions characterized by mtDNA abnormalities, and others in which mitochondrial ETC activity is directly involved, are caused by nuclear mutations (Table 2.16).

Definitive investigation of this group of disorders requires muscle biopsy with histochemical studies, electron microscopy, and biochemical studies on mitochondrial electron transport in mitochondria isolated fresh from the tissue (see Chapter 9). The presence of ragged-red fibers in skeletal muscle biopsies of the tissue stained by the modified Gomori trichrome stain (Figure 2.15) is a reflection of the proliferation and subsarcolemmal aggregation of mitochondria, which is characteristic of many of the mitochondrial myopathies. Electron microscopic examination often confirms the presence of abnormal square or rectangular paracrystalline inclusions between the inner and outer mitochondrial membranes, or globular inclusions in the matrix. The tissue often contains excess glycogen and fat, sometimes giving the

Table 2.14 Some common clinical features of
conditions caused by mitochondrial mutations

Present in most mitochondrial conditions
Persistent lactic acidosis
Myopathy (weakness, hypotonia)
Failure to thrive; short stature
Psychomotor retardation; dementia
Seizures

Present in many mitochondrial conditions
Ophthalmoplegia or other oculomotor abnormalities
Retinal pigmentary degeneration
Cardiomyopathy
Cerebellar ataxia (progressive or intermittent)
Sensorineural hearing loss
Cardiac arrhythmias
Diabetes mellitus
Stroke (in children)
Renal tubular dysfunction
Respiratory abnormalities (periodic apnea and tachypnea)

---

appearance of a 'lipid myopathy', such as is characteristic of the changes in patients
with fatty acid oxidation defects.

The identification of specific mitochondrial mutations is a growing part of the
investigation of mitochondrial disorders, including the mitochondrial myopathies.
However, this is not yet routinely available except in a handful of centers doing
basic research in the area.

Autonomic dysfunction

In a handful of inherited metabolic diseases, what appear to be abnormalities of
autonomic function are particularly prominent (Table 2.17). In some, such as Fabry
disease, the autonomic dysfunction may be the first indication of disease; in others,
attempts to control problems, such as intractable diarrhea, are the most challenging
aspects of the management of the diseases.

Psychiatric problems

Some inherited metabolic disorders in which chronic progressive encephalopathy is
prominent are characterized by severe behavior problems. For example, boys with

Table 2.15 Main clinical features of some relatively common mitochondrial syndromes resulting from mtDNA mutations

	KSS	MERRF	MELAS	NARP	LHON
Ophthalmoplegia	++++	0	0	0	0
Retinal degeneration	++++	0	0	++++	++++
Cerebellar dysfunction	+++	++++	0	+++	±
Psychomotor regression	++	++	+++	+	0
Myoclonus	0	++++	0	0	0
Seizures	+	+++	++++	++	0
Sensorineural deafness	+++	++	+	0	0
Cortical blindness ± hemiparesis (stroke)	0	0	++++	0	0
Renal tubular dysfunction	0	0	++	0	0
Cardiomyopathy	++	+	±	±	0
Cardiac conduction defects	++++	0	0	0	+
Short stature	+++	++	++++	0	0
Diabetes mellitus	0	0	+	++	0
Lactic acidosis	++	++	+++	±	0
Common mutations	Large rearrangements	TK*MERRF8344	TL1*MELAS3243	ATP6*NARP8993	ND4*LHON11778
Positive family history	±	+++	++	+++	+++

Abbreviations: KSS, Kearns-Sayre syndrome; MERRF, myoclonic epilepsy and ragged-red fiber disease; MELAS, mitochondrial encephalomyopathy, lactic acidosis, and stroke-like episodes; NARP, neurogenic weakness, ataxia, and retinitis pigmentosa; LHON, Leber's hereditary optic neuropathy; +, present; ±, variably present; 0, not present. The abbreviations for the common mtDNA mutations indicate the mitochondrial gene involved, the syndrome associated with the mutation, and the nucleotide number where the substitution has occurred. TK and TL1 refer to $tRNA^{Lys}$ and $tRNA^{Leu(UUR)}$, respectively.

Table 2.16 Some mitochondrial syndromes caused by nDNA mutations

Disease	Main clinical features	Molecular phenotype	Mode of inheritance	Genes involved
Leigh	Relapsing acute encephalopathy, progressive cerebral neurodegeneration, lactic acidosis, episodic tachypnea, hypotonia, seizures, ±cardiomyopathy, ±hepatocellular dysfunction, ±renal tubular dysfunction	Various mitochondrial ETC defects: Complex I, Complex II, Complex III, Complex IV (COX)	AR	Various
CPEO/KSS	Ophthalmoplegia, muscle weakness, sensorineural deafness, cardiomyopathy, cardiac conduction defects, peripheral neuropathy, ataxia	Large mtDNA deletions	AD or AR	
Pearson marrow-pancreas syndrome	Onset in infancy of failure to thrive, chronic diarrhea, lactic acidosis, siderblastic anemia, hypoparathyroidism; often evolves into KSS	Multiple mtDNA deletions		
MNGIE	Ophthalmoplegia, progressive leukodystrophy, dementia, myopathy, peripheral neuropathy, diarrhea, intestinal pseudo-obstruction, malabsorption	Thymidine phosphorylase deficiency; multiple mtDNA deletions, depletion, or both	AR	
Wolfram (DIDMOAD)[1]	Diabetes insipidus, diabetes mellitus, optic atrophy, sensorineural deafness, psychiatric disturbances (see Table 2.17)	Endoglycosidase H-sensitive membrane glycoprotein deficiency; multiple mtDNA deletions in some	AR	WFS1

(cont.)

Table 2.16 (*cont.*)

Disease	Main clinical features	Molecular phenotype	Mode of inheritance	Genes involved
Hepatocerebral MDS	Early-onset encephalopathy, oscillating eye movements, severe failure to thrive, hepatocellular failure, markedly elevated plasma α-fetoprotein, lactic acidosis, death in infancy	Deoxyguanosine kinse deficiency; mtDNA depletion in liver	AR	*DGUOK*
Myopathic MDS	Onset in early childhood of progressive skeletal myopathy, with death in first decade of life	Thymidine kinase deficiency; mtDNA depletion in muscle	AR	*TK2*
Friedreich ataxoa	Progressive gait ataxia, pes cavus, kyphoscoliosis, sensory neuropathy, dysarthria, nystagmus, sensorineural deafness, absent deep tendon reflexes, extensor plantar reflexes, cardiomyopathy, diabetes mellitus in some	Deficiency of frataxin	AR	*FRDA*
ARHSP	Progressive spastic paraplegia, sensory neuropathy, ragged-red fibres, with mental retardation, ataxia, retinitis pigmentosa, deafness, and ichthyosis in some	Primary paraplegin deficiency with secondary deficiencies of Complex I, II/III, and IV	AR	**SPG7**

Abbreviations: CPEO, chronic progressive external ophthalmoplegia; KSS, Kearns-Sayre syndrome; MNGIE, mitochondrial neurogastrointestinal encephalomyopathy and encephalopathy; ETC, electron transport chain; ARHSP, autosomal recessive hereditary spastic paraplegia; AR, autosomal recessive; AD, autosomal dominant; MDS, mitochondrial DNA depletion syndrome;

[1] In most cases of Wolfram syndrome, the mtDNA is intact.

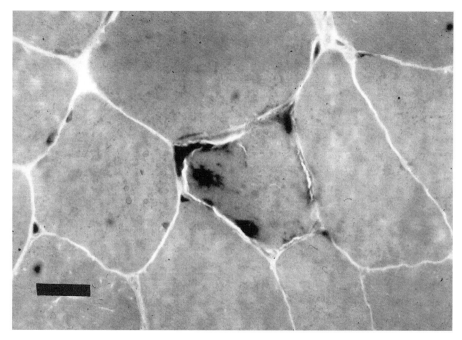

Figure 2.15 Photomicrograph of skeletal muscle stained by the modified Gomori trichrome method showing ragged-red fibers.
The bar represents 50 μm. (Courtesy of Dr. Venita Jay, Toronto, Canada.)

Hunter disease (MPS II) and children with Sanfilippo disease (MPS III) exhibit particularly severe hyperactivity, impulsiveness, short attention span, poor tolerance of frustration, aggressiveness, and sleeplessness. In Sanfilippo disease, the extraordinarily disruptive behavior may be what brings the patient to medical attention. The implacable irritability of infants with Krabbe globoid cell leukodystrophy is a prominent feature of the disease. Infants with hepatorenal tyrosinemia commonly exhibit acute episodes of extreme irritability, often accompanied by acute onset of reversible peripheral neuropathy, all attributable to the secondary porphyria which is a feature of the disease.

In many other inherited metabolic diseases, particularly late-onset disorders, the first indication of the onset of disease may be behavioral or personality changes (Table 2.18). The earliest signs of the disease in boys affected with X-linked adrenoleukodystrophy are often social withdrawal, irritability, obsessional behavior, and inflexibility. Patients with adult-onset metachromatic leukodystrophy may present with subtle evidence of chronic organic brain syndrome, such as anxiety, depression, emotional lability, social withdrawal, disorganized thinking, and poor memory. In late-onset variants of GM2 gangliosidosis, the patient may present with a frank psychosis characterized by severe agitation, obsessional paranoia,

Table 2.17 Inherited metabolic disease in which autonomic dysfunction is prominent

Disease	Clinical features	Diagnosis
Dopamine β-hydroxylase deficiency	Adolescent- or adult-onset severe orthostatic hypotension.	CSF neurotransmitter analysis: ↑HVA, normal 5HIAA, ↓MHPG, normal 3OMD, normal BH4, normal BH2, normal Neopterin
Neurovisceral porphyrias	Abdominal pain, vomiting, autonomic instability, hypertension, constipation, diarrhea, tachycardia, bladder dysfunction	See Chapter 9
Fabry disease	Severe, intermittent, paresthesias and acroparesthesias of hands and feet, hypohidrosis, chronic diarrhea, postural hypotension	Deficiency of lysosomal α-galactosidase A in plasma or leukocytes (males); increased urinary CTH (males or females); demonstration of *GLA* mutations (males or females)
MPS I, MPS II, MPS III	Chronic, frequent, loose stools, along with dysmorphic facies, dysostosis multiplex, hepatosplenomegaly, and mental retardation (see Chapter 6)	Deficiency of appropriate lysosomal enzyme activity in leukocytes or cultured skin fibroblasts
Occipital horn syndrome	Postural hypotension, marked hypotonia, chronic diarrhea, along with cutaneous hyperkeratosis, skeletal abnormalities (see Chapter 6)	Decreased concentrations of copper and ceruloplasmin in plasma
MNGIE	Early adult-onset recurrent diarrhea, intestinal pseudo-obstruction, cachexia, along with ophthalmoparesis, peripheral neuropathy, leukoencephalopathy	Deficiency of thymidine phosphorylase in leukocytes

Abbreviations: CSF, cerebrospinal fluid, HVA, homovanillic acid; 5HIAA, 5-hydroxyindoleacetic acid; MHPG, 3-methoxy-4-hydroxyphenylglycol; 3OMD, 3-O-methyldopa; BH4, tetrahydrobiopterin; BH2, 7,8-dihydrobiopterin; MPS, mucopolysaccharidosis; MNGIE, mitochondrial neurogastrointestinal encephalomyopathy; CTH, ceramide trihexoside.

Table 2.18 Some inherited metabolic diseases characterized by psychiatric or severe behavioral abnormalities

Disease	Psychiatric/behavioral abnormality
Children	
Sanfilippo disease (MPS III)	Extreme hyperactivity, impulsivity, poor tolerance of frustration, aggressiveness, sleeplessness
Hunter disease (MPS II)	Extreme hyperactivity, impulsivity, poor tolerance of frustration, aggressiveness, sleeplessness
X-linked ALD	Social withdrawal, irritability, obsessional behavior, and rigidity
Lesch-Nyhan syndrome	Severe self-mutilatory behavior
Adolescents and adults	
Late-onset MLD	Anxiety, depression, emotional lability, social withdrawal, disorganized thinking, poor memory, schizophrenia
Late-onset GM2 gangliosidosis	Acute psychosis with severe agitation, obsessional paranoia, hallucinations, stereotypic motor automatisms
Porphyria	Chronic anxiety and depression, and marked restlessness, insomnia, depression, paranoia, and sometimes, hallucinations (during acute crises)
Wilson disease	Anxiety, depression, schizophrenia, manic-depressive psychosis, antisocial behavior
Wolfram syndrome (DIDMOAD)	Depression, paranoia, auditory or visual hallucinations, violent behavior, dementia (in some), suicide
Cerebrotendinous xanthomatosis	Delusions, hallucinations, catatonia, dependency, irritability, agitation, and aggression
UCED	Periodic acute agitation, anxiety, hallucinations, paranoia
Homocystinuria (MTHF reductase deficiency)	Acute 'schizophrenia'
Homocystinuria (cystathionine β-synthase deficiency)	Acute onset of auditory and visual hallucinations, paranoia
Adult-onset NCL (Kuf disease)	Thought disorder, flat affect, paranoia with hallucinations, delusions, inappropriate behavior

Abbreviations: ALD, adrenoleukodystrophy; MLD, metachromatic leukodystrophy; UCED, urea cycle enzyme defects; DIDMOAD, diabetes insipidus-diabetes mellitus-optic atrophy-deafness; MTHF, methylenetetrahydrofolate; NCL, neuronal ceroid lipofuscinosis.

hallucinations, and stereotypic motor automatisms. Personality changes are a common feature of Wilson disease, but usually only after the development of other neurologic manifestations of the disease. Three of our older patients with HHH syndrome have experienced periodic episodes of acute hallucinatory states lasting up to a few hours. The episodes generally occurred during periods of hyperammonemia, and the frequency of attacks decreased with improved metabolic control; however, their occurrence did not correlate well with the severity of the hyperammonemia.

Psychiatric disturbance, including early signs of dementia, are a particularly common presentation for late-onset variants of conditions typically presenting as rapidly progressive psychomotor regression in more common, childhood-onset variants of the same diseases. In many cases, the pyschiatric problems may be the only, or at least the predominant, sign of disease for years. The characterization of the disturbances in this group of patients is still incomplete. However, signs that increase the suspicion of dementia caused by an inherited metabolic disorder include:

- onset before age 40 years
- a positive family history, especially in a sibling
- presence of hard neurological signs, specifically extrapyramidal abnormalities
- presence of white-matter abnormalites on MRI
- prominence of executive dysfunction on neuropsychological testing

Acute porphyria may present as an acute psychiatric emergency in patients with acute intermittent porphyria (AIP), the commonest inherited metabolic disorder of porphyrin biosynthesis everywhere except South Africa, where variegate porphyria affects 1 of every 250 individuals in the Afrikaans population. Typically, patients present with acute neurovisceral crises, with delirium, psychosis, autonomic instability (severe constipation, tachycardia, hypertension), abdominal pain, electrolyte disturbances, muscle weakness, and peripheral neuropathy, often when exposed to certain drugs, such as barbiturates, sulfonamides, or alcohol. However, the neuropsychiatric manifestations of the disease are extraordinarily protean, and the diagnosis of porphyria should be considered in any situation where the psychiatric symptoms include evidence of acute organic brain syndrome, resistance to conventional treatment, or association with exposure to known porphyrinogenic drugs. Although severe, acute, neurovisceral crises may cause death, only 20% of individuals who inherit AIP-causing mutations of the porphobilinogen deaminase gene actually develop any symptoms of the disease. Women are much more likely to become symptomatic than men, especially during the luteal phase of the menstrual cycle. The development of symptoms before puberty is unusual.

A summary of the metabolism of porphyrins and related inborn errors of porphyrin metabolism is presented in Figure 9.2 and Table 9.9. Some generalizations:

- the neurovisceral manifestations of porphyria are caused by accumulation of water-soluble, porphyrin precursors, porphobilinogen (PBG) and 5-aminolevulinic acid (ALA), not any of the more distal intermediates in heme biosynthesis;
- the cutaneous manifestations of the disease are caused by accumulation of metabolites distal to PBG or ALA;

- hereditary coproporphyria and variegate porphyria are often associated with neurovisceral symptoms because coprophyrinogen III and protoporphyrinogen IX inhibit PBG deaminase, causing secondary accumulation of PBG and ALA;
- the more distal porphyrin metabolites, such as coproporphyrinogens III and protoporphyrinogen IX, are less water-soluble than the more proximal metabolites, such as PBG and ALA, which is why the concentrations of these metabolites are higher in stool than in urine; and
- urinary porphyrin metabolites may only be present in excess for a few days, during the acute attack – fecal abnormalities tend to persist for several days, sometimes indefinitely.

An approach to the laboratory investigation of porphyria is presented in Chapter 9.

SUGGESTED READING

Aicardi, J. (1993). The inherited leukodystrophies clinical overview. *Journal of Inherited Metabolic Diseases*, **16**, 733–43.

Argov, Z. & Arnold, D. L. (2000). MR spectroscopy and imaging in metabolic myopathies. *Neurologic Clinics*, **18**, 35–52.

Assmann, B., Surtees, R. & Hoffmann, G. F. (2003). Approach to the diagnosis of neurotransmitter diseases exemplified by the differential diagnosis of childhood-onset dystonia. *Annals of Neurology*, **54** (suppl 6), S18–S24.

Batshaw, M. L. (1994). Inborn errors of urea synthesis. *Annals of Neurology*, **35**, 133–41.

Chaves-Carballo, E. (1992). Detection of inherited neurometabolic disorders. A practical clinical approach. *Pediatric Clinics of North America*, **39**, 801–20.

Crimlisk, H. L. (1997). The little imitator – porphyria: a neuropsychiatric disorder. *Journal of Neurology, Neurosurgery, and Psychiatry*, **62**, 319–28.

De Vivo, D. C. & Johnston, M. V. (eds) (2003). Pediatric neurotransmitter diseases. *Annals of Neurology*, **54** (Suppl 6), S1–S109.

DiMauro, S., Bresolin, N. & Papadimitriou, A. (1984). Fuels for exercise: Clues from disorders of glycogen and lipid metabolism. In *Neuromuscular Diseases*, ed. G. Serratgrice et al., pp. 45–50. New York: Raven Press.

DiMauro, S., Bonilla, E. & De Vivo, D. C. (1999). Does the patient have a mitochondrial encephalomyopathy? *Journal of Child Neurology*, **14** (Suppl 1), S23–35.

DiMauro, S. & Schon, E. A. (2003). Mitochondrial respiratory-chain diseases. *New England Journal of Medicine*, **348**, 2656–68.

Estrov, Y., Scaglia, F. & Bodamer, O. A. (2000). Psychiatric symptoms of inherited metabolic disease. *Journal of Inherited Metabolic Diseases*, **23**, 2–6.

Finsterer, J. (2004). Mitochondriopathies. *European Journal of Neurology*, **11**, 163–86.

Folstein, M. F., Folstein, S. E. & McHugh, P. R. (1975). "Mini-mental state". A practical method for grading the cognitive state of patients for the clinician. *Journal of Psychiatric Research*, **12**, 189–98.

Goebel, H. H. & Wisniewski, K. E. (2004). Current state of clinical and morphological features in human NCL. *Brain Pathology*, **14**, 61–9.

Haltia, M. (2003). The neuronal ceroid-lipofuscinoses. *Journal of Neuropathology and Experimental Neurology*, **62**, 1–13.

Hyland, K. (1999). Presentation, diagnosis, and treatment of the disorders of monoamine neurotransmitter metabolism. *Seminars in Perinatology*, **23**, 194–203.

Kahler, S. G. & Fahey, M. C. (2003). Metabolic disorders and mental retardation. *American Journal of Medical Genetics, Part C: Seminars in Medical Genetics*, **117**, 31–41.

Kaye, E. M. (2001). Update on genetic disorders affecting white matter. *Pediatric Neurology*, **24**, 11–24.

Kelly, P. J., Furie, K. L., Kistler, J. P., *et al.* (2003). Stroke in young patients with hyperhomocysteinemia due to cystathionine beta-synthase deficiency. *Neurology*, **60**, 275–9.

Kullmann, D. M. (2002). The neuronal channelopathies. *Brain*, **125**, 1177–95.

Leonard, J. V. & Schapira, A. H. (2000). Mitochondrial respiratory chain disorders I: mitochondrial DNA defects. *Lancet*, **355**, 299–304.

Leonard, J. V. & Schapira, A. H. (2000). Mitochondrial respiratory chain disorders II: neurodegenerative disorders and nuclear gene defects. *Lancet*, **355**, 389–94.

Lyon, G., Adams, R. D. & Kolodny, E. H. (1996). *Neurology of Hereditary Metabolic Diseases of Children*, 2nd ed. New York: McGraw-Hill.

Parker, C. C. & Evans, O. B. (2003). Metabolic disorders causing childhood ataxia. *Seminars in Pediatric Neurology*, **10**, 193–9.

Pavlakis, S. G., Kingsley, P. B. & Bialer, M. G. (2000). Stroke in children: genetic and metabolic issues. *Journal of Child Neurology*, **15**, 308–15.

Powers, J. M. & Moser, H. W. (1998). Peroxisomal disorders: genotype, phenotype, major neuropathologic lesions, and pathogenesis. *Brain Pathology*, **8**, 101–20.

Prasad, A. N. & Prasad, C. (2003). The floppy infant: contribution of genetic and metabolic disorders. *Brain & Development*, **27**, 457–76.

Rubio-Gozalbo M E, Dijkman K P, van den Heuvel L P, Sengers R C, Wendel U, Smeitink J A. (2000). Clinical differences in patients with mitochondriocytopathies due to nuclear versus mitochondrial DNA mutations. *Human Mutation*, **15**, 522–32.

Schiffmann, R. & van der Knaap, M. S. (2004). The latest on leukodystrophies. *Current Opinion in Neurology*, **17**, 187–92.

Skladal, D., Sudmeier, C., Konstantopoulou, V., *et al.* (2003). The clinical spectrum of mitochondrial disease in 75 pediatric patients. *Clinical Pediatrics (Philadelphia)*, **42**, 703–10.

Strub, R. L. & Black, F. W. (1999). *The mental status examination in neurology*, 4th ed. Philadelphia: F. A. Davis.

Surtees, R. (2000). Inherited ion channel disorders. *European Journal of Pediatrics*, **159** (Suppl 3), S199–S2003.

Tein, I. (1999). Neonatal metabolic myopathies. *Seminars in Perinatology*, **23**, 125–51.

Thunell, S., Harper, P., Brock, A. & Petersen, N. E. (2000). Porphyrins, porphyrin metabolism and porphyrias. II. Diagnosis and monitoring in the acute porphyrias. *Scandinavian Journal of Clinical Investigation*, **60**, 541–59

Tsujino, S., Nonaka, I. & DiMauro, S. (2000). Glycogen storage myopathies. *Neurologic Clinics*, **18**, 125–50.

Vedanarayanan, V. V. (2003). Mitochondrial disorders and ataxia. *Seminars in Pediatric Neurology*, **10**, 200–9.

3

Metabolic acidosis

Metabolic acidosis is a common presenting or coincident feature of many inherited metabolic diseases. In some cases, the acidosis is persistent, though so mild that the generally recognized clinical signs, such as tachypnea, are absent or so subtle that they are missed. In other cases, the patient presents with an episode of acute, severe, even life-threatening, acidosis, and the underlying persistence of the condition is only recognized after resolution of the acute episode. Diagnostically, the most frustrating presentation is infrequent bouts of recurrent, acute acidosis separated by long intervals of apparent good health during which diagnostic tests show no significant abnormality. This is a particularly challenging situation.

Buffers, ventilation, and the kidney

The hydrogen ion concentration, $[H^+]$, of body fluids is maintained within very narrow limits by a combination of buffers, acting immediately, pulmonary ventilation to restore the capacity of blood buffers, and renal mechanisms to eliminate excess H^+.

Quantitatively, the most important buffers in blood are the proteins, both the plasma proteins and hemoglobin. Alterations in the concentrations of these proteins, particularly hemoglobin, may seriously compromise the capacity of the body to cope with sudden accumulation of acid. The buffering contributed by the equilibrium between HCO_3^- and H_2CO_3 is important because the capacity of the system is rapidly restored by elimination of H_2CO_3 through conversion to CO_2 and expulsion of the excess CO_2 by increased pulmonary ventilation.

The buffering properties of the bicarbonate-carbonic acid system are shown by the familiar Henderson-Hasselbach equation:

$$pH = pK' + \log \frac{[HCO_3^-]}{[H_2CO_3] + CO_2(d)}$$

$pK' =$ a constant $= 6.10$ in arterial blood; $CO_2(d) =$ concentration of dissolved CO_2.

In the presence of carbonic anhydrase, H_2CO_3 is rapidly converted to H_2O and CO_2. The concentration of H_2CO_3 is, therefore, directly proportional to the concentration of CO_2, which is a function of the partial pressure of CO_2, the $PaCO_2$, in blood. The pH and $PaCO_2$ of blood are easily measured, and with that information, the $[H_2CO_3^-]$ can be calculated. The equation is often re-written to show the relationship between its components in terms of the variables that are easily measured:

$$pH = pK' + \log \frac{[HCO_3^-]}{S \times PaCO_2} \tag{3.1}$$

$PaCO_2 =$ partial pressure of CO_2 in arterial blood; $S =$ a constant.

Without having to recall any specific numbers, one can easily see that an increase in $[H^+]$, in the absence of any other change, would cause a decrease in pH. However, association of the H^+ with HCO_3^- to form H_2CO_3 causes a decrease in $[HCO_3^-]$ and increase in $PaCO_2$, tending to restore the pH. Removal of the excess CO_2 by increased ventilation permits the association of more H^+ with HCO_3^- to form more H_2CO_3, though the total CO_2 and, therefore, the total buffer capacity of the system, is decreased in the process. Restoring the buffer capacity of the system requires removal of the excess H^+ by some other mechanism. This critical function is carried out by the kidney.

The kidney plays two important roles in acid-base balance: it conserves HCO_3^- (and sodium), and it secretes H^+. In the proximal convoluted tubule, 99% of filtered HCO_3^- is reabsorbed, along with sodium, amino acids and peptides, glucose, and phosphate. Loss of HCO_3^-, as a result of damage to the proximal convoluted tubule, decreases the buffering capacity of the bicarbonate-carbonic acid system. In the distal convoluted tubule of the nephron, H^+ is secreted by a mechanism involving exchange with K^+ and the production and secretion of NH_4^+ and glutamine. Decreased H^+–K^+ exchange, with increased K^+ losses in the urine, is the reason chronic metabolic alkalosis causes potassium depletion.

Metabolic acidosis is diagnosed by measurement of blood gases. The typical changes are:

- Decreased arterial blood pH, caused by accumulation of H^+.
- Decreased plasma bicarbonate, as excess H^+ is buffered by HCO_3^- with a shift in the equilibrium between $H_2CO_3^-$ and H_2CO_3.
- Decreased $PaCO_2$, owing to compensatory hyperventilation.

When the accumulation of excess H^+ is relatively small, respiratory compensation is usually complete, restoring the blood pH to normal. However, with increasing H^+ accumulation, respiratory compensation becomes insufficient to restore the blood pH completely to normal. In practical terms, it is rarely possible to decrease the $PaCO_2$ below 16 mm Hg by increased respiratory effort alone. If respiratory compensation is incomplete, from associated pulmonary disease or from respiratory failure, a mixed metabolic respiratory acidosis develops, characterized by increased $PaCO_2$. Aggressive correction of metabolic acidosis, especially by administration of large amounts of sodium bicarbonate, is often accompanied by the development of respiratory alkalosis as result of persistence of central nervous system (CNS) acidosis after correction of the systemic acid-base disturbance. This is rarely a major problem except perhaps in the management of inborn errors of pyruvate oxidation, such as pyruvate carboxylase deficiency, in which CNS production of lactate may be enormous.

Is the metabolic acidosis the result of abnormal losses of bicarbonate or accumulation of acid?

A glance at the Henderson-Hasselbach equation shows that the drop in pH occurring with metabolic acidosis may occur as a result of either abnormal losses of bicarbonate, or abnormal accumulation of H^+, generally in association with some relatively non-volatile organic anion. One way to tell the difference is to calculate the concentration of unmeasured anion, the anion gap, which is the difference between the plasma $[Na^+]$ and the sum of the plasma $[Cl^-]$ and $[HCO_3^-]$. The normal anion gap is 10–15 mEq/L. Albumin is quantitatively the most important unmeasured anion in plasma. Lactate, acetoacetate, 3-hydroxybutyrate, phosphate, sulfate, and other minor anions also contribute to the normal anion gap. When metabolic acidosis occurs as a result of bicarbonate losses, either because of renal tubular dysfunction or gastrointestinal losses from diarrhea, the anion gap is usually normal, in spite of decreased $[HCO_3^-]$, owing to an increase in the plasma $[Cl^-]$. Hyperchloremic acidosis is, therefore, one of the hallmarks of metabolic acidosis occurring as a result of abnormal bicarbonate losses.

Metabolic acidosis caused by abnormal bicarbonate losses

A history of diarrhea is usually sufficient to distinguish hyperchloremic metabolic acidosis due to excessive gastrointestinal bicarbonate losses from that arising from renal tubular dysfunction. However, the situation may become confusing if the urine pH is discovered to be inappropriately high. The combination of acidosis and hypokalemia, owing to excessive gastrointestinal fluid and electrolyte losses, promotes renal ammonium production and excretion, increasing the urinary pH. By contrast, in patients with inappropriately high urinary pH as a result of renal tubular acidosis, the urine ammonium concentration is low. Urinary ammonium

Table 3.1 Inherited metabolic diseases associated with renal tubular acidosis (RTA)

Disease	Defect
Galactosemia	Galactose-1-phosphate uridyltransferase deficiency
Hereditary fructose intolerance	Fructose-1-phosphate aldolase deficiency
Hepatorenal tyrosinemia	Fumarylacetoacetase deficiency
Cystinosis	Defect in cysteine transport out of lysosomes
Glycogen storage disease, type I	Glucose-6-phosphase deficiency
Fanconi-Bickel syndrome	Defect in glucose and galactose transport
Congenital lactic acidosis	Cytochrome c oxidase deficiency
Wilson disease	Copper transporter defect
Vitamin D dependency	Cholecalciferol 1α-hydroxylase deficiency
Osteopetrosis with RTA	Carbonic anhydrase II deficiency
Lowe syndrome	Phosphatidylinositol-4,5-bisphosphate 5-phosphatase deficiency

concentrations, which are difficult to measure directly, can be estimated by calculating the urine net charge (UNC): $[Na^+ + K^+] – [Cl^-]$ in urine. A negative UNC is taken as an indication of the presence of ammonium, suggesting the acidosis is the result of abnormal gastrointestinal losses of bicarbonate (and potassium). This method for estimating urinary ammonium concentrations *does not apply* when the acidosis is the result of accumulation of organic anion.

The inappropriately high, though not necessarily alkaline, urinary pH in patients with proximal renal tubular dysfunction is the result of excessive urinary losses of bicarbonate. In addition to bicarbonate, the reabsorption of amino acids, glucose, phosphate, and urate (renal Fanconi syndrome) is also impaired. The urine may test positive for glucose and reducing substances, and chromatographic analysis shows generalized amino aciduria (see Chapter 9). The plasma phosphate and urate concentrations are also below normal.

Renal Fanconi syndrome is a common manifestation of several inherited metabolic diseases (Table 3.1). In some condition, such as cystinosis, Fanconi-Bickel syndrome, and Lowe syndrome, it may be a prominent clinical feature of the disease. In most, the clinical signs of disease are typically dominated by other problems, rather than to the acidosis or renal disease *per se*. For example, the renal tubular problems in patients with galactosemia or hepatorenal tyrosinemia are usually discovered incidentally; they are rarely the presenting problem. In GSD I, and in hereditary fructose intolerance, the metabolic acidosis caused by accumulation of lactic acid is much more prominent than that caused by renal tubular dysfunction.

Chronic metabolic acidosis, whether it is attributable to bicarbonate losses or to accumulation of anion, is commonly associated with failure to thrive. Patients are often reported to be 'sickly' and to have exaggerated difficulties with apparently trivial intercurrent illnesses. Developmental delay is common, but rarely severe, and it is often noted to affect gross motor skills more than speech or socialization. When it is severe and persistent, as it is in infantile cystinosis, metabolic acidosis arising from proximal renal tubular disease is invariably associated with marked growth retardation. Excessive renal tubular loss of phosphate causes rickets.

Metabolic acidosis resulting from accumulation of organic anion

Metabolic acidosis resulting from accumulation of organic anion, caused by inborn errors of organic acid metabolism, is usually persistent. Clinically, it is commonly associated with marked failure to thrive. In addition, persistent, mild metabolic acidosis is often punctuated by intermittent episodes of acute metabolic decompensation. Acute metabolic acidosis causes tachypnea, often without obvious dyspnea. Breathing is rapid and deep, but often it is apparently effortless, and the severity of the respiratory distress may not be appreciated. Secondary hypoglycemia and hyperammonemia, along with accumulation of organic anion, commonly produce acute encephalopathy with anorexia and vomiting, lethargy, ataxia, and drowsiness progressing to stupor and coma (see Chapter 2). The accumulation of organic anion is often accompanied by a peculiar odor of the sweat or urine.

Diagnostically the most important thing to do in patients presenting with metabolic acidosis and an increased anion gap is to identify the unmeasured anion. This is done by a combination of analysis of specific anions, such as lactate, 3-hydroxybutyrate and acetoacetate, and screening procedures, such as analysis of urinary organic acids (Figure 3.1) (see Chapter 9).

Lactic acidosis

Abnormal accumulation of lactic acid is by far the commonest cause of pathologic metabolic acidosis in children. In the majority of cases, it is caused by tissue hypoxia resulting from inadequate oxygen supply or poor circulation, so-called 'type A lactic acidosis'. It occurs in any situation in which the delivery of oxygen to tissues is impaired, such as shock, heart failure, congenital heart disease (especially that producing severe left outlet obstruction), or pulmonary hypertension. Lactic acidosis from hypoxemia may be very severe, with plasma lactate levels in excess of 30 mmol/L, and it is associated with an increase in the lactate to pyruvate ratio (L/P ratio) in plasma. The cause of the lactic acidosis is usually obvious, and the

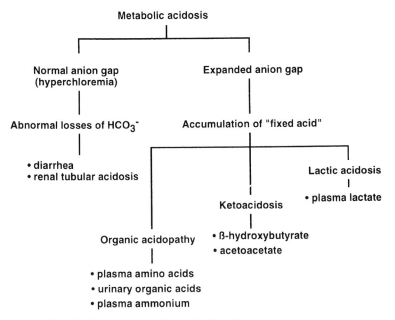

Figure 3.1   Approach to the investigation of metabolic acidosis.

acidosis is generally reversed within minutes to a few hours by correction of the hypoxic state. The lactic acidosis associated with cardiomyopathy presents a special diagnostic challenge because the cardiomyopathy itself may be due to a primary inherited defect in lactate metabolism (Chapter 5). A clinical classification of lactic acidosis is presented in Table 3.2.

Lactate is a 'dead-end' metabolite: it is eliminated metabolically by the same route it is formed – through the formation of pyruvate. In addition to H^+, the reaction involves two sets of substrates and products: pyruvate/lactate and $NADH/NAD^+$. The conversion is catalyzed by lactate dehydrogenase (LDH), which is ubiquitous and catalyzes the forward and reverse reactions equally well, so that the equilibrium concentration of lactate is directly related to the concentration of pyruvate and the ratio of the concentrations of NADH and NAD^+:

$$[Lactate]\alpha[Pyruvate] \times [H^+] \times \frac{[NADH]}{[NAD^+]}$$

It follows that lactate accumulation may occur as a result of pyruvate accumulation or NADH accumulation, both tending to push the reaction to the right, or as a result of H^+ accumulation.

Pyruvate accumulation

Pyruvate and lactate are the end products of glycolysis, the major source of energy when availability of oxygen is low and in tissues, like erythrocytes, that do not

Table 3.2 Clinical classification of lactic acidosis

Acquired	Inborn errors of metabolism
Hypoxemia	*Primary*
Circulatory collapse	Defects of pyruvate metabolism
Shock	PDH deficiency
Congestive heart failure	Pyruvate carboxylase deficiency
	Defects of NADH oxidation
Severe systemic disease	Mitochondrial ETC defects
Liver failure	
Kidney failure	*Secondary*
Diabetic ketoacidosis	Disorders of gluconeogenesis
Acute pancreatitis	GSD, type I
Acute leukemia	HFI
	PEPCK deficiency
Intoxication	Fructose-1,6-diphosphatase deficiency
Ethanol	Fatty acid oxidation defects
Methanol	Defects of biotin metabolism
Ethylene glycol	Biotinidase deficiency
Oral hypoglycemic drugs	Holocarboxylase synthetase deficiency
Acetylsalicylic acid	Defects of organic acid metabolism
	HMG-CoA lyase deficiency
Nutritional deficiency	Propionic acidemia
Thiamine deficiency	Methylmalonic acidemia
	Others

Abbreviations: PDH, pyruvate dehydrogenase; GSD, glycogen storage disease; HFI, hereditary fructose intolerance; PEPCK, phosphoenolpyruvate carboxykinase; HMG-CoA, 3-hydroxy-3-methylglutaryl-CoA.
Source: Modified from Lehotay & Clarke (1995).

contain mitochondria. Many of the reactions that make up the process of glycolysis are freely reversible and contribute well to gluconeogenesis, the process by which glucose is produced from pyruvate and amino acids (see Chapter 4). Although the sequence of reactions and the regulation of the rate and direction of metabolic flux are complicated, clinically important aspects of the process can be summarized in a few generalizations and the whole treated as a 'black box'. The key features of glycolysis are:

• It is a cytoplasmic process.
• Each molecule of glucose (six carbons), which is uncharged, is converted to two molecules of pyruvic acid (three carbons each), which are negatively charged.
• It results in the net production of two molecules of ATP per molecule of glucose.

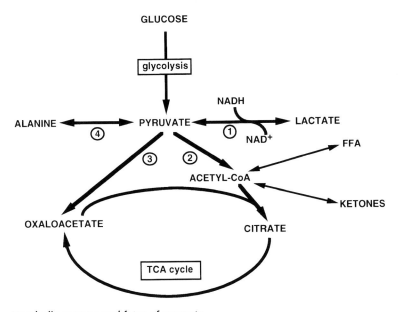

Figure 3.2   Metabolic sources and fates of pyruvate.
The enzymes involved in pyruvate metabolism are: **1**, lactate dehydrogenase; **2**, pyruvate dehydrogenase complex; **3**, pyruvate carboxylase; **4**, alanine aminotransferase.

- Overall flux is increased by an intracellular energy deficit and is decreased by signals indicating the concentrations of high energy compounds, like ATP, are adequate.
- It produces various intermediates, such as glycerol, required for the synthesis of compounds like triglycerides.

Among the inherited metabolic diseases, lactic acidosis due to pyruvate accumulation may occur as a result of *increased pyruvate production* by increased glycolytic flux. Increased pyruvate production is the mechanism of the lactic acidosis in patients with GSD I, or hereditary fructose intolerance, as a consequence of increased intracellular concentrations of stimulatory phosphorylated intermediates, like fructose-2,6-bisphosphate and fructose-1,6-bisphosphate, respectively.

Lactic acidosis also occurs as a consequence of *decreased oxidation of pyruvate.* Pyruvate, produced from glycolysis, or from the transamination of alanine, is either oxidized to acetyl-CoA, in a reaction catalyzed by the pyruvate dehydrogenase complex (PDH), or it is carboxylated to form oxaloacetate, in a reaction catalyzed by the biotin-containing enzyme, pyruvate carboxylase (PC) (Figure 3.2). Whether PDH or PC activity predominates at any particular moment is, as one might expect, determined by the energy needs of the cell. In general, PDH is stimulated by signals indicating an increased need for energy, such as low ATP/ADP ratios; PC is stimulated by indications, such as increased acetyl-CoA levels, that the concentration of TCA intermediates, particularly oxaloacetate, is too low to support continued operation of the cycle.

PDH deficiency

Persistent lactic acidosis is a prominent feature of PDH deficiency. PDH is a huge multicomponent enzyme complex made up of multiple units of four enzymes: pyruvate decarboxylase (E_1, 30 units), dihydrolipoyl transacetylase (E_2, 60 units), dihydrolipoamide dehydrogenase (E_3, 6 units), and protein X (6 units). Enzyme activity is regulated in part by phosphorylation (inactivation)-dephosphorylation (activation), reactions catalyzed by PDH kinase and PDH phosphatase, respectively. Most patients with PDH deficiency have mutations of the X-linked E_1 subunit of the pyruvate decarboxylase component of the enzyme complex. Nonetheless, males and females are equally represented, except among those patients with the relatively benign form of the disease, which is characterized by intermittent ataxia (see Chapter 2).

The clinical course of PDH deficiency is highly variable. The disease may present in the newborn period as severe persistent lactic acidosis (see Chapter 7) terminating in death within a few weeks or months. This variant of the disease is often associated with agenesis of the corpus callosum. Most children with PDH deficiency present later in infancy with a history of psychomotor retardation, hypotonia, failure to thrive, and seizures. The course of the disease is often punctuated by bouts of very severe lactic acidosis, often precipitated by intercurrent infections. Some show subtly dysmorphic facial features. Other patients present with classical Leigh disease (see Chapter 2).

Plasma lactate levels in PDH deficiency are persistently elevated, and the acidosis is generally made worse by ingestion of carbohydrate. However, the L/P ratio is characteristically normal. The plasma alanine level is elevated, a reflection of increased pyruvate concentrations. Urinary organic acid analysis in patients with $E_1\alpha$ defects is unremarkable apart from the presence of excess lactate and some 2-hydroxybutyrate, an organic acid found in the urine of patients with severe lactic acidosis, regardless of the cause. The diagnosis is confirmed by demonstrating PDH deficiency in cultured fibroblasts. Rarely, the PDH deficiency may be the result of a defect in the E_3 component (dihydrolipoamide dehydrogenase) of the enzyme complex. Clinically, affected patients are indistinguishable from patients with $E_1\alpha$ defects, though presentation in the newborn period has never been reported. Because both branched-chain 2-ketoacid dehydrogenase and 2-ketoglutarate dehydrogenase also contain the same E3 subunit as PDH, patients with E_3 defects have elevated plasma levels of branched-chain amino acids, though not as high as in maple syrup urine disease (MSUD), and the urinary organic acid analysis shows increased concentrations of 2-ketoglutarate, 2-hydroxyglutarate, and

2-hydroxyisovalerate. A small number of patients with classical Leigh disease have been found to have PDH phosphatase deficiency.

Although a few vitamin-responsive variants of PDH deficiency have been reported, treatment of this group of disorders is usually unsatisfactory. However, boys with the benign variant often do better on a high fat, low carbohydrate diet. The lactic acidosis in some patients is relieved to some extent by treatment with the pyruvate analogue, dichloroacetate, which increases PDH activity by inhibiting PDH kinase.

PC deficiency

Persistent lactic acidosis is also a prominent feature of PC deficiency. PC is a biotin-dependent enzyme that catalyzes the carboxylation of pyruvate to form oxaloacetate. It is dependent for activity on the presence of acetyl-CoA. In addition to its role in fueling the TCA cycle, PC catalyzes the first, and most important, reaction in gluconeogenesis (see Chapter 4).

PC deficiency is very rare. The most common variant of the disorder (type A) commonly presents in the first few months of life with a history of psychomotor retardation and signs of intermittent acute metabolic acidosis. Despite the central role PC plays in gluconeogenesis, hypoglycemia is not as a rule a prominent feature of the disease. The majority of patients in North America have been Amerindian. The L/P ratio is normal. The plasma alanine and proline levels are elevated. Urinary organic acid analysis shows elevated concentrations of lactate and 2-ketoglutarate.

Patients with the severe form of PC deficiency (type B) present in the newborn period with persistently severe lactic acidosis culminating in death within a few months. In contrast to type A patients, the L/P ratio is elevated. In addition to the biochemical abnormalities found in type A disease, affected infants are moderately hyperammonemic, and the concentrations of citrulline, lysine, and proline are increased in plasma. The diagnosis is confirmed by measuring PC activity in peripheral blood leukocytes or in fibroblasts.

Multiple carboxylase deficiency

Multiple carboxylase deficiency, either because of holocarboxylase synthetase deficiency or biotinidase deficiency, is associated with lactic acidosis, which is the result of deficiency of PC, one of the four biotin-dependent enzymes affected in the disease. Holocarboxylase synthetase deficiency is rare and usually presents within the first few weeks of birth with signs of acute metabolic acidosis accompanied by hyperammonemia. Feeding problems, failure to thrive, hypotonia, psychomotor retardation, peculiar odor, and seizures are also common and prominent features of the disease. Biotinidase deficiency is more common than

Table 3.3 Urinary organic acids in multiple carboxylase deficiency

	Enzyme deficiency	
3-Methylcrotonyl-CoA carboxylase	Propionyl-CoA carboxylase	Pyruvate carboxylase
3-Methylcrotonate	Propionate	**Lactate**
3-Methylcrotonylglycine	**3-Hydroxypropionate**	3-Hydroxybutyrate
3-Hydroxyisovalerate	**Methylcitrate**	Acetoacetate
	Tiglylglycine	

Note: Bold type indicates those compounds that are usually present or present in high concentrations in the disease.

holocarboxylase synthetase deficiency, and clinical presentation is generally later in infancy. Presentation is usually with psychomotor delay, hypotonia, myoclonic seizures, and acute metabolic acidosis. Most patients also have a seborrheic skin rash and at least partial alopecia; many have conjunctivitis, fungal infections, and other evidence of impaired resistance to infection. Some show evidence of optic atrophy, sensorineural hearing loss, and ataxia.

The urinary organic acid profile in these disorders reflects the deficiencies of the three biotin-dependent mitochondrial carboxylases involved (Table 3.3). The organic aciduria is variable, particularly in biotinidase deficiency, in which the organic acid pattern in urine may be normal. The diagnosis of biotinidase deficiency can be confirmed by enzyme assay on dried blood spots using synthetic chromogenic or fluorogenic substrates; the determination of holocarboxylase synthetase is based on the effect of biotin treatment on the activity of the mitochondrial carboxylases in peripheral blood leukocytes or cultured fibroblasts. Both forms of multiple carboxylase deficiency respond to treatment with large doses of oral biotin, 10–20 mg per day, though the response and ultimate outcome tends to be better for infants with holocarboxylase synthetase deficiency.

NADH accumulation

NADH production, like pyruvate production, is increased by any process that increases glycolytic flux. Ignoring for the moment problems of intracellular compartmentation and the complex matter of NADH transport within the cell, the principal route of NADH disposal by oxidation is by intramitochondrial electron transport linked to ATP generation – the main energy-producing process in the body. In this process, the final electron acceptor is oxygen, and any condition causing local or systemic hypoxia will cause NADH accumulation and lactic acidosis.

NADH accumulation, whether the result of increased production or decreased oxidation, causes lactic acidosis by pushing the pyruvate-lactate equilibrium toward lactate production. Therefore, defects of NADH oxidation, including inborn errors of the mitochondrial electron transport chain (ETC), are typically characterized by increased L/P ratios in blood and CSF. The laboratory investigation of mitochondrial defects is discussed in Chapter 9.

A rapidly growing number of patients with disease caused by ETC defects is being reported. Although many are associated with lactic acidosis as a result of NADH accumulation, the acidosis is generally not severe and is rarely the problem that brings the patient to medical attention. Instead, most present with one of more of: psychomotor retardation, skeletal myopathy, cardiomyopathy, hepatocellular dysfunction, or retinal degeneration, although other conditions have been associated with mitochondrial mutations, including diabetes mellitus and other endocrinopathies (see Chapter 2). There is considerable overlap in the relationship between the type of mutation, or the ETC complex affected, and the clinical pattern of disease among patients with mitochondrial ETC defects. For example, Leigh disease has been found associated with defects in Complex I, Complex IV, Complex V, as well as PC deficiency and PDH deficiency. In this situation, the clinical presentation provides very little insight into the nature of the underlying genetic defect.

Ketoacidosis

Increased fatty acid oxidation results in the production of large amounts of acetyl-CoA (see Chapter 4). Excess acetyl-CoA is converted in the liver to ketones (3-hydroxybutyrate and acetoacetate) which are transported via the circulation to be taken up and oxidized by peripheral tissues, including the brain (Figure 3.3). This is one of the most important adaptations to starvation because the ability of tissues, such as the brain, which normally derive much of their energy from glucose oxidation, to utilize ketones for energy, spares the glucose for use by tissues, such as erythrocytes, which cannot derive energy from non-glucose energy substrates. Defects in ketone utilization cause ketoacidosis.

Ketoacidosis, sometimes severe, is a prominent secondary phenomenon in several inherited metabolic diseases, such as MSUD, organic acidopathies (e.g., methylmalonic acidemia, propionic acidemia, isovaleric acidemia, holocarboxylase synthetase deficiency), glycogen storage diseases (e.g., GSD type III, hepatic phosphorylase deficiency, phosphorylase kinase deficiency, glycogen synthase deficiency), and disorders of gluconeogenesis (e.g., pyruvate carboxylase deficiency, fructose-1, 6-diphosphatase deficiency, phosphoenolpyruvate carboxykinase deficiency). Primary disorders of ketone utilization are rare.

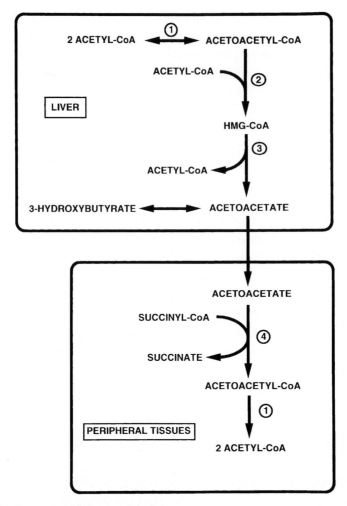

Figure 3.3   Summary of ketone metabolism.
The reactions involved in ketone production and oxidation are: **1**, acetoacetyl-CoA thiolase; **2**, 3-hydroxy-3-methylglutaryl-CoA (HMG-CoA) synthetase; **3**, HMG-CoA lyase; **4**, succinyl-CoA:3-ketoacid CoA transferase (SCOT).

Mitochondrial acetoacetyl-CoA thiolase deficiency (β-ketothiolase deficiency)

β-Ketothiolase deficiency is characterized by the onset between one and two years of age of episodic attacks of severe ketoacidosis and encephalopathy, generally precipitated by intercurrent illness or fasting, sometimes associated with hyperammonemia. The response to treatment with intravenous glucose is characteristically brisk, and between episodes of metabolic decompensation, patients are typically completely well. Urinary organic acid analysis at the time of metabolic decompensation shows the presence of 2-methyl-3-hydroxybutyrate, 2-methylacetoacetate, 2-butanone, and tiglylglycine – all derived from the intermediary metabolism of

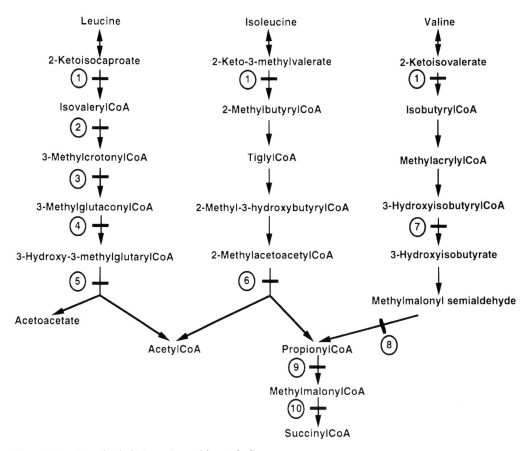

Figure 3.4   Branched-chain amino acid metabolism.
The various enzymes shown are: **1**, branched-chain 2-ketoacid decarboxylase; **2**, isovaleryl-CoA dehydrogenase; **3**, 3-methylcrotonyl-CoA carboxylase; **4**, 3-hydroxyl-3-methylglutaryl-CoA (HMG-CoA) synthetase; **5**, HMG-CoA lyase; **6**, 2-methylacetoacetate thiolase; **7**, 3-hydroxyisobutyryl-CoA deacylase; **8**, methylmalonyl semialdehyde dehydrogenase; **9**, propionyl-CoA carboxylase; **10**. methylmalonyl-CoA mutase.

isoleucine (Figure 3.4), as well as huge amounts of 3-hydroxybutyrate and acetoacetate. Definitive diagnosis requires demonstration of specific deficiency of potassium-stimulated enzyme activity, preferably using 2-methylacetoacetyl-CoA as substrate. Cytosolic acetoacetyl-CoA thiolase deficiency is very rare. It is characterized by severe psychomotor retardation and hypotonia, a reflection perhaps of the importance of the enzyme in sterol and isoprenoid biosynthesis.

Succinyl-CoA:3-ketoacid CoA transferase (SCOT) deficiency

Only a handful of patients with SCOT deficiency have ever been studied in detail. All presented early in life with life-threatening bouts of severe ketoacidosis. Unlike patients with β-ketothiolase deficiency, who may be to all appearances completely normal between episodes of ketoacidosis, patients with SCOT deficiency are persistently ketotic between episodes of metabolic decompensation. The urinary organic acid analysis shows large amounts of 3-hydroxybutyrate and acetoacetate.

Organic aciduria

The development of rapid, accurate, and technically relatively easy and inexpensive techniques for the analysis of low molecular weight organic acids in physiologic fluids, like urine, has led to the discovery of a large number of new inherited metabolic diseases. A number of these present as acute, chronic, or acute-on-chronic metabolic acidosis, and urinary organic acid analysis is a logical and important aspect of the diagnostic investigation. However, for some organic acidopathies, clinical signs of metabolic acidosis may be so subtle that they are completely obscured by symptoms referable to the nervous system, heart, liver, kidneys, or other systems. To limit the application of organic acid analysis to patients who have frank metabolic acidosis with increased anion gaps would invariably miss patients affected with some of these disorders.

The clinical spectrum of the known disorders of organic acid metabolism spans a wide range of presentations involving almost every system in the body. In many cases, the urinary organic acid profile is typical of the disease, and diagnosis is relatively easy. In others, the abnormalities may be quite subtle or only present intermittently. Table 3.4 presents disorders of organic acid metabolism organized according to the principal pathologic urinary organic acid abnormalities. The clinical aspects of many of the conditions listed are discussed in other parts of the book more appropriate to the nature of the clinical presentation.

Some of the conditions merit specific discussion either because they are relatively common, the interpretation of the clinical and laboratory findings may be difficult, or they serve to illustrate some general principle.

Methylmalonic acidemia (MMA)

MMA is a relatively common disorder of organic acid metabolism. However, the metabolism of methylmalonic acid is complex, involving the interaction of a number of distinct gene products and environmental factors (Figure 3.5). Deficiency or a defect in any one of them might produce methylmalonate accumulation. Classical MMA is caused by complete deficiency of methylmalonyl-CoA mutase (mut), which normally catalyzes the rearrangement of methylmalonyl-CoA to succinyl-CoA. It commonly presents in the newborn period in a manner clinically indistinguishable from propionic acidemia (see Chapter 7) with severe metabolic acidosis, acute encephalopathy, hyperammonemia, neutropenia, and thrombocytopenia.

Table 3.4 Organic acidurias

Urinary organic acids	Enzyme defect	Distinguishing clinical features
2-Ketoisocaproate, 2-hydroxyisocaproate, 2-keto-3-methylvalerate, 2-ketoisovalerate, 2-hydroxyisovalerate	Branched-chain 2-ketoacid decarboxylase	MSUD: Acute encephalopathy, ketosis, psychomotor retardation
Lactate, 2-ketoglutarate, 2-ketoisocaproate, 2-hydroxyisocaproate, 2-keto-3-methylvalerate, 2-ketoisovalerate, 2-hydroxyisovalerate	Lipoamide dehydrogenase	Psychomotor retardation, chronic lactic acidosis with acute exacerbations
3-Methylglutaconate, 3-hydroxyisovalerate, 3-methylglutarate, 3-hydroxybutyrate, acetoacetate	3-Methylglutaconyl-CoA hydratase	3-Methylglutaconic aciduria, type I: mild psychomotor retardation, hypoglycemia, ketoacidosis
3-Methylglutaconate, 3-methylglutarate, 2-ethylhydracrylate	Tafazzin (TAZ)	Barth syndrome (3-methylglutaconic aciduria, type II): X-linked cardiomyopathy, skeletal myopathy, chronic neutropenia
3-Methylglutaconate, 3-methylglutarate	Unknown	Costeff optic atrophy syndrome: (3methylglutaconic aciduria, type III): optic atrophy, severe psychomotor retardation, choreoathetosis, spasticity, seizures
3-Methylglutaconate, 3-methylglutarate, lactate, TCA cycle intermediates	Mitochondrial ATP-synthase	3-Methylglutaconic aciduria, type IV: severe multi-organ disease, congenital malformations, clinically heterogeneous, including Pearson mitochondrial DNA deletion syndrome
3-Hydroxy-3-methylglutarate, 3-methylglutaconate, 3-methylglutarate, 3-hydroxyisovalerate	HMG-CoA lyase	Episodic severe metabolic acidosis with encephalopathy, hypoglycemia $\pm$ hyperammonemia
Mevalonate	Mevalonate kinase	Psychomotor retardation, dysmorphism, cataracts, hepatosplenomegaly, lymphadenopathy, anemia, chronic diarrhea, arthralgia, fever, skin rash
Isovalerylglycine, 3-hydroxyisovalerate, lactate, 3-hydroxybutyrate, acetoacetate	Isovaleryl-CoA dehydrogenase	Severe metabolic acidosis, hyperammonemia, neutropenia, thrombocytopenia, odor of sweaty feet
2-Methyl-3-hydroxybutyrate, 2-methylacetoacetate, 2-butanone, 3-hydroxybutyrate, acetoacetate, tiglylglycine	Mitochondrial acetoacetyl-CoA thiolase	Episodic severe ketoacidosis
3-Methylcrotonate, 3-methylcrotonylglycine, 3-hydroxyisovalerate	3-Methylcrotonyl-CoA carboxylase	Episodic severe ketoacidosis, hypoglycemia

Metabolites	Enzyme defect	Clinical features
3-Methylcrotonate, 3-methylcrotonylglycine, 3-hydroxyisovalerate, propionate, 3-hydroxypropionate, methylcitrate, tiglylglycine, lactate, 3-hydroxybutyrate and acetoacetate	(a) Holocarboxylase synthetase or (b) Biotinidase	(a) Metabolic acidosis, hyperammonemia, thrombocytopenia, peculiar odor, seizures, ataxia, (skin rash, alopecia) (b) Psychomotor delay, hypotonia, myoclonic seizures, metabolic acidosis, seborrheic skin rash, alopecia
Ethylmalonate, methylsuccinate, butyrylglycine, isovalerylglycine, 2-methylbutyrylglycine	A mitochondrial matrix protein (*ETHE1*) with uncertain function	Ethylmalonic encephalopathy Spastic diplegia, orthostatic acrocyanosis, chronic diarrhea, psychomotor retardation, lactic acidosis
Ethylmalonate, isobutyrylglycine, isovalerylglycine, 2-methylbutyrylglycine	Cytochrome *c* oxidase	Psychomotor retardation, encephalopathy, ataxia, spasticity
L-2-Hydroxyglutarate	Unknown	Ataxia, dysarthria, psychomotor retardation, ± seizures
D-2-Hydroxyglutarate	D-2-Hydroxyglutarate dehydrogenase	Psychomotor retardation, seizures
Methylmalonate, methylcitrate, 3-hydroxybutyrate, acetoacetate	Methylmalonyl-CoA mutase or Cobalamin defects	Severe metabolic acidosis, hyperammonemia, neutropenia, thrombocytopenia
3-Hydroxyisobutyrate, lactate	3-Hydroxyisobutyryl-CoA dehydrogenase	Episodic ketoacidosis, facial dysmorphism, cerebral dysgenesis, hypotonia, failure to thrive
4-Hydroxybutyrate, 3,4-dihydroxybutyrate	Succinic semialdehyde dehydrogenase	Psychomotor retardation, hypotonia, ataxia, choreoathetosis
Fumarate	Fumarase	Psychomotor retardation
Propionate, 3-Hydroxypropionate, propionylglycine, methylcitrate, tiglylglycine, 3-hydroxybutyrate, acetoacetate	Propionyl-CoA carboxylase	Severe metabolic acidosis, hyperammonemia, neutropenia, thrombocytopenia
Malonate	Malonyl-CoA decarboxylase	Psychomotor retardation ± cardiomyopathy
L-Glycerate, oxalate	D-Glycerate dehydrogenase	Urolithiasis, urinary tract infections, renal colic
Oxalate, glycolate	Alanine: glyoxylate aminotransferase (type I)	Urolithiasis, nephrocalcinosis, peripheral neuropathy, anemia, arthropathy, progressive renal failure
Medium-chain dicarboxylic acids (adipate, suberate, sebacate), 5-hydroxyhexanoate, 7-hydroxyoctanoate, hexanoylglycine, phenylpropionylglycine, octanoylcarnitine	Medium-chain acyl-CoA dehydrogenase	Recurrent Reye-like encephalopathy, sudden unexpected death

(cont.)

Table 3.4 (cont.)

Urinary organic acids	Enzyme defect	Distinguishing clinical features
Ethylmalonate, methylsuccinate, adipate, butyrylglycine	Short-chain acyl-CoA dehydrogenase	Skeletal myopathy, cardiomyopathy, failure to thrive, metabolic acidosis
Medium-chain dicarboxylic acids, dodecanedioate, tetradecanedioate	Long-chain acyl-CoA dehydrogenase	Cardiomyopathy, skeletal myopathy, exercise intolerance with myoglobinuria, Reye-like episodes of acute encephalopathy
Medium-chain dicarboxylic acids, 3-hydroxydodecanedioate, 3-hydroxydodecenedioate, 3-hydroxytetradecanedioate, 3-hydroxytetradecenedioate	Trifunctional protein (long-chain 3-hydroxyacyl-CoA dehydrogenase)	Cardiomyopathy, variable skeletal myopathy, intermittent acute hepatocellular dysfunction, peripheral neuropathy
Glutarate, 3-hydroxyglutarate	Glutaryl-CoA dehydrogenase	Progressive dystonia, choreoathetosis, intermittent ketoacidosis and acute encephalopathy
Glutarate, 2-hydroxyglutarate, ethylmalonate, adipate, suberate, sebacate, dodecanedioate, isovalerylglycine, hexanoylglycine	Electron transfer flavoprotein (ETF) or ETF dehydrogenase	Severe: Facial dysmorphism, cerebral dysgenesis, cystic kidneys, or Mild: Intermittent severe ketoacidosis, hyperammonemia, acute encephalopathy, failure to thrive
5-Oxoproline (pyroglutamate)	Glutathione synthetase	Hemolytic hypochromic, microcytic anemia
4-Hydroxycyclohexylacetate	4-Hydroxyphenyl-pyruvate oxidase	Hawkinsinuria: autosomal dominant intermittent metabolic acidosis in infancy
N-Acetylaspartate	Aspartoacylase	Canavan syndrome: Severe, progressive psychomotor retardation, macrocephaly, seizures
Orotate	(a) UMP synthase or (b) Various defects in urea biosynthesis	(a) Megaloblastic anemia, urolithiasis, failure to thrive, psychomotor retardation (b) See Chapter 2
Uracil, thymine	Dihydropyrimidine dehydrogenase	Uncertain. Increased susceptibility to 5-fluorouracil toxicity

Abbreviations: MSUD, maple syrup urine disease; TCA, tricarboxylic acid; HMG-CoA, 3-hydroxy-3-methylglutaryl-CoA; ETF, electron transfer flavoprotein.

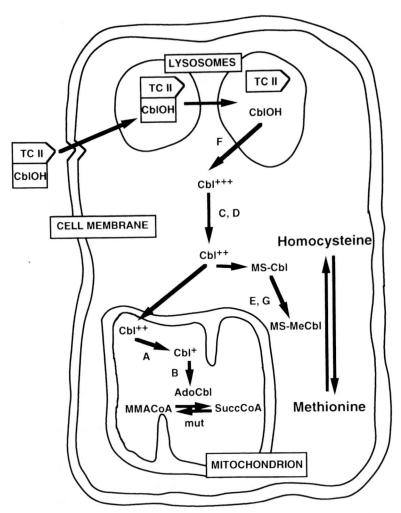

Figure 3.5   Relationship between cobalamin, methylmalonic acid (MMA), and homocysteine metabolism.

The letters, A to F, refer to the locations of the metabolic defects of the different complementation groups of inherited defects in cobalamin metabolism. Abbreviations: Cbl, cobalamin; TC II, transcobalamin II; MS-Cbl, methionine synthase-bound cobalamin; MMACoA, methylmalonyl-CoA; SuccCoA, succinyl-CoA; AdoCbl, adenosylcobalamin; mut, methylmalonyl-CoA mutase.

Late-onset variants of the disease, in which residual mutase activity is high, are common. Generally, the later the onset, the milder the disease; some individuals with MMA as a result of *mut* mutations show no symptoms at all.

Methylmalonyl-CoA mutase is one of only two human enzymes known to require cobalamin (vitamin B_{12}) for activity. MMA caused by defects in the intramitochondrial processing or adenosylation of cobalamin (*cblA* and *cblB* variants, respectively) and defects affecting the affinity of mutase for adenosylcobalamin, is often somewhat milder than disease caused by complete mutase deficiency, and it is often responsive to treatment with pharmacologic doses of vitamin B_{12}. In every other respect, it is clinically indistinguishable from classical MMA.

Methionine synthase (MS) is the other enzyme in the body that requires cobalamin for activity. In this case, the active species of the cofactor is methylcobalamin. Defects in the processing of MS-Cbl (*cblE* and *cblG* variants) cause homocystinemia and homocystinuria, but not MMA. Patients with *cblE* or *cblG* disease present early in life with psychomotor retardation, feeding difficulties and failure to thrive, hypotonia, cerebral atrophy, and megaloblastic anemia that is hematologically indistinguishable from that caused by nutritional vitamin B_{12} deficiency. In contrast to the marked elevation of plasma methionine concentrations in classical homocystinuria due to cystathionine β-synthase deficiency, the methionine levels in patients with *cblE* or *cblG* defects are, as one would expect, decreased below normal.

Defects in the transport, intracellular uptake, lysosomal processing, release from lysosomes, or reduction of Cbl^{+++} to Cbl^{++} are characterized biochemically by both MMA and homocyst(e)inemia and homocystinuria. All these defects are associated with megaloblastic anemia, variable psychomotor retardation, and failure to thrive, some with onset in early infancy and others only emerging in later life. Patients with hereditary defects in cobalamin processing (*cblC*, *cblD* and *cblF* variants) generally have more severe disease than those with defects in cobalamin absorption and transport (e.g., transcobalamin II deficiency). Developmental retardation, failure to thrive, seizures, and megaloblastic anemia are prominent, along with MMA and homocystinuria. Although symptoms of feeding difficulty and hypotonia often develop in the first few weeks of life (especially in *cblC* disease), urinary methylmalonic acid levels are never as high as in MMA due to mut deficiency, and acute metabolic acidosis with hyperammonemia does not occur, even in patients with early-onset variants of these cobalamin defects. The clinical variability among patients with different cobalamin defects is considerable, making classification of the defects on clinical grounds alone unreliable. As a rule, definitive classification requires complementation studies on cultured skin fibroblasts (see Chapter 9).

Over the years, we have encountered a number of infants presenting in the first few months of life with MMA, megaloblastic anemia, and homocystinuria with normal or low plasma methionine levels, as a result of dietary vitamin B_{12} deficiency. In every case, the mother was a strict vegan and the infant was breast fed. The cause of the metabolic abnormalities in each case was confirmed by demonstrating that plasma vitamin B_{12} levels were well below normal. We have also seen a breast-fed infant who presented at 6 months of age with a history of marked developmental delay, hypotonia, lethargy, and methylmalonic aciduria associated with vitamin B_{12} deficiency caused by previously unrecognized maternal pernicious anemia.

3-Hydroxy-3-methylglutaryl-CoA (HMG-CoA) lyase deficiency

HMG-CoA lyase catalyzes the last step in the intramitochondrial catabolism of the amino acid, leucine (Figure 3.4). The products of the reaction, acetoacetate and acetyl-CoA, are important energy substrates, particularly during illness or fasting. Patients with HMG-CoA lyase deficiency may present in the newborn period, in a manner resembling neonatal propionic acidemia or MMA, with severe metabolic acidosis, vomiting, lethargy and drowsiness progressing to coma, poor feeding, hypoglycemia in most, and hyperammonemia in many. However, HMG-CoA lyase deficiency is different from the other organic acidopathies presenting with similar symptoms because of the absence of ketonuria. The disease presenting for the first time in older infants often resembles Reye syndrome or a fatty acid oxidation defect, such as medium-chain acyl-CoA dehydrogenase (MCAD) deficiency (see Chapter 2). The findings of enlargement of the liver and abnormal liver function tests add to the potential for diagnostic confusion. However, urinary organic acid analysis characteristically shows abnormalities typical of the disease, particularly during metabolic crises: massive excretion of 3-hydroxy-3-methylglutarate and 3-methylglutaconate, and large amounts of 3-hydroxyisovalerate and 3-methylglutarate. Lactic acidosis and marked increases in urinary glutaric acid and adipic acid levels are often seen during very severe metabolic crises. Plasma carnitine levels are decreased and the proportion of esterified carnitine is increased as a result of the formation of 3-methylglutarylcarnitine; neither HMG or 3-methylglutaconate form carnitine esters in patients with this disease. Treatment is effective in decreasing the frequency and severity of episodes of acute metabolic decompensation. In spite of apparently adequate treatment, with a high carbohydrate, low protein diet supplemented with carnitine, some patients develop cardiomyopathy, which may be fatal.

Glutaric aciduria

Glutaric aciduria type I (GA I), caused by deficiency of mitochondrial glutaryl-CoA dehydrogenase, usually presents in early infancy as a neurologic syndrome (see Chapter 2). After some weeks or months of apparently normal development, affected infants suddenly develop the first of recurrent episodes of marked hypotonia, dystonia, opisthotonus, grimacing, fisting, tongue thrusting and seizures. Partial recovery is followed by progressive neurologic deterioration and periodic episodes of ketoacidosis, vomiting and acute encephalopathy, usually precipitated by intercurrent infections. In some patients, the neurologic abnormalities

Table 3.5 Flavoprotein dehydrogenases for which ETF/ETF dehydrogenase is the electron acceptor

Mitochondrial fatty acid β-oxidation
Very long-chain acyl-CoA dehydrogenase
Long-chain acyl-CoA dehydrogenase
Medium-chain acyl-CoA dehydrogenase
Short-chain acyl-CoA dehydrogenase
Leucine oxidation
Isovaleryl-CoA dehydrogenase
Valine and isoleucine oxidation
2-Methylbutyryl-CoA dehydrogenase
Lysine, hydroxylysine, and tryptophan oxidation
Glutaryl-CoA dehydrogenase
Choline oxidation
Dimethylglycine dehydrogenase
Sarcosine dehydrogenase

Abbreviations: ETF, electron transfer flavoprotein.

remain relatively stationary with gross motor retardation, chronic choreoathetosis, dystonia, and hypotonia, with apparent preservation of intellect. CNS imaging studies typically show early cortical atrophy and attenuation of white matter and basal ganglia (see Figure 2.14). Some patients present with acute Reye-like disease without the extrapyramidal neurologic signs. During acute metabolic decompensation, laboratory studies show metabolic acidosis and ketosis, hypoglycemia, hyperammonemia, and mild hepatocellular dysfunction. Besides marked increases in glutaric acid concentration, urinary organic acid analysis shows the presence of 3-hydroxyglutarate, considered pathognomonic of the disease, and sometimes glutaconic acid during severe ketoacidosis. Between episodes of metabolic decompensation, the urinary organic acids may be normal or only mildly abnormal. Plasma carnitine levels are decreased.

Glutaric aciduria type II (GA II), which is also called multiple acyl-CoA dehydrogenase deficiency, is caused by deficiency of either electron transport flavoprotein (ETF), the intramitochondrial electron acceptor for a number of acyl-CoA dehydrogenases, or ETF dehydrogenase (Table 3.5). The condition may present in one of three ways:

- Very severe, neonatal disease, characterized by facial dysmorphism, muscular defects of the abdominal wall, hypospadias (in males), cystic disease of the kidneys, hypotonia, hepatomegaly, hypoketotic hypoglycemia, metabolic acidosis, and hyperammonemia (see Chapters 6 and 7).

- Severe neonatal disease without dysmorphism, but with hypotonia, hepato-megaly, hypoketotic hypoglycemia, metabolic acidosis, and hyperammonemia.
- Mild disease characterized by later-onset episodic acute metabolic acidosis, failure to thrive, hypoglycemia, hyperammonemia, and encephalopathy.

The severe variants are often associated with a peculiar odor of sweaty feet similar to that encountered in infants with severe isovaleric acidemia. Plasma amino acid analysis shows elevations of several amino acids, especially proline and hydrox-yproline. Urinary organic acid analysis in infants with severe variants of the dis-ease characteristically shows very large amounts of glutarate, ethylmalonate, and the dicarboxylic acids, adipate, suberate, and sebacate, in addition to isovalerate, isovalerylglycine, 2-hydroxyglutaraate, hexanoylglycine, and 5-hydroxyhexanoate. The mild form of GA II is often called ethylmalonic-adipic aciduria, referring to the predominant urinary organic acid abnormalities. However, the urinary organic acids may be normal between episodes of metabolic decompensation.

Secondary glutaric aciduria is much more common than glutaric aciduria due to primary disorders of glutaric acid metabolism, like GA I and GA II. It is commonly found in relatively large concentrations in infants with mitochondrial ETC defects, presumably a reflection of 'sick mitochondria'. We have also seen massive glutaric aciduria in a boy with late-onset, but severely decompensated propionic acidemia. It has been reported in 2-ketoadipic aciduria (α-aminoadipic acidemia), probably as a result of nonenzymic decarboxylation of 2-ketoadipate. It is also one of the dicarboxylic acids appearing in the urine of infants on medium-chain triglyceride formulas.

Dicarboxylic aciduria

Increased concentrations of the medium-chain dicarboxylic acids, adipic (6-carbon), suberic (8-carbon), and sebacic (10-carbon) acids, is one of the most prominent laboratory abnormalities in patients with inherited disorders of mito-chondrial fatty acid β-oxidation, such as medium-chain acyl-CoA dehydrogenase (MCAD) deficiency. These disorders usually present as acute neurologic or hepatic syndromes, rather than as metabolic acidosis (see Chapters 2 and 4).

Medium-chain dicarboxylic aciduria is also a common secondary feature of several other conditions. The levels of adipic, suberic, and sebacic acids in the urine are generally increased under any circumstances in which fatty acid utilization is increased beyond the capacity for mitochondrial β-oxidation, such as during starvation and in patients with diabetes mellitus. It is also commonly seen in patients on the anticonvulsant, valproic acid, which inhibits fatty acid β-oxidation, and in newborn infants. When the dicarboxylic aciduria is the result of increased fatty acid oxidation, it is routinely associated with marked ketosis and the excretion of large amounts of 3-hydroxybutyrate (3-HOB) and acetoacetate. The ratio of 3-HOB to adipate is generally >2.0. By contrast, in patients with mitochondrial fatty acid β-oxidation defects, the urinary ketone concentrations are characteristically low, and the 3-HOB/adipate ratio is <2.0. Unfortunately, in very young infants, or in infants on formulas containing medium-chain triglycerides, the relationship breaks down; many apparently healthy newborn infants, particularly low birth-weight premature infants, excrete amounts of medium chain dicarboxylic acids comparable to the levels seen in asymptomatic infants with fatty acid oxidation defects. Analyses of urinary acylglycines and acylcarnitines, and especially measurements of plasma acylcarnitines by tandem MSMS, are particularly helpful in distinguishing infants with genetic defects in fatty acid metabolism.

Ethylmalonic aciduria

Ethylmalonate and adipate are particularly prominent in the urine of patients with the mild variant of multiple acyl-CoA dehydrogenase deficiency (GA II). However, ethylmalonate is excreted in a wide variety of other circumstances, some associated with severe systemic inherited metabolic diseases, others being quite benign.

Increased concentrations of ethylmalonate, along with methylsuccinate, may be the only urinary organic abnormalities in patients with short-chain acyl-CoA dehydrogenase (SCAD) deficiency. Ethylmalonic aciduria, without methylsuccinate, is also found in patients with cytochrome *c* oxidase deficiency. The combination of lactic acidosis, ethylmalonic, and methylsuccinic aciduria, along with the excretion of butyrylglycine, isovalerylglycine, and 2-methylbutyrylglycine, is characteristic of ethylmalonic encephalopathy, characterized clinically by severe psychomotor retardation, spasticity, chronic diarrhea, petechiae, and orthostatic acrocyanosis. The disease is caused by mutations in *ETHE1*, the gene coding for a mitochondrial matrix protein of uncertain function.

D-Lactic acidosis

Infants or young children with gastrointestinal abnormalities, such as blind loops, involving bowel stasis, sometimes develop attacks of severe metabolic acidosis, often associated with acute encephalopathy, with increased anion gap. Plasma lactate, 3-hydroxybutyrate, and acetoacetate levels may be completely normal. However, organic acid analysis shows the presence of large amounts of lactic acid in the urine. The acidosis in these cases is not the result of an inborn error of metabolism; it is caused by accumulation of D-lactate, a product of bacterial carbohydrate metabolism that is readily absorbed from the gut. The routine measurement of lactate in blood is by an enzymic method, employing LDH, which is specific for L-lactate, the usual product of carbohydrate metabolism in humans. Urinary organic acid analysis is generally carried out by chromatographic techniques, such as gas chromatography-mass spectrometry (GC-MS), which do not differentiate the

Table 3.6 Some common causes of spurious or artefactual organic aciduria

Organic acid	Underlying condition or disease
D-Lactic acid	Intestinal bacterial over-growth. May be sufficient to cause metabolic acidosis and encephalopathy
Methylmalonic, ethylmalonic, and 3-hydrocypropionic acids	Very young infants with gastroenteritis; may be associated with methemoglobinemia
Medium-chain dicarboxylic acids (adipic>suberic>sebacic)	Valproic acid administration. The pattern often resembles that seen in patients with defects in mitochondrial fatty acid oxidation.
Medium-chain dicarboxylic acids (sebacic>suberic>adipic)	Ingestion of formulas containing medium-chain triglycerides. The relationship between the organic acids varies according to the fatty acid composition of the medium-chain triglyceride.
Adipic acid	Ingestion of large amounts of Jello® containing adipic acid additive. The elevation of adipate may be large, but the absence of any other organic acid abnormality suggests the underlying dietary etiology.
Long-chain 3-hydroxydicarboxylic acids	Acetaminophen intoxication; severe hepatocellular disease.
Pivalic acid	Pivampicillin or pivmecillinam administration.
Octenylsuccinc acid	Formulas containing octenylsuccinate-modified cornstarch as emulsifying agent.
Methylmalonic acid	A prominent feature of dietary vitamin B_{12} deficiency.
Azelaic and pimelic acids	Extracts from plastic storage containers.
2-Hydroxybutyric acid	Occurs with severe lactic acidosis, irrespective of the cause.
5-Oxoproline (pyroglutamic acid)	Acetaminophen or vigabatrin ingestion.

D-isomer of lactate from the L-isomer. The marked discrepancy between the results of lactate measurements by the two techniques provides the clue to the origin of the acidosis. Treatment with oral, non-absorbed, antimicrobials usually produces rapid resolution of the acidosis, though recurrence of the problem is common.

Adventitious organic aciduria

In addition to expanding tremendously the number of identified inherited metabolic diseases, the widespread application of urinary organic acid analysis has also posed some challenging problems in interpretation owing to the effects of age, bowel flora, intercurrent illness, and medications, on urinary organic acid excretion. Some of the more common causes of urinary organic artifacts are shown in Table 3.6.

SUGGESTED READING

Fall, P. J. (2000). A stepwise approach to acid-base disorders. Practical patient evaluation for metabolic acidosis and other conditions. *Postgraduate Medicine*, **107**, 249–50, 253–4, 257–8 passim.

Goldstein, M. B., Bear, R., Richardson, R. M. A., Marsden, P. A. & Halperin, M. L. (1986). The urine anion gap: a clinically useful index of ammonium excretion. *American Journal of Medical Science*, **292**, 198–202.

Lehotay, D. & Clarke, J. T. R. (1995). Organic acidurias and related abnormalities. *Critical Reviews in Clinical Laboratory Sciences*, **32**, 377–429.

Mitchell, G. A., Kassovska-Bratinova, S., Boukaftane, Y., *et al.* (1995). Medical aspects of ketone body metabolism. *Clinical and Investigative Medicine*, **18**, 193–216.

Niaudet, P. & Rotig, A. (1996). Renal involvement in mitochondrial cytopathies. *Pediatric Nephrology*, **10**, 368–73.

Ogier de Baulny, H. & Saudubray, J. M. (2002). Branched-chain organic acidurias. *Seminars in Neonatology*, **7**, 65–74.

Rabier, D., Bardet, J., Parvy, Ph., *et al.* (1995). Do criteria exist from urinary organic acids to distinguish β-oxidation defects? *Journal of Inherited Metabolic Diseases*, **18**, 257–60.

Rotig, A. (2003). Renal disease and mitochondrial genetics. *Journal of Nephrology*, **16**, 286–92.

Stacpoole, P. W. (1997). Lactic acidosis and other mitochondrial disorders. *Metabolism*, **46**, 306–21.

Thorburn, D. R. & Dahl, H. H. (2001). Mitochondrial disorders: genetics, counseling, prenatal diagnosis and reproductive options. *American Journal of Medical Genetics*, **106**, 102–14.

Uribarri, J., Oh, M. S. & Carroll, H. J. (1998). D-lactic acidosis. A review of clinical presentation, biochemical features, and pathophysiologic mechanisms. *Medicine (Baltimore)*, **77**, 73–82.

4

Hepatic syndrome

Liver involvement of some kind is a presenting feature of a number of inherited metabolic diseases. The metabolic activities of the liver span a vast catalogue of functions important to the metabolism of the entire body. It is surprising, therefore, that the repertoire of responses to injury is limited, and inborn errors of metabolism manifesting as hepatic syndrome are commonly difficult to distinguish from many acquired conditions, such as infections, intoxications, developmental abnormalities, and neoplasia. One approach to the diagnosis of inherited metabolic diseases presenting as hepatic syndrome is to consider four possible presentations, recognizing that there is considerable overlap between them. They are:
• jaundice;
• hepatomegaly;
• hypoglycemia;
• hepatocellular dysfunction.

Jaundice

Jaundice is caused by accumulation of unconjugated or conjugated bilirubin, which may occur as a result of increased production, impaired metabolism, or biliary obstruction. Bilirubin is a porphyrin pigment derived from the degradative metabolism of the heme of hemoglobin.

Unconjugated hyperbilirubinemia

Pure unconjugated hyperbilirubinemia is characteristic of disorders associated with increased bilirubin production. Mature erythrocytes have no mitochondria. They derive virtually all the energy needed to maintain ion gradients, intracellular nucleotide concentrations, membrane plasticity, the iron of hemoglobin in the reduced state, and other functions, from glycolysis and the hexose monophosphate shunt. Not surprisingly, specific hereditary deficiencies of any of the enzymes involved commonly present with hemolytic anemia. Some are also associated with neurologic symptoms, such as severe psychomotor retardation (e.g., triosephosphate isomerase deficiency) or myopathy (e.g., phosphofructokinase deficiency) (see Chapter 2). The hyperbilirubinemia caused by hemolysis is characteristically unconjugated, and it is not generally accompanied by any clinical or biochemical evidence of hepatocellular dysfunction.

The commonest inborn error or erythrocyte metabolism presenting as jaundice is X-linked recessive glucose-6-phosphate dehydrogenase (G6PD) deficiency, a defect in the first reaction of the hexose monophosphate shunt. Carriers of the gene show relative resistance to malaria accounting for the high prevalence of the mutation in areas of the world where it is endemic. Acute hemolysis is typically precipitated by intercurrent illness or exposure to oxidizing drugs, such as sulfonamides and antimalarials, though it may occur spontaneously in the newborn period. The commonest inborn error of glycolysis presenting as unconjugated hyperbilirubinemia is pyruvate kinase (PK) deficiency which, like G6PD deficiency, may present in the newborn period with severe nonspherocytic hemolytic anemia.

Unconjugated hyperbilirubinemia is also a feature of some primary disorders of bilirubin metabolism. Normal bilirubin metabolism involves uptake by hepatocytes, conjugation with glucuronic acid, and excretion in bile. At least some individuals with Gilbert syndrome, a common (3% of the population), benign disorder of bilirubin metabolism associated with mild persistent unconjugated hyperbilirubinemia, generally presenting after puberty, appear to have a defect in bilirubin uptake along with partial deficiency of bilirubin UDP-glucuronosyltransferase (BGT). The absence of any evidence of hemolysis or hepatocellular dysfunction is typical of this condition.

Severe neonatal unconjugated hyperbilirubinemia caused by specific BGT deficiency is characteristic of Crigler-Najjar syndrome. It is commonly associated with unconjugated bilirubin levels >500 μmol/L in the absence of hemolysis, infection, or significant hepatocellular dysfunction. Phototherapy and exchange transfusions are ineffective, and affected infants invariably develop severe kernicterus. Some patients, classified as Crigler-Najjar syndrome type 2 (also called Arias syndrome), respond to administration of phenobarbital (4 mg/kg/day) with a dramatic drop in plasma bilirubin levels. Patients with Crigler-Najjar syndrome are not usually difficult to distinguish from patients with breast milk jaundice, which is milder, later in onset, and can be shown to be associated with breast feeding.

It is important to remember that the hyperbilirubinemia in infants with classical galactosemia is often initially unconjugated, converting only after a period of some days to the conjugated hyperbilirubinemia that is widely regarded as characteristic of the disease. Even early in the course of the disease, galactosemia is associated with evidence of significant hepatocellular dysfunction, which sets it apart from

Crigler-Najjar syndrome. Galactosemia is discussed in more detail in the section 'Hepatocellular dysfunction'.

Conjugated hyperbilirubinemia

Conjugated hyperbilirubinemia as a manifestation of inherited metabolic disease is more common than unconjugated hyperbilirubinemia because it includes those diseases, like galactosemia, hepatorenal tyrosinemia, and hereditary fructose intolerance, in which hepatocellular dysfunction is prominent (see 'Hepatocellular dysfunction').

Mixed conjugated and unconjugated hyperbilirubinemia in the absence of any other evidence of hepatocellular dysfunction or hemolysis, with onset in later childhood, is typical of Rotor syndrome or Dubin-Johnson syndrome caused by benign defects in the intrahepatic biliary excretion of bilirubin glucuronide. The two conditions are differentiated from each other by differences in urinary porphyrins. The former is associated with a marked increase in urinary excretion of coproporphyrin I and III with <80% being the I isomer; in Dubin-Johnson syndrome, the urinary coproporphyrin levels may be normal, but the I isomer accounts for >80% of the total (normal about 25%).

Hepatomegaly

Asymptomatic hepatomegaly is common in children, and the decision about who to investigate, and how intensively, is sometimes difficult. The hepatomegaly associated with inherited metabolic diseases is generally persistent and nontender. If the liver is so soft that the edge is difficult to palpate, enlargement is likely to be due to accumulation of triglyceride, a typical feature of GSD (glycogen storage disease) type I. At the other extreme, a hard and irregular liver edge, often associated with only modest enlargement of the organ, is characteristic of cirrhosis, such as is characteristic of hepatorenal tyrosinemia (hereditary tyrosinemia, type I). When it is enlarged as a result of lysosomal storage, the liver is usually firm, but not hard.

Is the spleen also enlarged? A history of hematemesis or the presence of ascites or abdominal venous dilatation, would suggest that splenomegaly is caused by portal hypertension resulting from cirrhosis. However, the spleen may be enlarged by infiltration or accumulation of the same cells or metabolites causing enlargement of the liver. Besides sharing the portal circulation, the liver and spleen both contain components of the reticuloendothelial system (RES). Conditions causing expansion of the RES, either as a result of cellular proliferation or storage within RES cells (i.e., macrophages), commonly present with clinical enlargement of both organs. This is characteristic, for example, of many of the lysosomal storage diseases (see Chapter 6).

Glycogen storage disease, type III (GSD III) commonly presents as asymptomatic hepatomegaly discovered incidentally in the course of routine physical examination. The spleen may also be enlarged, but the splenomegaly is mild compared with the enlargement of the liver. Glycogen accumulation in this condition is caused by deficiency of a debrancher enzyme that converts the branch-points in glycogen into linear molecules for further hydrolysis by phosphorylase. The enlargement of the liver may be marked. It is generally firm and nontender, with a sharp, smooth, edge that is easy to palpate. In most patients, hypoglycemia does not occur, or it occurs only after prolonged fasting. However, in a significant minority, it may present in early infancy and be as severe as the hypoglycemia seen in patients with GSD I. Severe early infantile GSD III may also be associated with failure to thrive and hyperlipidemia, further blurring the clinical differentiation from GSD I. However, lactic acidosis and hyperuricemia do not occur, or are very mild, in patients with GSD III. Moreover, the condition is associated with ketosis during fasting and with moderate increases in liver aminotransferases (AST and ALT), which, as a rule, do not occur in GSD I. Liver biopsy shows increased glycogen with variable interlobular fibrosis, but very little fat. Rarely, the fibrosis progresses to frank cirrhosis, producing portal hypertension and liver failure. As adults, many patients develop evidence of muscle involvement, including cardiomyopathy in some. This is characterized by proximal muscle weakness, depressed deep tendon reflexes, and elevation of plasma creatine phosphokinase (see Chapter 2).

Patients with GSD III will show a rise in plasma glucose in response to ingestion of galactose, fructose, or amino acids, indicating that gluconeogenesis is intact. They also show a significant increase in plasma glucose in response to glucagon administered two to four hours after feeding, but they do not respond after 10–12 hours of fasting when all the hepatic linear glycogen accessible to phosphorylase activity has been depleted. Confirmation of the diagnosis requires measurement of debrancher enzyme activity in fresh liver obtained by biopsy.

Hepatic phosphorylase deficiency (GSD VI) is often clinically indistinguishable from GSD III, though it is much less common, and involvement of skeletal muscle and the heart does not occur. Phosphorylase deficiency can be demonstrated histochemically on tissue obtained by biopsy.

Phosphorylase b kinase deficiency is more common than GSD VI. The most common variant appears to be transmitted as an X-linked recessive disorder. Clinically, it is often indistinguishable from GSD III. However, unlike patients with GSD III, patients with this type of glycogen storage disease show only minimal increases in plasma glucose in response to glucagon after fasting of any duration. Liver biopsy shows increased glycogen, which may be more dispersed in appearance than in GSD III. There is often some interlobular fibrosis, though cirrhosis is rare. Confirmation of the diagnosis is best done by direct enzyme analysis of fresh liver, although some patients show deficiency of the enzyme in red blood cells. Involvement of skeletal muscle occurs in a small proportion of patients, in which the condition appears to be transmitted as an autosomal recessive. Isolated involvement of skeletal muscle or the myocardium is very rare (see Chapters 2 and 5). Mutation analysis is also often helpful in confirming the diagnosis.

Hypoglycemia

Hunger, apprehension, jitters, irritability, and sweating are common early symptoms of hypoglycemia in older patients. Unless the cause of the symptoms is recognized and treated, this is followed by disturbance of consciousness with drowsiness progressing rapidly to stupor and coma accompanied by convulsions. Idiosyncratic presentations dominated by behavioural abnormalities are common. In very young infants, the early signs may be subtle with nothing more than irritability, sweating, and somnolence. A seizure may be the first recognized indication of the problem, and hypoglycemia should be considered in any infant presenting for the first time with convulsions. Treatment with intravenous glucose should not be delayed.

The differential diagnosis of hypoglycemia is made easier by some understanding of the normal mechanisms for maintaining normal plasma glucose concentrations during fasting. During the intervals between meals, the plasma concentration is supported by two general mechanisms:

- Mechanisms directed at producing glucose (glycogen breakdown and gluconeogenesis);
- Mechanisms that decrease peripheral glucose utilization by providing alternative energy substrates (fatty acid and ketone oxidation).

Hypoglycemia may occur as a result of primary or secondary defects in glucose production (deficiency of supply), or as a result of defects in fatty acid or ketone oxidation (over-utilization).

Ways to increase glucose production

Glycogen is a high-molecular weight, highly branched polymer of glucose. During feeding it is formed by polymerization of glucose, derived primarily from dietary carbohydrate. During fasting, the process is reversed with glucose being released by phosphorylase-catalyzed hydrolysis of glycogen. Glycogen is an excellent form of immediately available glucose. However, storage in the liver involves the simultaneous storage of large amounts of water, and the total amount of glycogen that can be accommodated is, therefore, actually relatively small. As a result, within only 24–48 hours of fasting, the glycogen in the liver becomes totally depleted as it is rapidly converted into glucose to meet the needs of tissues, like the brain, having high energy requirements.

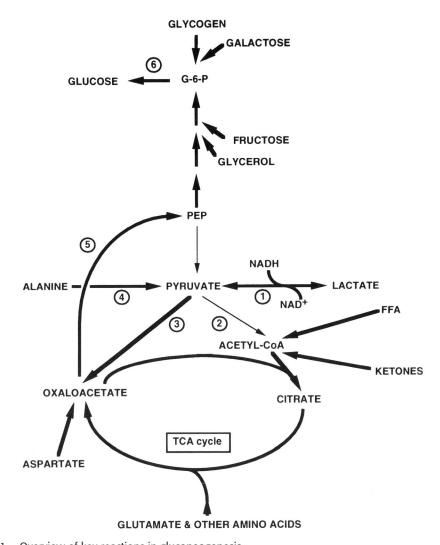

Figure 4.1   Overview of key reactions in gluconeogensis.
The various enzymes involved in key reactions of gluconeogensis are: **1**, lactate dehydrogenase (LDH); **2**, pyruvate dehydrogenase complex (PDH); **3**, pyruvate carboxylase (PC); **4**, alanine aminotransferase (ALT); **5**, phosphoenolpyruvate carboxykinase (PEPCK); **6**, glucose-
6-phosphatase.

The synthesis of glucose from nonglucose substrates (gluconeogenesis) occurs
coincidentally with glycogenolysis during fasting, and it is ultimately capable of sup-
plying much more glucose over a longer period of time. The process (Figure 4.1),
which takes place predominantly in the cytosol, is functionally the reverse of
glycolysis. One of the most important regulatory steps in the process is the carboxylation of pyruvate to form oxaloacetate (catalyzed by pyruvate carboxylase)

within mitochondria. The oxaloacetate formed by the reaction is then converted to phosphoenolpyruvate in a reaction catalyzed by mitochondrial phosphoenolpyruvate carboxykinase (PEPCK). The PEP diffuses out of the mitochondria into the cytoplasm where it is converted to glucose in a series of reactions that mirror the same steps in glycolysis.

Oxaloacetate is also transported out of mitochondria into the cytoplasm by the 'malate shuttle'. Cytosolic oxaloacetate is converted to PEP by cytosolic PEPCK, which is genetically distinct from the mitochondrial isozyme. There is some evidence that mitochondrial PEPCK is particularly important in the synthesis of glucose from pyruvate derived from lactate, and that cytosolic PEPCK is more important in gluconeogenesis involving oxaloacetate and pyruvate derived from amino acid metabolism.

Other important gluconeogenic substrates, such as galactose, fructose, and glycerol, feed into the process at different steps between PEP and glucose-6-phosphate. The final step in *both* glycogenolysis and gluconeogenesis is glucose-6-phosphatase-catalyzed hydrolysis of glucose-6-phosphate to form free glucose.

A critical aspect of gluconeogenesis is an adjustment made to preserve and re-utilize the carbon skeleton of glucose, rather than having it lost irretrievably as a result of oxidation all the way to CO_2. This process, which is called the Cori cycle (Figure 4.2), involves the simultaneous synthesis of glucose from pyruvate in the liver (gluconeogenesis) and partial oxidation of glucose to pyruvate (glycolysis) in the periphery, primarily in muscle. The partial oxidation of a single molecule of glucose by glycolysis yields only a fraction of the ATP that could be derived from total oxidation to CO_2 and water. However, the capacity to re-synthesize glucose, using energy derived largely from fatty acid oxidation, more than compensates for the relative inefficiency: the trade-off is expanded capacity in exchange for decreased efficiency.

Ways to decrease peripheral glucose utilization

The capacity to derive energy from mitochondrial fatty acid β-oxidation is a critically important mechanism for sparing glucose. The storage efficiency of energy as triglyceride is much greater than as hepatic glycogen. Long after liver glycogen has been depleted by starvation, the body continues to draw on the triglyceride in adipose tissue to provide an alternative to glucose for energy production. The process decreases the need for glucose production to a minimum, sparing it for various biosynthetic processes and for use by tissues, like red blood cells, that cannot meet their energy needs any other way. Organs, like the brain, which do not derive significant amounts of energy from fatty acid β-oxidation within the tissue itself, oxidize ketones produced by fatty acid oxidation in the liver. The relationship between hepatic ketogenesis and peripheral ketone utilization is reviewed in Chapter 3.

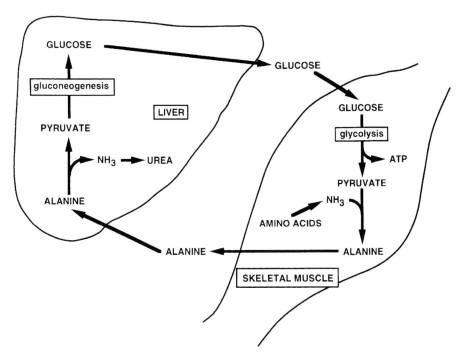

Figure 4.2   The Cori cycle.

During starvation, increased secretion of epinephrine and glucagon stimulates hormone-sensitive lipase in adipose tissue to break down triglyceride into free fatty acids and glycerol. The glycerol is taken up by the liver and converted into glucose by gluconeogenesis (Figure 4.1). The fatty acids are transported in the circulation bound to albumin to tissues like liver and muscle where they are taken up, activated by esterification with coenzyme A, and transported into mitochondria, by a process dependent on availability of carnitine. In mitochondria, they undergo β-oxidation with the production of energy in the form of ATP. In the liver, the principal inter-mediate in the process, acetyl-CoA, is converted to ketones (3-hydroxybutyrate and acetoacetate) for export via the circulation to tissues, such as the brain, able to regenerate acetyl-CoA and complete the oxidation of the compound to pro-duce ATP. Defects in ketone utilization are characterized by intermittent, severe ketoacidosis (Chapter 3).

Free fatty acids and their coenzyme A esters are toxic. When the mobilization of fatty acids is increased, or the capacity for mitochondrial β-oxidation is exceeded, for whatever reason, any excess fatty acid is converted back to triglyceride, or it is oxidized by nonmitochondrial systems, such as microsomal ω-oxidation and peroxisomal β-oxidation (see Figure 4.5). Mitochondrial fatty acid β-oxidation depends critically on the availability of adequate amounts of carnitine. Although

Table 4.1 Causes of secondary carnitine deficiency

Decreased biosynthesis
Chronic liver disease
Chronic renal disease
Extreme prematurity
Inadequate intake (nutritional)
Prolonged TPN in premature infants
Severe protein calorie malnutrition
Intestinal malabsorption
Vegetarian diet
Increased losses
Renal tubular dysfunction
Renal failure (uremia)
Hemodialysis
Organic acidopathies (PA, MMA, etc.)
Treatment with valproic acid
UCED treated with sodium benzoate

Abbreviations: TPN, total parenteral nutrition; UCED, urea cycle enzyme defects; PA, propionic acidemia; MMA, methylmalonic acidemia.
Source: See Pons & De Vivo (1995).

carnitine is synthesized endogenously, and generally occurs in ample quantities in the diet, secondary deficiency is quite common (Table 4.1). No primary disorder of carnitine biosynthesis has yet been found. However, carnitine deficiency does occur as a result of genetic defects in its cellular transport. This may take the form of systemic carnitine deficiency, characterized clinically by recurrent attacks of Reye-like encephalopathy with hypoketotic hypoglycemia or as severe cardiomyopathy. Skeletal myopathy also occurs in patients with transport defects, apparently limited to the uptake of carnitine by muscle.

Carnitine also provides an alternative to coenzyme A (CoASH) in the esterification of organic acid intermediates of amino acid metabolism. Exchanging the coenzyme A of organic acyl-CoA ester with carnitine frees CoASH. CoASH is required by many processes in intermediary metabolism, particularly related to gluconeogenesis and ammonium metabolism. In patients with inborn errors of organic acid metabolism, such as methylmalonic acidemia, acylcarnitine esters accumulate and are excreted in the urine causing secondary carnitine depletion.

Within the mitochondrial matrix, fatty acyl-CoA undergoes β-oxidation. The process involves four enzymic steps operating in a cycle to shorten a fatty acyl-CoA chain by two carbons with the release of one molecule of acetyl-CoA per turn (see Figure 9.11). Several of the steps in fatty acid transport and oxidation are catalyzed by enzymes having different substrate chain-length specificities. The most important of these from the standpoint of inherited disorders of fatty acid oxidation is the first step, catalyzed by four different fatty acyl-CoA dehydrogenase enzymes: very long-chain acyl-CoA dehydrogenase (VLCAD), long-chain acyl-CoA dehydrogenase (LCAD), medium-chain acyl-CoA dehydrogenase (MCAD), and short-chain acyl-CoA dehydrogenase (SCAD).

The electrons derived from the various fatty acyl-CoA dehydrogenase reactions are transferred to a common electron transport flavoprotein (ETF) which is oxidized in turn by a reaction catalyzed by ETF dehydrogenase. ETF dehydrogenase catalyzes the transfer of electrons to coenzyme Q, part of Complex II of the mitochondrial electron transport chain (see Figure 9.12). Mutations affecting the amount of function of ETF or ETF dehydrogenase cause multiple acyl-CoA dehydrogenase deficiency (GA II). See also Chapters 3.

An approach to the differential diagnosis of hypoglycemia

Hypoglycemia is a common nonspecific problem in severely ill neonates and young infants, regardless of the cause of the illness. Sometimes, whether the hypoglycemia is the cause, or a nonspecific result, of illness can be difficult at first to determine. Regardless of the cause, correction of hypoglycemia without delay is at least as important as making a specific diagnosis. As a rule, when it is associated with severe systemic disease, such as sepsis, it is relatively easy to control by administration of glucose at a rate at, or slightly greater than, the normal basal glucose oxidation rate (4–6 mg/kg/min in neonates and 3–5 mg/kg/min in older infants and children). Figure 4.3 shows an overview of one approach to the diagnosis of hypoglycemia, focusing primarily on that caused by inborn errors of metabolism.

The presence of nonglucose reducing substances in the urine is characteristic of untreated classical galactosemia and hereditary fructose intolerance (HFI). This is simple to determine at the bedside. Testing a few drops of urine with Benedict's reagent or with Clinitest tablets is positive in the presence of glucose, galactose, or fructose. However, dipping the same urine with Clinistix is usually negative in these conditions, indicating that the reducing substance is not glucose. Both diseases are generally associated with other prominent clinical problems. As a rule, patients with galactosemia have other evidence of hepatocellular dysfunction, and HFI is associated with marked lactic acidosis. The glycosuria in these conditions typically clears rapidly after removal of the toxic sugars from the diet. Therefore, a negative test does not eliminate the possibility of one of these disorders, particularly if the patient has been on intravenous glucose for more than a few hours.

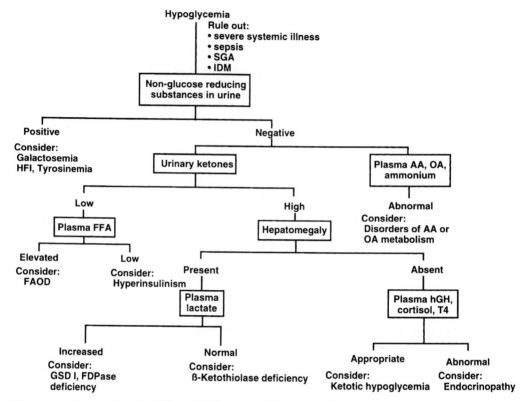

Figure 4.3   Approach to the differential diagnosis of hypoglycemia.
Abbreviations: SGA, small for gestational age; IDM, infant of diabetic mother; HFI, hereditary
fructose intolerance; AA, amino acids; OA, organic acids; FFA, free fatty acids; FAOD, fatty
acid oxidation defect; hGH, human growth hormone; T4, thyroxine; GSD, glycogen storage
disease; FDPase, fructose-1,6-diphosphatase.

Because hypoglycemia is a common secondary metabolic consequence of various inborn errors of amino acid and organic acid metabolism, the investigation should include analysis of urinary organic acids and plasma amino acids and ammonium.

Primary defects in glucose production

The normal physiologic response to decreased glucose production is increased mitochondrial fatty acid β-oxidation and the production of ketones. Accordingly, urinary tests for ketones, another bedside test, provide an indirect indication of whether hypoglycemia is the result of inadequate production or over-utilization of glucose. The hypoglycemia caused by insulin-induced over-utilization of glucose is characteristically associated with very low plasma and urine ketone concentrations (hypoketotic hypoglycemia). However, in some disorders of glucose production, such as GSD I and PEPCK deficiency, ketogenesis is often suppressed, and plasma and urinary ketone levels, though elevated, may be inappropriately low for the degree of hypoglycemia. The history of the relationship of the hypoglycemia to feeding is often helpful here. On the one hand, hypoketotic hypoglycemia developing within several minutes of feeding, particularly if it is severe, is typical of hyperinsulinism. On the other hand, patients with defects in glycogen breakdown, gluconeogenesis, or fatty acid oxidation tend to tolerate short-term fasting much better. A significant exception is GSD I, and rare cases of GSD III, in which hypoglycemia may develop within two to three hours of feeding.

GSD I may present with hypoglycemia in the newborn period. However, it is typically not difficult to control and the liver may not be particularly enlarged. In fact, a normal three-hourly feeding schedule is generally sufficient to suppress symptomatic hypoglycemia. Affected infants usually come to attention at three to five months of age when prolonging the interval between feeds, or associated intercurrent illness, precipitates an episode of severe hypoglycemia, often heralded by a seizure or coma. Some infants come to attention as a result of failure to thrive, others because of massive hepatomegaly discovered incidentally during physical examination. Occasionally, an infant with GSD I is brought to medical attention as a result of tachypnea caused by lactic acidosis. Affected children are usually pale and pasty-looking with characteristic facies, often described as 'cherubic' because of the doll-like appearance caused by the chubby cheeks. Truncal obesity and marked abdominal protuberance contrast with the typically thin extremities. Recurrent nosebleeds are common as a result of a secondary defect in platelet function; platelet numbers are usually normal.

In addition to hypoglycemia, laboratory examination typically shows lactic acidosis, hyperuricemia, hypertriglyceridemia, and hypophosphatemia. Serial measurements of plasma glucose show that the tolerance of fasting is poor, often less than three hours. The hypoglycemia is characteristically unresponsive to administration of glucagon. A distinguishing feature of GSD I is a significant rise in plasma lactate in response to glucagon. The kidneys are typically enlarged, and mild renal tubular dysfunction is common, though rarely clinically significant.

The basic defect in GSD I is deficiency of the production of glucose from glucose-6-phosphate, the final common pathway for glycogenolysis and gluconeogenesis (Figure 4.1). The most common variant of the disease (type Ia) is caused by deficiency of the microsomal enzyme, glucose-6-phosphatase. The enzyme is only expressed in liver and kidney, and definitive diagnosis requires enzyme analysis of one or other tissue, usually liver. Liver biopsy shows massive glycogen accumulation, including glycogen within the nucleus of hepatocytes (Figure 4.4). In addition, there is marked accumulation of macrovesicular fat, but typically no fibrosis, evidence of biliary obstruction, or inflammation. Deficiency of glycose-6-phosphatase can

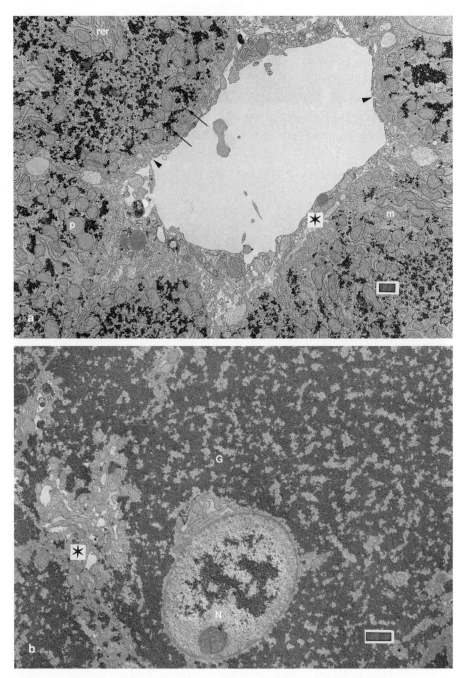

Figure 4.4   Electron micrograph of normal liver (a) and liver in glycogen storage disease (b).
Figure **a**, shows normal liver. Portions of several normal hepatocytes surrounding a sinu-
soidal blood space are shown. The black deposits (arrows) in the cytoplasm of liver cells are
glycogen aggregates. Mitochondria (m), peroxisomes (p) and rough endoplasmic reticulum
(rer) can also be seen. Note the endothelial cell processes (*) and fenestra (arrowheads).
The bar represents 1 μm. Figure **b**, shows liver from a patient with glycogen storage disease,
type Ia. Massive stores of electron dense glycogen particles (G) occupy the cytoplasm and
displace mitochondria and other organelles (*) to the periphery of the cells. Glycogen can
also be seen in the nucleus (N). The bar represents 1 μm. (Courtesy of Dr. M. J. Phillips.)

often be demonstrated histochemically. However, the diagnosis should generally be confirmed by specific enzyme analysis on fresh liver obtained by biopsy.

The non-type Ia variants of GSD I are caused by deficiency in the microsomal transport of glucose-6-phosphate (type Ib), phosphate (type Ic), or glucose (type Id). Types Ib and Ic are clinically indistinguishable from type Ia. However they are also associated with persistent neutropenia, and affected children typically have histories of recurrent pyogenic infections and pyorrhea.

Treatment of all types of GSD I is aimed primarily at preventing hypoglycemia by administration of frequent low-fat feeds, containing as little fructose and galactose as possible. This is supplemented by intermittent ingestion of uncooked cornstarch during the day and tube feeding with formula during the night. The neutropenia in patients with non-type Ia disease responds well to treatment with granulocyte-colony stimulating factor (G-CSF).

Fasting hypoglycemia and marked hepatomegaly associated with early-onset, renal tubular dysfunction, characterized by polyuria, hypophosphatemic rickets, hyperchloremic metabolic acidosis, and severe growth retardation, is typical of Fanconi-Bickel syndrome. This condition is caused by mutations in the *GLUT2* gene, coding for the liver-type glucose transporter. Hepatic glucose-6-phosphatase activity is normal.

The combination of hypoglycemia, marked hepatomegaly, and lactic acidosis is also characteristic of other defects of gluconeogenesis, such as hereditary fructose intolerance, fructose-1,6-diphosphatase deficiency, PEPCK deficiency, and sometimes pyruvate carboxylase (PC) deficiency.

In patients with hereditary fructose intolerance (HFI), the development of symptoms is clearly related to the ingestion of fructose or sucrose, often presenting with intractable vomiting, sometimes severe enough to suggest pyloric obstruction. Fructose ingestion often precipitates symptomatic hypoglycemia. More prolonged exposure results in failure to thrive, chronic irritability, hepatomegaly, abdominal distension, edema, and jaundice. Milder variants of the disease are common. Affected patients may complain of nothing more than sugar intolerance (bloating, abdominal discomfort, diarrhea).

In addition to hypoglycemia, marked lactic acidosis, hyperuricemia, and hypophosphatemia, affected patients have evidence of hepatocellular dysfunction (elevated aminotransferases, increased plasma methionine and tyrosine levels, prolonged prothrombin and partial thromboplastin times, hypoalbuminemia, hyperbilirubinemia), and renal tubular dysfunction (hyperchloremic metabolic acidosis, generalized amino aciduria). The diagnosis is confirmed by demonstrating deficiency of aldolase B (fructose-1,6-bisphosphate aldolase) in fresh liver with fructose-1-phosphate and fructose-1,6-bisphosphate as substrates. Activities with both substrates are typically markedly decreased, although the effect with fructose-1-phosphate as substrate is more pronounced. Fructose tolerance tests in patients with HFI are dangerous and should only be conducted under carefully controlled circumstances in patients who are in good general condition. Mutation analysis is often helpful, though failure to demonstrate a mutation does not rule out the disease, especially if analysis focuses on the small number of common mutations. HFI may present clinically indistinguishable from congenital disorder of glycosylation syndrome, type Ib, caused by deficiency of phosphomannose isomerase. In fact, analysis of the glycosylation pattern of plasma transferrin by isoelectric focussing may produce evidence of hypoglycosylation that is identical to that seen in CDG Ib (see Figure 6.13). However, a few weeks on a fructose-restricted diet not only results in marked clinical improvement of infants with HFI, the isoelectric focusing pattern returns to normal.

Fructose-1,6-diphosphatase deficiency may be difficult to differentiate from GSD Ia. In both diseases, the liver may be greatly enlarged. In fructose-1,6-diphosphatase deficiency, however, the response to glucagon is preserved. Definitive diagnosis requires measurement of the enzyme in fresh liver obtained by biopsy. Mitochondrial PEPCK deficiency is a very rare hereditary defect in gluconeogenesis associated with severe hypoglycemia, lactic acidosis, hepatomegaly, renal tubular dysfunction, hypotonia, and deteriorating liver function. Liver biopsy shows microvesicular steatosis and inflammatory changes. The diagnosis can be made by demonstrating deficiency of the enzyme in fibroblasts in which the mitochondrial isozyme predominates.

Over-utilization of glucose

The glucose utilization rate can be measured directly by infusions of stable isotope-labeled glucose, but this is generally impractical except in centers actively involved in research on glucose metabolism. However, glucose oxidation rates can be estimated indirectly by determining the *minimum* rate of glucose administration needed to maintain euglycemia. This is relatively easy in neonates who are often receiving intravenous glucose. In older infants and children, the absence of ketones in the urine or depressed plasma 3-hydroxybutyrate levels during hypoglycemia is usually a strong indication that glucose utilization is increased. Increased glucose utilization (i.e., hypoketotic hypoglycemia) occurs either as a result of hyperinsulinism, or as a result of a primary or secondary defect in fatty acid oxidation. The two situations are distinguishable by measurement of plasma free fatty acid levels. One of the most powerful physiologic effects of insulin is inhibition of hormone-sensitive lipase in adipose tissue. Low free fatty acid levels during hypoglycemia are a strong indication that insulin levels are abnormally elevated. Be contrast, in patients with impaired fatty acid oxidation, free fatty acid levels are typically elevated. One way to quantitate this is to calculate the ratio of free fatty acids to 3-hydroxybutyrate

Table 4.2 Approach to hypoketotic hypoglycemia

Tolerance of fasting (in hours)	Possible causes	Laboratory findings
Less than 1	Hyperinsulinism	Low plasma FFA levels with normal FFA/3-HOB ratio; high insulin/3-HOB ratio; high insulin/glucose ratio.
1–6	GSD type 1; other defects in gluconeogenesis	High plasma FFA levels with increased FFA/3-HOB ratio; lactic acidosis.
8–24	Fatty acid oxidation defects; systemic carnitine deficiency	High plasma FFA levels with very high FFA/3-HOB ratio; organic aciduria; low plasma carnitine levels

Abbreviations: FFA, free fatty acids; 3-HOB, 3-hydroxybutyrate; GSD, glycogen storage disease.

(or to 3-hydroxybutyrate + acetoacetate). Hypoketotic hypoglycemia caused by hyperinsulinism is associated with a normal ratio (<2.0), while that associated with fatty acid oxidation defects is typically elevated (>3.0). In disorders of gluconeogenesis, including GSD I, the ratio is also often elevated as a result of secondary inhibition of ketogenesis. However the timing of the hypoglycemia and other laboratory findings (Table 4.2) usually make differentiation of the conditions relatively straight forward.

In the face of relative or absolute decrease in the capacity for mitochondrial fatty acid β-oxidation, fatty acids are oxidized by nonmitochondrial oxidative pathways to produce medium-chain (6- to 10-carbon length) dicarboxylic acids (Figure 4.5). This occurs when increased fatty acid oxidative flux exceeds the normal capacity for mitochondrial β-oxidation, or when normal mitochondrial fatty acid β-oxidation is impaired. The first is typically associated with marked ketonuria and moderate medium-chain dicarboxylic aciduria. The ratio of adipate to 3-hydroxybutyrate in urine is generally <0.5. By contrast, patients with defects in mitochondrial fatty acid β-oxidation characteristically have hypoketotic hypoglycemia and marked medium-chain dicarboxylic aciduria owing to increased nonmitochondrial fatty acid oxidation. The adipate/3-hydroxybutyrate ration is >0.5. Therefore, a urinary adipate/3-hydroxybutyrate ratio >0.5 is suggestive, though not diagnostic of a mitochondrial fatty acid β-oxidation defect (see Chapter 3).

Inherited disturbances of fatty acid oxidation, such as systemic carnitine deficiency and MCAD deficiency, often present as acute or recurrent Reye-like syndrome: vomiting, lethargy, drowsiness, stupor, seizures, hepatomegaly, hypoglycemia, and hyperammonemia. These patients are particularly important to recognize because treatment is simple and effective. Moreover, since the metabolic

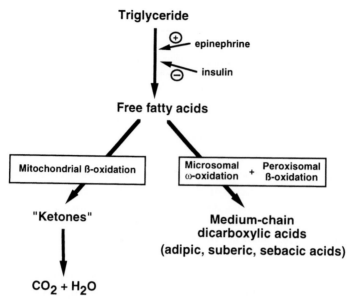

Figure 4.5   Overview of fatty acid metabolism.

defects are hereditary, the siblings of affected children are at high risk for being similarly affected.

The diagnosis of fatty acid oxidation defects can usually be confirmed by demonstrating the presence of high concentrations of C-6 to C-10 dicarboxylic acids (adipic, suberic, and sebacic acids) in the urine, the presence of characteristic acylcarnitines in plasma, and the present of depressed free carnitine concentrations in plasma during acute metabolic decompensation. Since the organic acid abnormalities often disappear when the child is apparently healthy, diagnosis may be difficult if urine and blood samples are not saved from the time when the patient was acutely ill.

Hypoglycemia is a prominent secondary metabolic phenomenon in all mitochondrial fatty acid β-oxidation defects. However, each of the disorders is also associated with other problems arising from primary and secondary effects of the respective enzyme or transport deficiencies (Table 4.3). These are described in other chapters dealing with the most prominent clinical aspects of various defects, such as acute encephalopathy, chronic myopathy, or cardiomyopathy.

What was once called "leucine-sensitive hypoglycemia" has recently been shown in many infants to be a condition caused by mutations of the glutamate dehydrogenase gene (*GLUD1*) resulting in relative insensitivity of the enzyme to normal inhibition by GTP. Infants with this condition usually present in the first year of life with a history of recurrent hypoketotic hypoglycemia, elevated plasma insulin levels, and persistent hyperammonemia. Affected children generally show unexpected

Table 4.3 Relationship between metabolic defects and clinical manifestations of mitochondrial fatty acid β-oxidation defects

Pathophysiology	Clinical effects
Accumulation of intermediates of fatty acid oxidation (substrate accumulation)	Organic aciduria, acute encephalopathy, hepatocellular dysfunction, cardiac arrhythmias.
Inability to meet the energy needs of tissues that are highly dependent on fatty acid oxidation for energy (deficiency of product)	Skeletal myopathy, cardiomyopathy
Requirement for tissues to draw on glucose oxidation to meet energy needs (secondary metabolic abnormalities)	Hypoglycemia
Secondary carnitine depletion (resulting from accumulation and excretion of acylcarnitines)	Hypoglycemia, hyperammonemia, myopathy, cardiomyopathy

tolerance of fasting. By contrast, ingestion of high-protein foods often precipitates hypoglycemic attacks. Plasma ammonium levels correlate poorly with dietary protein intake, often remaining elevated despite aggressive dietary protein restriction and high carbohydrate intake. Affected infants and children often respond well to treatment with diazoxide.

Hepatocellular dysfunction

Inherited metabolic diseases presenting as acute hepatocellular dysfunction present a particularly challenging diagnostic problem. The resemblance of some of them to acquired disorders, particularly viral infections and intoxications, is so close that discrimination on clinical grounds alone is next to impossible. Furthermore, hepatocellular dysfunction, regardless of the underlying cause, is associated with secondary metabolic abnormalities that are often difficult to distinguish from the abnormalities observed in primary metabolic disorders. For example, increased concentrations of tyrosine in plasma are a common nonspecific metabolic manifestation of severe liver disease. Hypertyrosinemia is also typical of hepatorenal tyrosinemia. To make matters even more confusing, hepatorenal tyrosinemia commonly presents in early infancy as severe liver failure.

One way to approach this category of inborn errors of metabolism is to organize them according to age of onset. Inherited metabolic diseases characterized by severe liver disease may present in early infancy, later in childhood, or in adulthood (Table 4.4).

The presentation of inherited metabolic diseases with onset in the newborn period or early infancy as acute hepatocellular disease is characterized in most

Table 4.4 Inherited metabolic diseases presenting as severe hepatocellular dysfunction organized according to age of onset

Disease	Defect	Distinguishing features
Onset in the first few months of life		
Galactosemia	GALT	Severe hyperbilirubinemia; hemolytic anemia; coagulopathy
Hepatorenal tyrosinemia	Fumarylacetoacetate hydrolase	Prominent coagulopathy; extreme elevation of AFP; succinylacetone in urine
LCHAD deficiency	Trifunctional protein (LCHAD)	'Hepatitis'; cardiomyopathy; dicarboxylic aciduria
α_1-antitrypsin deficiency	α_1-antitrypsin	Jaundice; failure to thrive; portal hypertension; GI hemorrhages
HFI	Aldolase B	Lactic acidosis; hypoglycemia; hyperuricemia
GSD, type IV	Glycogen brancher enzyme	Early, severe cirrhosis; myopathy
Wolman disease	Acid lipase	Severe failure to thrive; steatorrhea; calcification of adrenals
Disorders of bile acid metabolism	Various disturbances of bile acid synthesis	"Neonatal hepatitis"
Mitochondrial DNA depletion syndrome	mtDNA depletion caused by deoxyguanosine kinase deficiency	Severe hepatocellular dysfunction, myopathy, lactic acidosis
CDG syndrome	Various defects in glycoprotein biosynthesis	Failure to thrive, chronic vomiting and diarrhea, ±seizures, ±psychomotor retardation (see Chapter 6)
Onset later in infancy or early childhood		
GSD, type III	Glycogen debrancher enzyme	Skeletal myopathy
Gaucher disease, type III	Glucocerebrosidase	Massive hepatosplenomegaly; storage cells in marrow (see Fig 8.5).
Niemann-Pick disease, type C	Intracellular cholesterol trafficking	Neurodegenerative disease; storage cells in marrow; hepatosplenomegaly
CPT I deficiency	CPT I	Hypoketotic hypoglycemia; elevated plasma carnitine levels
Onset in adolescence		
Wilson disease	Copper transporter ATPase	Acute 'hepatitis'; hemolysis; neuropsychiatric disturbances
CESD	Acid lipase	Hepatosplenomegaly; hypercholesterolemia
Adult onset		
Niemann-Pick disease, type B	Acid sphingomyelinase	Hepatosplenomegaly; storage cells in marrow; pulmonary infiltrates

Abbreviations: AFP, alpha-fetoprotein; HFI, hereditary fructose intolerance; CDG, congenital disorders of glycosylation; CPT, carnitine palmitoyltransferase; CESD, cholesterol ester storage disease; GALT, galactose-1-phosphate uridyltransferase; GSD, glycogen storage disease; LCHAD, long-chain 3-hydroxyacyl-CoA dehydrogenase.

cases by some combination of failure to thrive, mild to severe hyperbilirubinemia, hypoglycemia, hyperammonemia, elevated aminotransferases, bleeding diathesis, edema, and ascites. Classical galactosemia is the prototypic example, and it is discussed in detail in Chapter 7.

Persistent jaundice with marked conjugated hyperbilirubinemia, elevated aminotransferases hepatosplenomegaly, and failure to thrive, dating from the first few weeks of life, is often the first indication of hepatic disease due to α_1-antitrypsin deficiency. Cholestasis may be severe enough to cause acholic stools resembling those seen in infants with extrahepatic biliary atresia. Infants with α_1-antitrypsin deficiency may be virtually asymptomatic until they present at a few months of age with cirrhosis, with portal hypertension, abdominal distension, ascites, marked enlargement of the liver and spleen, and upper gastrointestinal hemorrhage from esophageal varices. Despite the apparently aggressive nature of the disease, survival for many years with severe liver disease is not unusual. Liver biopsy shows typical PAS-positive, diastase-resistant inclusions within the endoplasmic reticulum of hepatocytes. Conventional electrophoresis of plasma proteins on cellulose acetate usually shows absence or marked deficiency of the alpha-1 protein peak. The diagnosis is confirmed by demonstrating the characteristic PI type ZZ phenotype on PI typing of plasma α_1-antitrypsin by isoelectric focusing or agarose gel electrophoresis of plasma proteins. Alternatively, the diagnosis can be confirmed by demonstrating homozygosity for the *PI**Z allele by PCR amplification of genomic DNA from peripheral blood.

Infants with hepatorenal tyrosinemia may present early in infancy with acute hepatic failure progressing rapidly to death (see Chapter 7). More often, they present at a few months of age with a history of failure to thrive, with intermittent episodes of marked anorexia, irritability, and drowsiness generally associated with intercurrent illness. As a rule, they show only mild hyperbilirubinemia. The liver may not be particularly large, but it is usually hard and irregular to palpation, an indication of the extent of the fibrosis occurring early in the disease. Some ascites is common at presentation. Hypotonia and depressed deep tendon reflexes are an indication of peripheral neuropathy.

Affected infants usually show moderate to severe anemia and thrombocytopenia. Hypoglycemia is common, but plasma ammonium levels are usually not severely elevated. The aminotransferases may be only moderately elevated, but the coagulopathy is characteristically severe and typically associated with dysfibrinogenemia (reptilase time greater than the thrombin time). The renal tubular acidosis is more severe than that seen in infants with galactosemia. It is often associated with phosphate losses sufficient to cause rickets. Plasma amino acid analysis typically shows increased levels of tyrosine, methionine, and phenylalanine. However, the levels may not be much higher than those seen in patients with other types of severe hepatocellular disease; they are often not particularly helpful in making the diagnosis of tyrosinemia. But plasma α-fetoprotein (AFP) levels are characteristically extremely high. In fact, there are only a few situations in which comparable AFP levels are seen: hepatoblastoma, neonatal hemochromatosis, and resolving viral hepatitis are the main ones. Urinary organic acid analysis usually, though not always, shows the presence of succinylacetone, derived from fumarylacetoacetate accumulating proximal to the enzyme defect. If a diagnosis of hepatorenal tyrosinemia is strongly suspected, urinary organic acid analysis, including analysis of oxime derivatives (see Chapter 9), should be repeated at least three to four times. Definitive diagnosis is made by measuring fumarylacetoacetate hydrolase (FAH) activity in leukocytes, erythrocytes, fibroblasts, or liver tissue obtained by biopsy. Treatment with dietary tyrosine restriction often produces prompt clinical and metabolic improvement. However, plasma methionine levels often rise to levels exceeding 1 mmol/L during the early phases of treatment. The treatment of this condition has been revolutionized by the introduction of NTBC, an inhibitor of p-hydroxyphenylpyruvic acid dioxygenase (see Chapter 10).

Early-onset cirrhosis is also a prominent feature of glycogen storage disease, type IV (GSD IV). However, unlike α_1-antitrypsin deficiency, many patients also show evidence of neuromuscular involvement with hypotonia, weakness, muscle wasting and depressed deep tendon reflexes. In fact, the disease in patients presenting later in life with milder variants of the condition is characterized by progressive skeletal myopathy, sometimes involving the myocardium (see Chapter 5). The course of typical early–onset disease is usually very aggressive, and survival beyond a few months is uncommon. Liver biopsy typically shows advanced cirrhosis and the presence in hepatocytes of characteristic inclusions comprised of abnormal glycogen. The diagnosis is confirmed by measurement of glycogen brancher enzyme activity in leukocytes, fibroblasts, or tissue.

Some children with the subacute neuronopathic variant of Gaucher disease (type 3) present in the first few years of life with massive hepatosplenomegaly and early evidence of chronic hepatic failure. In addition to massive enlargement of the liver and spleen, affected children show marked failure to thrive, protuberance of the abdomen, anemia, edema, ascites, and a bleeding diathesis out of proportion to the thrombocytopenia caused by hypersplenism. Death often occurs within a few years, before the underlying neuronopathic nature of the disease becomes obvious. Bone marrow aspirates show the presence of typical storage cells (see Chapter 6). The diagnosis is confirmed by demonstrating deficiency of β-glucosidase in leukocytes or fibroblasts.

Severe failure to thrive, associated with chronic diarrhea, massive hepatomegaly, marked hypotonia, and developmental delay, with onset in the 1–3 months of life is characteristic of Wolman disease. Calcification of the adrenal glands, usually visible on plain radiographs of the abdomen or by ultrasound examination, is virtually pathognomonic of the disease in young infants with this clinical appearance. The plasma cholesterol concentration is elevated. The diagnosis is confirmed by demonstration of profound acid lipase deficiency in cultured skin fibroblasts. This disease is invariably fatal within a few months.

Chronic diarrhea, with marked failure to thrive, hepatomegaly, hepatocellular dysfunction, coagulopathy and hypoalbuminemia, is also characteristic of some infants with hereditary fructose intolerance (HFI). Infants with HFI may be clinically indistinguishable from infants with congenital disorders of glycosylation (CDG), type Ib, caused by deficiency of the enzyme, phosphomannose isomerase (PMI). Distinguishing between the two diseases is made difficult by the observation that the isoelectric focusing pattern of plasma transferrin in many infants with HFI is indistinguishable from that seen in patients with CDG Ib. The abnormality in HFI is reversed, generally within a few weeks, with treatment by dietary fructose restriction.

Another condition that is often clinically indistinguishable, at least initially, from Wolman disease is early-onset mitochondrial DNA depletion syndrome. This autosomal recessive disorder is characterized by hepatomegaly, severe generalized weakness and hypotonia, persistent, often severe, lactic acidosis, encephalopathy, and variable renal tubular dysfunction. Hypoglycemia is not usually severe or difficult to treat. The age of onset and course of the disease are highly variable. The diagnosis is supported by muscle biopsy and histochemical staining for cytochrome *c* oxidase (COX), which typically shows marked predominance of COX-negative muscle fibers. The disease is caused by deficiency of deoxyguanosine kinase (dGK). The enzyme defect is not expressed in cultured skin fibroblasts; confirmation of the diagnosis requires measurement of enzyme activity in muscle or liver, or the demonstration of mutations in the *DGUOK* gene. The disease is invariably fatal, though survival into middle childhood may occur in patients with milder variants of the disease.

Onset of clinically significant liver disease before age five years in patients with Wilson disease is unusual, though not unknown. Patients with this condition may present with hepatic syndrome, neurologic syndrome, or severe intravascular hemolysis. Some patients present with acute hepatitis, with jaundice, anorexia, general malaise, pale stools, and dark urine. The symptoms and routine laboratory findings are indistinguishable from those of acute viral hepatitis. Recovery is the rule, and the underlying defect often goes undetected at this stage. The absence of serologic evidence of viral infection, along with the presence of mild hemolytic anemia, should alert the clinician to the possibility of the disease.

Some patients, usually adolescents, present with an acute icteric hepatitis progressing over a period of several days to weeks to frank liver failure, with severe

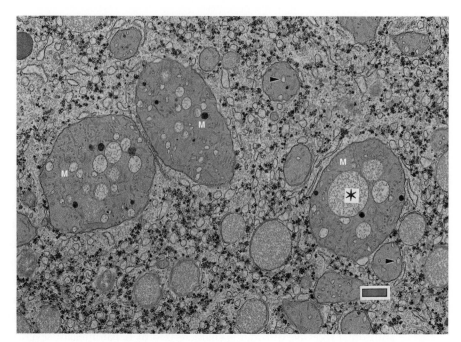

Figure 4.6   Electron micrograph of liver in Wilson disease.
Greatly enlarged mitochondria (M) containing microcystic inclusions (*) and smaller dilated cristae in normal sized mitochondria (arrowheads) are shown. The latter is the most constant abnormality seen in liver of patients with Wilson disease. The bar represents 1 mm. (Courtesy of Dr. M. J. Phillips.)

jaundice, hepatic coma, severe coagulopathy, ascites, renal failure, and death. The course of the illness and age of the patient often raises questions about severe viral hepatitis or intoxication. However, the presence of severe non-immune hemolytic anemia, caused by sudden release of copper from dying liver cells, is typical of this fulminant form of Wilson disease.

Presentation as 'chronic active hepatitis' may occur among adolescents and young adults with Wilson disease, with fatiguability, general malaise, anorexia, and hyper-bilirubinemia, and tender enlargement of the liver. Sometimes the disease presents insidiously, with signs of slowly progressive cirrhosis, including edema, gyneco-mastia, ascites, clubbing, or spider nevi. Some patients may have pathognomonic Kayser-Fleischer rings in the corneas. Laboratory studies show elevated aminotrans-ferases and γ-globulin, decreased plasma albumin, and prolonged prothrombin time. Liver biopsy shows abnormalities typical of chronic active hepatitis, in addi-tion to steatosis and periportal glycogenated nuclei, which are more suggestive of Wilson disease. Ultrastructural studies typically show mitochondrial abnormalities characteristic of the disease (Figure 4.6).

Presentation of Wilson disease as a neuropsychiatric disorder is common, par-ticularly among older adolescents and young adults. The clinical aspects of this

Table 4.5 Investigation of liver function

Tests of cholestasis	*Investigation of inborn errors of metabolism*
Bilirubin, conjugated and unconjugated	Copper and ceruloplasmin
Alkaline phosphatase (ALP)	α-Fetoprotein
γ-Glutamyltranspeptidase (GGT)	α_1-Antitrypsin (PI phenotyping)
Bile acids	Plasma amino acids
	Urinary organic acids
Tests of active liver cell damage	Red cell GALT activity
Aspartate aminotransferase (AST)	Various lysosomal enzyme assays
Alanine aminotransferases (ALT)	
Tests of synthetic functions	
Albumin	
PT and PTT	
Coagulation factors VII, V	
Ammonium	

Abbreviations: PT, prothrombin time; PTT, partial thromboplastin time; GALT, galactose-1-phosphate uridyltransferase.

presentation are discussed in Chapter 2. Most patients with neurologic Wilson disease also show some evidence of hepatic dysfunction.

Confirmation of the diagnosis may be difficult. In Wilson disease, plasma copper and ceruloplasmin levels are usually low. However, copper levels may be normal or elevated in patients with fulminant liver failure, and ceruloplasmin levels often overlap with those of patients with other types of liver disease. Urinary copper excretion is usually increased in Wilson disease, especially after administration of penicillamine. This is the basis of a diagnostic procedure widely used when the results of other studies are ambiguous. Diagnosis is also facilitated by the identification of disease-associated mutations in the *ATP7B* gene.

Investigation

Liver function tests

Initial investigation might include a selection of studies to assess cholestasis, active liver cell damage, synthetic functions of the liver, and some selected studies that might be indicated by the nature of the hepatic presentation (Table 4.5).

Fasting tests

Carefully monitored fasting is one of the few provocative tests still widely used to screen for defects in carbohydrate or fat metabolism. It is undertaken to evaluate the integrity of glycogenolysis, gluconeogenesis, and fatty acid oxidation in the adaptation to starvation.

Any provocative testing should be conducted very carefully to avoid acute metabolic decompensation, which might have disastrous results. Fasting as a provocative procedure should only be undertaken under controlled and closely monitored circumstances. Testing should be done when the patient is free of inter-current illness.

In the investigation of severe hypoglycemia, or hypoglycemia occurring after only a few hours of fasting, such as is characteristic of GSD I, the entire procedure can generally be completed in a few hours. After any feeding of the day, a secure intravenous is established with 0.9% NaCl infusing at a slow rate to maintain the line. The blood glucose is monitored periodically with the use of bedside test trips or glucometer until it drops to 2 mmol/L, until the child becomes symptomatic (usually with irritability, restlessness, sweating, or drowsiness), or until four to six hours have elapsed, depending on the age of the patient. At the termination of the fast, a sample of blood is obtained for measurement of blood glucose, lactate, free fatty acids, 3-hydroxybutyrate, acetoacetate, insulin, and growth hormone. Glucagon (1 mg) is then administered intramuscularly, and blood samples are obtained at 10, 20, and 30 minutes for analysis of glucose and lactate. In the event the child becomes severely symptomatic or refuses oral feedings at the end of the test, a bolus of glucose solution (500 mg/kg) should be administered intravenously and followed by a continuous glucose infusion.

In the absence of a clear history of hypoglycemia, or if the history indicates the child is able to tolerate at least several hours of starvation, fasting is begun from the evening feeding the day before: at 2200 hours in children <18 months and at 1800 hours in patients >18 months of age. The blood glucose should be monitored periodically at the bedside during the night. At 0800 hours, an intravenous of 0.9% NaCl is established and baseline analyses done of plasma glucose, lactate, free fatty acids, 3-hydroxybutyrate, acetoacetate, ammonium, and free and total carnitine. After the patient has voided for the first time in the morning, all urine passed during the rest of the period of fasting is collected for urinary ketone and organic acid analysis. Blood glucose levels are monitored by bedside testing at hourly intervals. When the blood glucose falls to 2 mmol/L, the child becomes symptomatic, or after a total of 16 hours of fasting in children <18 months and 22 hours in children >18 months of age, which ever comes first, blood is obtained for repeat analysis of the baseline studies.

Provocative fasting as a test for defects in fatty acid oxidation has been abandoned by many centers because it is potentially dangerous. Alternative testing procedures include carnitine or phenylpropionate loading coupled with analysis of acylcar-nitines or phenylpropionate, respectively, in urine. Loading in this situation is done only to ensure that the patient has adequate stores of carnitine, or is produc-ing sufficient amounts of phenylpropionate in the gut, to produce the characteristic abnormalities in urine. Investigation of this group of disorders has been facilitated enormously by the introduction of tandem MSMS analysis of plasma acylcarnitines. The analysis can be done on a few drops of blood soaked into a piece of filter paper, dried, and mailed to laboratories with the appropriate equipment and expertise.

SUGGESTED READING

Bonnefont, J. P., Specola, N. B., Vassault, A., *et al.* (1990). The fasting test in pediatrics: application to the diagnosis of pathological hypo- and hyperketotic states. *European Journal of Pediatrics,* **150**, 80–5.

Clayton, P. T. (2002). Inborn errors presenting with liver dysfunction. *Seminars in Neonatology,* **7**, 49–63.

Cornblath, M. & Ichord, R. (2000). Hypoglycemia in the neonate. *Seminars in Perinatology,* **24**, 136–49.

Elpeleg, O. N. (1999). The molecular background of glycogen metabolism disorders. *Journal of Pediatric Endocrinology & Metabolism,* **12**, 363–79.

Guzmán, M. & Geelen, M. J. H. (1993). Regulation of fatty acid oxidation in mammalian liver. *Biochimica et Biophysica Acta,* **1167**, 227–41.

Holme, E. & Lindstedt, S. (1995). Diagnosis and management of tyrosinemia type I. *Current Opinions in Pediatrics,* **7**, 726–32.

Ibdah, J. A., Bennett, M. J., Rinaldo, P., *et al.* (1999). A fetal fatty-acid oxidation disorder as a cause of liver disease in pregnant women. *New England Journal of Medicine,* **340**, 1723–31.

Ibdah, J. A., Yang, Z. & Bennett, M. J. (2000). Liver disease in pregnancy and fetal fatty acid oxidation defects. *Molecular Genetics and Metabolism,* **71**, 182–9.

Jevon, G. P. & Dimmick, J. E. (1998). Histopathologic approach to metabolic liver disease: Part 1. *Pediatric and Developmental Pathology,* **1**, 179–99.

Lteif, A. N. & Schwenk, W. F. (1999). Hypoglycemia in infants and children. *Endocrinology and Metabolism Clinics of North America,* **28**, 619–46.

Morris, A. A., Taanman, J. W., Blake, J., *et al.* (1998). Liver failure associated with mitochondrial DNA depletion. *Journal of Hepatology,* **28**, 556–63.

Ozand, P. T. (2000). Hypoglycemia in association with various organic and amino acid disorders. *Seminars in Perinatology,* **24**, 172–93.

Pollitt, R. J. (1995). Disorders of mitochondrial long-chain fatty acid oxidation. *Journal of Inherited Metabolic Diseases,* **18**, 473–90.

Pons, R. & De Vivo, D. C. (1995). Primary and secondary carnitine deficiency syndromes. *Journal of Child Neurology,* **10** (Suppl. 2), 208–24.

Rinaldo, P., Yoon, H. R., Yu, C., Raymond, K., Tiozzo, C. & Giordano G. (1999). Sudden and unexpected neonatal death: a protocol for the postmortem diagnosis of fatty acid oxidation disorders. *Seminars in Perinatology,* **23**, 204–10.

Saudubray, J. M., Martin, D., de Lonlay, P., *et al.* (1999). Recognition and management of fatty acid oxidation defects: a series of 107 patients. *Journal of Inherited Metabolic Diseases,* **22**, 488–502.

Suchy, J. F. (ed.) (1994). *Liver Disease in Children.* St. Louis: Mosby-Year Book, Inc.

Talente, G. M., Coleman, R. A., Alter, S., *et al.* (1994). Glycogen storage disease in adults. *Annals of Internal Medicine,* **120**, 218–26.

Treem, W. R. (2000). New developments in the pathophysiology, clinical spectrum, and diagnosis of disorders of fatty acid oxidation. *Current Opinions in Pediatrics,* **12**, 463–8.

Wanders, R. J., Vreken, P., den Boer, M. E., Wijburg, F. A., van Gennip, A. H. & Ijlst, L. (1999). Disorders of mitochondrial fatty acyl-CoA beta-oxidation. *Journal of Inherited Metabolic Diseases,* **22**, 442–87.

5

Cardiac syndromes

Until recently, the contribution of inherited metabolic diseases to conditions presenting primarily with symptoms of cardiac disease would have been considered to be small, and devoting an entire chapter of a clinical text like this to them would have been considered unusual. However, over the past 15 years, presentation as serious cardiac disease has become associated in particular with two types of inherited metabolic disorders, inborn errors of fatty acid oxidation and mitochondrial electron transport chain (ETC) defects. Clinically significant cardiac involvement is also now recognized to be a serious complication, if not the present problem, in patients with some inherited metabolic diseases in which it was previously unknown, rare, or trivial.

Cardiomyopathy

Many of the inherited metabolic disorders in which cardiac disease is particularly prominent present as cardiomyopathy (Table 5.1). The clinical characteristics of the cardiomyopathy itself are often not much help in determining whether it is the result of an inborn error of metabolism or some nonmetabolic condition, such as infection or intoxication. Moreover, even among the inherited metabolic diseases, the clinical characteristics of the cardiac involvement are usually not characteristic enough to suggest a specific diagnosis without further investigation.

In most inherited metabolic diseases presenting with cardiomyopathy, echocardiography shows some thickening of the left ventricular wall. However, in some, notably in patients with systemic carnitine deficiency, the marked enlargement of the heart seen on radiographs of the chest is principally the result of dilatation. Cardiac enlargement and dilatation is commonly accompanied by arrhythmias. Severe, intractable disturbances of cardiac rhythm, such as ventricular tachycardia, are particularly prominent in some of the fatty acid oxidation disorders, especially in carnitine-acylcarnitine translocase deficiency. Valvular abnormalities, such as

Table 5.1 Inherited metabolic diseases in which cardiomyopathy is prominent

Disease	Other clinical features
Disorders of glycogen metabolism and glycolysis	
Pompe disease (GSD II)*	Profound skeletal myopathy presenting in early infancy; early death
GSD III (debrancher enzyme deficiency)	Hepatomegaly, variable hypoglycemia, mild hepatocellular dysfunction
GSD IV (brancher enzyme deficiency)*	Hepatic involvement may initially be mild in variants with major cardiac involvement
Phosphorylase *b* kinase deficiency*	Cardiomyopathy many be the only problem
Triosephosphate isomerase deficiency	Chronic hemolytic anemia, progressive dystonia, spasticity; early death
Disorders of fatty acid metabolism	
Systemic carnitine deficiency*	Skeletal myopathy, acute encephalopathy, hypoketotic hypoglycemia, hepatocellular dysfunction, hepatomegaly, hypotonia
LCAD deficiency*	Skeletal myopathy, exercise intolerance with myoglobinuria, acute encephalopathy, hypoketotic hypoglycemia, hepatocellular dysfunction, hepatomegaly, hypotonia
VLCAD deficiency*	Skeletal myopathy, acute encephalopathy, hypoketotic hypoglycemia, hyperammonemia, hepatomegaly, hypotonia, exercise intolerance with myoglobinuria
LCHAD* or trifunctional protein deficiency*	Skeletal myopathy, hepatocellular dysfunction, peripheral neuropathy, retinitis pigmentosa
Short-chain L-3-hydroxyacyl-CoA dehydrogenase deficiency	Late-onset skeletal myopathy, exercise- or illness-induced myoglobinuria
Carnitine-acylcarnitine translocase deficiency	Early-onset acute encephalopathy, hypotonia, hyperammonemia, seizures, hepatomegaly and hepatocellular dysfunction, cardiac arrhythmias
Organic acidopathies	
Propionic acidemia*	Intermittent acute metabolic acidosis, ketosis, hyperammonemia, neutropenia
Methylmalonic acidemia	Intermittent acute metabolic acidosis, ketosis, hyperammonemia, neutropenia
HMG-CoA lyase deficiency	Intermittent acute metabolic acidosis, ketosis, hyperammonemia, neutropenia
Mitochondrial acetoacetyl-CoA thiolase (β-ketothiolase) deficiency	Intermittent acute metabolic acidosis, ketosis, hyperammonemia
Glutaric aciduria type II (multiple acyl-CoA dehydrogenase deficiency)	Facial dysmorphism, congenital malformations, hypotonia, hepatomegaly, hypoketotic hypoglycemia, metabolic acidosis, hyperammonemia
Amino acidopathies	
Hepatorenal tyrosinemia	Acute hepatocellular dysfunction, hypoglycemia, renal tubular acidosis, porphyria
Alkaptonuria†	Dark urine, calcification of cartilage, arthritis
Homocystinuria†	Marfanoid habitus, psychomotor retardation, dislocation of lens, thromboembolic phenomena

Mitochondrial cardiomyopathies

Kearns-Sayre syndrome*	PEO, retinal degeneration, cerebellar ataxia, growth failure, sensorineural hearing impairment, heart block
Lethal infantile cardiomyopathy*	Cardiac dysrhythmias (e.g., WPW syndrome); early death
Leigh disease (subacute necrotizing encephalomyelopathy)	Psychomotor retardation, hypotonia, failure to thrive, breathing abnormalities, oculomotor disturbances, seizures, lactic acidosis (see Chapter 2)
Hypertrophic cardiomyopathy and myopathy*	Skeletal myopathy, diabetes mellitus, cataracts, cardiac dysrhythmia (e.g., WPW syndrome)
Barth syndrome*	Skeletal myopathy, chronic neutropenia, 3-methylglutaconic aciduria
Benign infantile mitochondrial myopathy and cardiomyopathy	Weakness, hypotonia, respiratory failure, severe lactic acidosis, cardiomyopathy, variable course
MELAS	Psychomotor retardation, growth failure, seizures, stroke-like episodes, lactic acidosis (see Chapter 2)
MERRF	Cerebellar ataxia, skeletal myopathy, psychomotor retardation, myoclonus, seizures

Glycosphingolipidoses, mucopolysaccharidoses, and glycoproteinoses

Fabry disease*	Chronic and recurrent neuritic pain in hands and feet, peculiar skin lesions (angiokeratomata), corneal opacities, progressive renal failure, cardiac dysrhythmias, premature cerebrovascular disease
Hurler disease (MPS IH)*	Facial dysmorphism, hepatosplenomegaly, dysostosis multiplex, progressive psychomotor retardation, corneal clouding, MPSuria (see Chapter 6)
Hunter disease (MPS II)	Facial dysmorphism, hepatosplenomegaly, dysostosis multiplex, progressive psychomotor retardation, MPSuria (see Chapter 6)
Maroteaux-Lamy disease (MPS VI)	Short stature, dysostosis multiplex, corneal clouding, normal intelligence, MPSuria
GM1 gangliosidosis*	Facial dysmorphism, hepatosplenomegaly, ± dysostosis multiplex, oligosacchariduria
GM2 gangliosidosis	Chronic progressive encephalopathy, seizures, cherry-red spots in retina, blindness
Gaucher disease	Hepatosplenomegaly, anemia, thrombocytopenia, bone crises (see Chapter 6)
Niemann-Pick disease	Hepatosplenomegaly, chronic progressive encephalopathy
I-cell disease	Hurler-like appearance, hepatosplenomegaly, dysostosis multiplex
Juvenile neuronal ceroid-lipofuscinosis	Psychomotor regression, seizures, progressive visual impairment (see Chapter 2)
CDG syndrome	Psychomotor retardation, inverted nipples, abnormal subcutaneous fat pads (disappear with age), strabismus, ataxia with cerebellar atrophy, joint contractures, hyporeflexia

Abbreviations: MPS, mucopolysaccharidosis; MPSuria, mucopolysacchariduria; GSD, glycogen storage disease; LCAD, long-chain acyl-CoA dehydrogenase; LCHAD, VLCAD, very-long-chain acyl-CoA dehydrogenase; long-chain 3-hydroxyacyl-CoA dehydrogenase; HMG-CoA, 3-hydroxy-3-methylglutaryl-CoA; WPW, Wolff-Parkinson-White; MELAS, mitochondrial encephalomyopathy, lactic acidosis, and stroke-like episodes; MERRF, myoclonic epilepsy and ragged-red fiber disease; CDG, congenital disorders of glycosylation.

* Cardiomyopathy may be dominant or only clinical problem.

† Cardiomyopathy probably the result of chronic ischemic heart disease.

mitral insufficiency and mitral valve prolapse, are also common consequences of cardiomyopathy, regardless of the underlying cause.

From the standpoint of making a specific clinical diagnosis of inherited metabolic cardiomyopathy, regardless of the underlying defect, the most important features of the various conditions in which it occurs are the associated non-cardiac findings. The myocardium is muscle, and most inherited metabolic conditions affecting cardiocytes also affect skeletal muscle, at least to some extent. The presence of clinically significant myopathy is, therefore, an important clue to the metabolic nature of the underlying defect. In some cases, such as glycogen storage disease, type II (GSD II or Pompe disease), the skeletal myopathy is profound; in others, like long-chain 3-hydroxyacyl-CoA dehydrogenase (LCHAD) deficiency, it may be relatively subtle and difficult to differentiate from nonspecific weakness and hypotonia owing to the severity of the heart disease. Skeletal muscle biopsy is often helpful, if not diagnostic, in many of these disorders, particularly the mitochondrial myopathies (see Chapter 2).

The presence of hepatomegaly may be a clue to a systemic defect in glycogen or fatty acid metabolism (see Chapter 4), bearing in mind that enlargement of the liver, often with some evidence of hepatocellular dysfunction, is a prominent nonspecific sign of heart failure in young infants. Marked hepatomegaly without evidence of severe hepatocellular dysfunction is a characteristic of all the hepatic glycogen storage diseases, except GSD IV (brancher enzyme deficiency) in which cirrhosis generally occurs early and clinically significant cardiomyopathy is relatively rare. It is of some interest, particularly in the light of the discovery of patients with late-onset disease apparently limited to the heart, that children with GSD IV without apparent heart involvement may develop fatal dilated cardiomyopathy some years after the hepatic disease is cured by liver transplantation. Cardiomyopathy is a relatively common, though rarely clinically significant, problem in patients with GSD III (debrancher enzyme deficiency).

The presence of severe hepatocellular dysfunction is a classic characteristic of fatty acid oxidation defects (FAOD), including many patients with systemic carnitine deficiency, at least during metabolic decompensation (see Chapter 4). In fact, patients with systemic carnitine deficiency, long-chain acyl-CoA dehydrogenase (LCAD) or LCHAD deficiency are about equally split between those presenting as a hepatic syndrome and those presenting as cardiomyopathy. Interestingly, cardiomyopathy does not occur in patients with medium-chain acyl-CoA dehydrogenase (MCAD) deficiency. As a rule, among patients with other fatty acid oxidation defects, the older the patient, the more likely they are to present with cardiomyopathy. However, even in these, evidence of hepatocellular dysfunction is generally obvious. This includes enlargement of the liver, elevated transaminases, and decreased plasma carnitine levels with increased ratio of esterified to free carnitine. In LCAD deficiency, LCHAD deficiency and trifunctional protein deficiency, urinary organic acid analyses done when the patient acutely ill show the presence of medium- and long-chain dicarboxylic acids and, in LCHAD deficiency, long-chain (C12 and C14) 3-hydroxy monocarboxylic and dicarboxylic acids (see Chapter 3). The organic acid abnormalities are characteristically evanescent and may not be present by the time urine is collected for analysis. Analysis of plasma acyl-carnitine profiles, by tandem mass spectrometry, are usually abnormal, even when the patient is clinically well, and the pattern of abnormalities is often diagnostic of the specific defect. Confirmation of the diagnosis may require the demonstration of a defect in fatty acid oxidation in fibroblasts, coupled with the identification of the presence of disease-associated mutations in the relevant gene. In patients with cardiomyopathy associated with multiple acyl-CoA dehydrogenase deficiency (glutaric aciduria type II; GA II), hepatocellular dysfunction, skeletal myopathy, and metabolic acidosis are generally more prominent than the cardiac involvement. However, occasionally, cardiomyopathy develops as an early and fatal complication.

Hepatosplenomegaly is a prominent and diagnostically important associated finding in patients with cardiomyopathies occurring in mucopolysaccharide or other storage conditions. Patients with Hurler disease (MPS IH) may present at three to five months of age in frank congestive heart failure, as a result of infiltration of the myocardium with glycosaminoglycan. Although the liver and spleen are typically palpably enlarged, these signs, along with the characteristic coarse facial appearance and dysostosis multiplex, are subtle at this age, and they may be missed. Severe cardiomyopathy in the other neurovisceral storage diseases, such as Niemann-Pick disease, is rare, and the presence of the associated neurologic and somatic abnormalities is usually obvious. What is important to bear in mind here is that sudden deterioration of a patient with one of these conditions may be the result of cardiomyopathy.

Neurologic abnormalities (including skeletal myopathy) are characteristic of the multisystem involvement that is typical of the mitochondrial myopathies in which cardiomyopathy may dominate the presentation (see Chapter 2). The cardiomyopathy in patients with mitochondrial ETC defects is almost always hypertrophic, and it is often associated with conduction abnormalities and arrhythmias. In some instances, the non-cardiac manifestations of a mitochondrial cytopathy may be insignificant. Because the disorder often affects members of every generation, shows transmission from parents to offspring, and affects both sexes equally, the cardiomyopathy may be concluded to be the result of an autosomal dominant genetic defect. However, a carefully recorded family history in these cases will show that

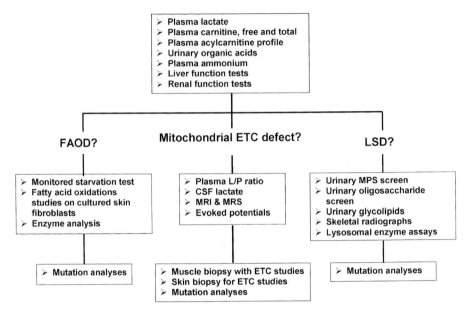

Figure 5.1 Investigation of metabolic cardiomyopathy.

the disorder is transmitted in a matrilineal manner, from mothers to offspring, but never through fathers. This pattern of inheritance is typical of mtDNA mutations (see Chapter 1).

Initial investigation of possible inherited metabolic cardiomyopathy

Because of the clinical overlap in the cardiac manifestations of various inherited metabolic diseases, the initial diagnostic laboratory workup of a patient presenting with cardiomyopathy should include the examination of several possibilities (Figure 5.1).

Endocardial biopsy is sometimes helpful in the differential diagnosis of the cardiomyopathies occurring as a result of inborn errors of metabolism. In addition to the routine assessment of inflammatory changes and a search for viral particles, specimens should be examined by electron microscopy for evidence of submicroscopic mitochondrial lesions. Specific microscopic changes may be subtle and obscured by the presence of secondary pathological changes, such as endocardial fibroelastosis. Three types of microscopic change are particularly helpful in suggesting the presence of an inborn error of metabolism, but they are not invariably present:

Evidence of intralysosomal storage of macromolecules is typical of lysosomal storage diseases, and the histochemical and ultrastructural characteristics of the stored material provide guidance for further, more specific diagnostic investigation. In conditions like GSD II, Fabry disease, and late-onset neuronal ceroid-lipofuscinosis, the histochemical and electron microscopic changes are generally sufficiently typical to suggest the specific diagnosis. In others, like Niemann-Pick disease, the changes are either nonspecific or too dispersed to be reliably identifiable in the small samples of tissue obtainable by this technique.

The presence of significant amounts of microvesicular neutral lipid, demonstrable by Oil Red O or Sudan Black B staining of frozen sections, or by electron microscopy, is characteristic of disorders of fatty acid oxidation, such as systemic carnitine deficiency, LCHAD deficiency, trifunctional protein deficiency, and Barth syndrome. The changes in the myocardium of patients with fatty acid oxidation defects may be subtle. One of our patients with confirmed LCHAD deficiency showed only modest inflammatory change in an endocardial biopsy; there was no evidence of neutral lipid accumulation.

The presence of markedly increased numbers of mitochondria, which are characteristically aggregated immediately under the sarcolemma and are often enlarged and structurally abnormal, is characteristic of the cardiomyopathy associated with mitochondrial ETC defects. In some cases, mitochondrial proliferation is so great that it causes enlargement of muscle fibers, producing the appearance of histiocyte-like cells, sometimes called oncocytic or 'histiocytoid' cardiomyopathy. Abnormal intracellular accumulation of glycogen and neutral fat is also a feature of mitochondrial cardiomyopathies. In other cases, some increase in the number of mitochondria and the accumulation of some glycogen and neutral fat occurs as nonspecific changes with chronic hypoxemia. Marked accumulation of cytosolic glycogen in cardiocytes may be the only clue to the nature of the underlying disease in infants with a particularly virulent variant of phosphorylase *b* kinase deficiency, apparently limited to the heart, presenting in the newborn period with dilated or hypertrophic cardiomyopathy and progressing rapidly to death. Some patients with variants of GSD IV (brancher enzyme deficiency) also present with cardiac glycogenosis with only subtle hepatic involvement.

Glycogen storage disease, type II (GSD II or Pompe disease)

The massive hypertrophic cardiomyopathy of Pompe disease (GSD II) is rarely confused with other causes of cardiomyopathy in infants. Radiographs of the chest typically show massive cardiomegaly (Figure 5.2). The ECG shows huge QRS complexes, marked left-axis deviation, shortening of the PR interval, and T-wave inversion (Figure 5.3). The liver is often palpably enlarged as a result of congestive heart failure, not hepatic glycogen storage. Skeletal muscle involvement is generally obvious (see Chapter 2). The diagnosis is confirmed by demonstrating profound deficiency of α-glucosidase (acid maltase) in leukocytes of fibroblasts. Urinary oligosaccharide

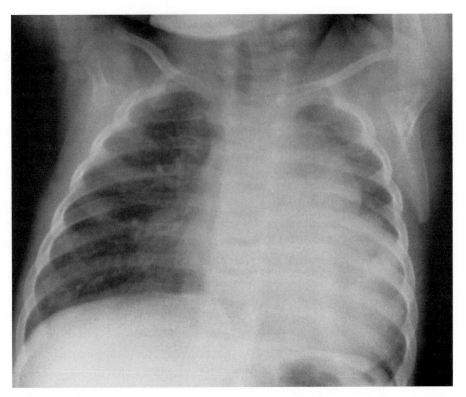

Figure 5.2   Radiograph of the chest in a 3-month-old infant with Pompe disease (GSD II).

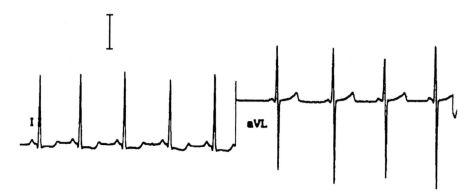

Figure 5.3   ECG of infant with Pompe disease. The bar represents 2μv.

analysis often shows abnormalities, but these are not sufficiently specific to establish the diagnosis. Although the cardiac disease is severe, death is usually the result of respiratory failure because of the skeletal myopathy. The results of preliminary clinical trials indicate that the course of the disease may be dramatically altered by enzyme replacement therapy.

Primary systemic carnitine deficiency

Patients with primary systemic carnitine deficiency coming to attention in the first few months of life often present with hypoketotic hypoglycemia, hyperammonemia, and other evidence of hepatocellular dysfunction (see Chapter 4); the cardiomyopathy may not be particularly prominent, though it is usually present. In contrast, cardiomyopathy is often the primary problem in children presenting with the disease after a year of age. The cardiomyopathy is usually progressive, and it is associated with weakness and hypotonia resulting from skeletal muscle involvement. Plasma carnitine levels are markedly decreased as a result of a generalized defect in carnitine transport. Carnitine levels may be nonspecifically depressed in patients with cardiomyopathy, regardless of the underlying cause. However, in patients with primary systemic carnitine deficiency, plasma levels are generally extremely low ($<10\ \mu mol/L$), and the response to treatment with large doses of oral L-carnitine is usually dramatic, with significant improvement in myocardial function occurring within several days. The diagnosis is confirmed by mutation analysis of the *OCTN2* gene.

In the other FAOD, carnitine depletion is generally secondary to increased excretion as acylcarnitines. The esterified carnitine fraction is increased in plasma. The acylcarnitine pattern, determined by tandem mass spectrometry, is abnormal and usually characteristic of the specific disorder, particularly in the case of FAOD resulting from deficiency of one of the acyl-CoA dehydrogenases

Severe secondary carnitine depletion is also a characteristic feature of many inborn errors of organic acid metabolism (see Chapter 3), some of which may present as cardiomyopathy. Therefore, the investigation of any infant or child presenting in this manner should also include analysis of urinary organic acids. In children with primary systemic carnitine deficiency, the urinary organic acid profile is generally normal.

Fabry disease

Cardiac involvement in patients with Fabry disease is usually associated with diagnostically important noncardiac signs, such as the peculiar skin lesions (Figure 5.4), severe neuritic pain in the hands and feet and proteinuria, which dominate the clinical presentation of the disease. However, in some, the cardiac findings are the only clinically significant manifestations of the disease. Left ventricular hypertrophy and mitral insufficiency, as a result of accumulation of globotriaosylceramide (GL-3) in the myocardium and mitral valve, are common findings in adolescents and young adult males with this X-linked disorder of glycolipid metabolism. Conduction abnormalities (progressive shortening of the PR interval) and arrhythmias (intermittent supraventricular tachycardia) are also common, though rarely severe.

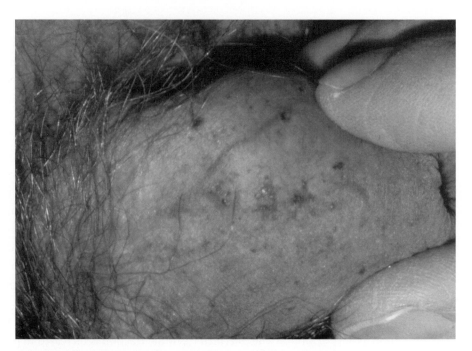

Figure 5.4   Typical angiokeratomata on the penis of a man with Fabry disease.

Mitochondrial cardiomyopathies

Cardiomyopathy is a feature of many of the mitochondrial myopathies discussed in Chapter 2. In some, cardiac involvement is subtle compared with the devastating effect of the disease on the nervous system. However, in others, involvement of the heart is prominent; in some, it may be the only manifestation of disease (Table 5.2).

In those conditions in which it is the only manifestation of disease, the cardiomyopathy is often, though not always, hypertrophic. It may be associated with persistent, mild lactic acidosis, sensorineural hearing loss, diabetes mellitus, or subtle evidence of skeletal myopathy. The family history often includes a number of relatives who have died suddenly of heart failure in early adulthood, and examination of the pedigree shows that the relationship between those affected is consistent with the matrilineal inheritance of mtDNA. In most of the mitochondrial conditions in which cardiomyopathy is the dominant or only manifestation of disease, the onset of heart disease is usually in early adulthood. The course of the disease is often very rapid, culminating in death within weeks or even days. In infants with severe mitochondrial cardiomyopathy, associated severe neurological involvement is common and the course of the disease is typically short.

Even in the absence of clinically apparent skeletal myopathy, skeletal muscle biopsy often shows evidence of mitochondrial proliferation, i.e., ragged-red fibers.

Table 5.2 mtDNA point mutations associated with cardiomyopathy

Mutation	Gene	Clinical features
A3243	tRNA$^{Leu(UUR)}$	MELAS; PEO; diabetes mellitus/deafness; cardiomyopathy
A3260G	tRNA$^{Leu(UUR)}$	Myopathy; cardiomyopathy
C3303T	tRNA$^{Leu(UUR)}$	Cardiomyopathy
A4269G	tRNA^{Ile}	Encephalomyopathy; cardiomyopathy
A4295G	tRNA^{Ile}	Cardiomyopathy
A4300G	tRNA^{Ile}	Cardiomyopathy
C4320T	tRNA^{Ile}	Cardiomyopathy
G8363A	tRNA^{Lys}	MERRF/deafness/cardiomyopathy
T9997C	tRNA^{Gly}	Cardiomyopathy
T8993G	ATPase 6	NARP/MILS; cardiomyopathy
A1555G	12S rRNA	Deafness/aminoglycoside-induced deafness; cardiomyopathy

Abbreviations: MERRF, myoclonus epilepsy and ragged-red fiber disease; MELAS, mitochondrial encephalomyopathy, lactic acidosis, and stroke-like episodes; NARP, neurogenic weakness, ataxia, and retinitis pigmentosa; MILS, maternally inherited Leigh syndrome.
Source: Table is from DiMauro & Hirano (1998).

Biochemical abnormalities can also often be demonstrated in skeletal muscle. Endomyocardial biopsy usually shows structural abnormalities of mitochondria and evidence of mitochondrial proliferation, in addition to accumulation of neutral fat and glycogen. mtDNA mutation analysis is helpful (Table 5.2 and Table 9.14.), though the absence of a mtDNA mutation does not, of course, rule out the possibility that the cardiomyopathy is the result of a defect in mitochondrial energy metabolism.

Some of the general clinical characteristics of various inherited metabolic cardiomyopathies are summarized in Table 5.3. The table shows how identification of non-cardiac manifestations of disease in patients with cardiomyopathy helps to guide diagnostic thinking and relevant laboratory investigation.

Arrhythmias

Arrhythmias are a common, relatively nonspecific complication of the cardiomyopathy in patients with inherited metabolic diseases regardless of the underlying metabolic disorder. Varying degrees of heart block or other conduction defects and associated dysrrhythmias, such as Wolff-Parkinson-White pre-excitation syndrome, occur in a variety of otherwise unrelated inherited metabolic cardiomyopathies. Kearns-Sayre syndrome (a mitochondrial cytopathy), Fabry disease

Table 5.3 Some clinical characteristics of various inherited metabolic cardiomyopathies

	Cardiomyopathy	Nervous system	Liver	Muscle	Kidney	Other
FAOD	Dilated, arrhythmias	±	+++	+–++	0	Hypoketotic hypoglycemia, hyperammonemia
Organic acidopathies	Dilated	±	0	±	0	Marked metabolic acidosis
Mitochondrial ETC defects	Hypertrophic or dilated	+++	0–++	++–+++	0–++ Renal tubular dysfunction	Lactic acidosis
Storage diseases	Hypertrophic	±	Enlarged, but function normal	0–++++	0	Dysostosis multiplex, splenomegaly
CDG syndrome	Dilated or hypertrophic, pericardial effusion	Cerebellar atrophy	+–+++	±	Cystic disease	Facial dysmorphism, lipodystrophy, failure to thrive

Abbreviations: FAOD, fatty acid oxidation defects; ETC, electron transport chain; CDG, congenital disorders of glycosylation.

(a lysosomal storage disease), carnitine-acylcarnitine translocase (CACT) deficiency (a fatty acid oxidation defect), and propionic acidemia (an organic acidopathy), are just a few. However, in some conditions, disturbances of cardiac rhythm are particularly prominent, even fatal. Heart block is particularly common in patients with Kearns-Sayre syndrome, and it may develop before the characteristic non-cardiac features of the disease are recognized.

Intractable tachyarrhythmias, including supraventricular or ventricular tachycardia, are common in young infants with various fatty acid oxidations defects (FAOD), especially with CACT deficiency, carnitine palmitoyltransferase II (CPT-II) deficiency, trifunctional protein deficiency, or very long-chain fatty acyl-CoA dehydrogenase (VLCAD) deficiency. The mechanism of the arrhythmias is unclear, though accumulation of long-chain acylcarnitines has been suggested to contribute to the problem. Treatment with L-carnitine is generally regarded to be an important part of the management of fatty acid oxidation defects. However, in the light of the possible role of acylcarnitine accumulation as a cause of the arrhythmias occurring in these diseases, some have challenged this recommendation, especially in patients with intractable tachyarrhythmias. Despite these fears, the administration of carnitine has not been reported to be overtly toxic in patients with arrhythmias caused by FAOD. In patients who are carnitine depleted, as shown by subnormal plasma carnitine concentrations, carnitine supplementation may actually be important to restore intramitochondrial free coenzyme A concentrations, by exchanging carnitine for the coenzyme A of fatty acyl-CoA esters accumulating as a result of the enzyme defect.

Coronary artery disease

Familial hypercholesterolemia

Premature coronary artery disease is the hallmark of familial hypercholesterolemia (FH). The condition is caused by defects in the uptake and metabolism of circulating cholesterol, the most common being mutations affecting the amount or the properties of the cell surface receptor for plasma low density lipoprotein (LDL). The lipids in plasma are transported in association with specific apoproteins (Table 5.4). LDL uptake occurs by LDL receptor-mediated endocytosis and fusion of the endosome with lysosomes where the cholesterol is de-esterified and the apoprotein is broken down to its constituent amino acids. The unesterified cholesterol exits the lysosome and enters the cytosol where it is used for the synthesis of membranes. It also down-regulates the local production of LDL receptor and the activity of 3-hydroxy-3-methylglutaryl-CoA (HMG-CoA) reductase, the most important enzyme in the regulation of cholesterol biosynthesis. LDL receptor defects cause

Table 5.4 Plasma lipoproteins

Lipoprotein	Apoproteins	Protein (% of dry wt)	Lipids (% of dry wt)			Function
			TG	PL	C+CE	
Chylomicrons	**Apo B-48, C-I, C-II** Apo A-I, A-IV, C-III, E	1	90	5	4	Transport of absorbed triglyceride from gut. Triglyceride is hydrolyzed by endothelium-bound LPL in adipose tissue and muscle; Apo A and Apo C transferred to HDL. Chylomicron remnants taken up by liver.
VLDL	**Apo B-100, C-I, C-II & C-III** Apo A-I, A-II, E	8	55	19	20	Transport of triglyceride synthesized in liver to adipose tissue and muscle; Apo C transferred to HDL. About half the VLDL is converted into LDL in liver.
LDL	**Apo B-100** Apo C-I, C-II, C-III, E	20	5	20	55	Transport of cholesterol from the liver to peripheral tissues.
HDL	**Apo A-I, A-II** Apo C-I, C-II, C-III, E	50	5	27	21	Transport of cholesterol from peripheral tissues to liver.

Abbreviations: VLDL, very low-density lipoproteins; LDL, low-density lipoproteins; HDL, high-density lipoproteins; TG, triglyceride; PL, phospholipid; C+CE, sum of cholesterol and cholesterol ester. Bold type indicates principal apoprotein species.

Source: Data are from Bachorik & Kwiterowich (1991).

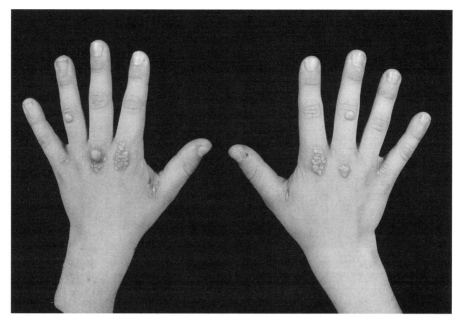

Figure 5.5   Tuberous xanthomas on the hands of a seven-year-old boy with familial hypercholesterolemia.

impaired uptake of the lipoprotein resulting in enhanced intracellular biosynthesis of the lipid, as well as retention of the cholesterol-rich lipoprotein in the circulation. The result is marked increases in the concentration of LDL-cholesterol in plasma and early development of atherosclerosis.

FH is one of the most common mendelian genetic diseases, affecting about one of every 500 individuals in Western countries like the U.S. It is transmitted as an autosomal dominant condition. Heterozygotes generally present in their late twenties or thirties with coronary artery disease, often fatal myocardial infarction. Homozygotes have severe hypercholesterolemia and often present in early childhood, or even as infants, with ischemic heart disease, including myocardial infarction, and evidence of cholesterol accumulation in other tissues, particularly in skin. Myocardial infarction in infants is manifested by tachypnea, sweating, pallor, and the appearance of apprehension. In older children, cholesterol in the skin and other tissues produces typical tuberous xanthomas on the extensor surfaces of the extremities (Figure 5.5), arcus senilis, xanthelasma, subcutaneous nodules, and thickening of the Achilles tendons. Patients with this condition usually have a strong family history of premature ischemic heart disease. Measurements of fasting plasma lipids typically reveals total cholesterol levels in excess of 6.5 mmol/L in heterozygotes and 15 mmol/L in homozygotes. The excess cholesterol is accountable

Table 5.5 Familial hyperlipidemias

Lipid abnormality	Type	Primary defect	Associated clinical features	Secondary disorders
Exogenous hyperlipidemia (↑↑Chylomicrons)	I	Familial LPL deficiency Apo C-II deficiency	Eruptive xanthomatosis, lipemia retinalis, acute pancreatitis, dyspnea, recent memory loss	Dysglobulinemias SLE
Endogenous hyperlipidemia (↑VLDL)	IV	(a) Familial hypertriglyceridemia (b) FCH (c) Tangier disease	(a) Eruptive xanthomatosis, lipemia retinalis, acute pancreatitis, dyspnea, recent memory loss (b) Premature coronary artery disease (c) Enlarged orange tonsils, splenomegaly, peripheral neuropathy	Many conditions, including GSD type I, uremia, nephrotic syndrome, diabetes mellitus*, alcoholism*, estrogens*, glucocorticoids*, stress*
Mixed hyperlipidemia (↑VLDL + Chylomicrons)	V	Familial hypertriglyceridemia Familial LPL deficiency	Eruptive xanthomatosis, lipemia retinalis, acute pancreatitis, dyspnea, recent memory loss	The same conditions as cause secondary type IV hyperlipidemia
Hypercholesterolemia (↑↑LDL)	IIa	FH FCH	Premature coronary artery disease, tuberous xanthomas, tendinous xanthomas, arcus senilis	Nephrotic syndrome, hypothyroidism, dysglobulinemias, Cushing syndrome, AIP
Combined hyperlipidemia (↑LDL + VLDL)	IIb	FCH	Premature coronary artery disease	Nephrotic syndrome, hypothyroidism, dysglobulinemias, Cushing syndrome, glucocorticoids*, stress*
Remnant hyperlipidemia (β-VLDL)	III	Familial dysbetalipoproteinemia	Tuberous and tuberoeruptive xanthomas, planar xanthomas, premature coronary artery disease, peripheral vascular disease	Hypothryoidism, SLE

Abbreviations: VLDL, very low–density lipoproteins; LDL, low–density lipoproteins; SLE, systemic lupus erythematosis; FCH, familial combined hyperlipopro-teinemia; AIP, acute intermittent porphyria; LPL, lipoprotein lipase; FH, familial hypercholesterolemia; GSD, glycogen storage disease.

* Conditions which by themselves do not cause hyperlipidemia, but often aggravate a primary hyperlipidemia.

Source: Data taken from Havel & Kane (1995)

by increased levels of LDL; VLDL (very low-density lipoprotein) levels are generally only modestly elevated, and high-density lipoprotein (HDL) levels are often decreased.

Abnormalities of plasma lipids are features of a number of primary disorders of lipoprotein metabolism, many of which are associated with an increased risk of premature coronary artery disease (Table 5.5). The investigation of hyperlipidemia requires careful attention to the circumstances of testing and consideration of the large number of conditions in which secondary hyperlipidemia occurs. In general, secondary hyperlipidemia is much more common than primary disorders of plasma lipoprotein metabolism. Plasma lipid analyses should be done on blood obtained after an over-night fast and after at least three days abstention from alcohol. Lipid analyses should include measurement of total triglycerides, total cholesterol, LDL-cholesterol, and HDL-cholesterol (see Chapter 9). Note should be made of any medications, dietary fat intake, obesity, and history of medical conditions, such as diabetes, kidney disease, and hypothyroidism. Testing should routinely include tests of thyroid, liver, and kidney function.

Tuberous xanthomatosis is seen in patients with sitosterolemia, a disorder of plant sterol metabolism, which is characterized by premature coronary atherosclerosis, intermittent hemolysis or chronic hemolytic anemia, and recurrent arthritis of the knees and ankles. In patients with sitosterolemia, the plasma apo B-100 concentrations may be elevated, but the plasma cholesterol is either normal or only moderately increased. Tendinous xanthomatosis is one of the primary clues to the diagnosis of cerebrotendinous xanthomatosis, a disorder characterized clinically by the onset in adolescence of progressive neurologic deterioration (see Chapter 2).

Premature coronary artery disease is a major feature of Fabry disease in which accumulation of globotriaosylceramide (GL-3) in the walls of small arteries and arterioles predisposes to coronary atherosclerosis, myocardial ischemia, and myocardial infarction. Stroke may also occur as a result of cerebrovascular involvement. The same deposition in vessels of the skin and mucous membranes causes the pathognomonic skin lesions of the disease, angiokeratoma corporis diffusum.

SUGGESTED READING

Antonicka, H., Mattman, A., Carlson, C. G., *et al.* (2003). Mutations in COX15 produce a defect in the mitochondrial heme biosynthetic pathway, causing early-onset fatal hypertrophic cardiomyopathy. *American Journal of Human Genetics*, **72**, 101–14.

Barth, P. G., Wanders, R. J., Vreken, P., Janssen, E. A., Lam, J. & Baas F. (1999). X-linked cardioskeletal myopathy and neutropenia (Barth syndrome) (MIM 302060). *Journal of Inherited Metabolic Diseases*, **22**, 555–67.

Bonnet, D., de Lonlay, P., Gautier, I. *et al.* (1998). Efficiency of metabolic screening in childhood cardiomyopathies. *European Heart Journal*, **19**, 790–93.

Bonnet, D., Martin, D., de Lonlay, P. *et al.* (1999). Arrhythmias and conduction defects as presenting symptoms of fatty acid oxidation disorders in children. *Circulation*, **100**, 2248–53.

Breslow, J. L. (2000). Genetics of lipoprotein abnormalities associated with coronary artery disease susceptibility. *Annual Review of Genetics*, **34**, 233–54.

Cederbaum, S. D., Koo-McCoy, S., Tein, I. *et al.* (2002). Carnitine membrane transporter deficiency: a long-term follow up and OCTN2 mutation in the first documented case of primary carnitine deficiency. *Molecular Genetics and Metabolism*, **77**, 195–201.

Dangel, J. H. (1998). Cardiovascular changes in children with mucopolysaccharide storage diseases and related disorders – clinical and echocardiographic findings in 64 patients. *European Journal of Pediatrics*, **157**, 534–8.

Fosslien, E. (2003). Mitochondrial medicine – cardiomyopathy caused by defective oxidative phosphorylation. *Annals of Clinical & Laboratory Science*, **33**, 371–95.

Gehrmann, J., Sohlbach, K., Linnebank, M. *et al.* (2003). Cardiomyopathy in congenital dosrders of glycosylation. *Cardiology in the Young*, **13**, 345–51.

Gilbert-Barness, E. (2004). Review: metabolic cardiomyopathy and conduction system defects in children. *Annals of Clinical Laboratory Science*, **34**, 15–34.

Guertl, B., Noehammer, C. & Hoefler, G. (2000). Metabolic cardiomyopathies. *International Journal of Experimental Pathology*, **81**, 349–72.

Holmgren, D., Wahlander, H., Eriksson, B. O., Oldfors, A., Holme, E. & Tulinius, M. (2003). Cardiomyopathy in children with mitochondrial disease; clinical course and cardiological findings. *European Heart Journal*, **24**, 280–8.

Lev, D., Nissenkorn, A., Leshinsky-Silver, E. *et al.* (2004). Clinical presentations of mitochondrial cardiomyopathies. *Pediatric Cardiology*, **25**, 443–50.

Linhart, A., Magage, S., Palecek, T. & Bultas, J. (2002). Cardiac involvement in Fabry disease. *Acta Paediatrica Suppl.*, **91**, 15–20.

Parini, R., Menni, F., Garavaglia, B. *et al.* (1998). Acute, severe cardiomyopathy as main symptom of late-onset very long-chain acyl-coenzyme A dehydrogenase deficiency. *European Journal of Pediatrics*, **157**, 992–5.

Sachdev, B., Takenaka, T., Teraguchi, H. *et al.* (2002). Prevalence of Anderson-Fabry disease in male patients with late onset hypertrophic cardiomyopathy. *Circulation*, **105**, 1407–11.

Saudubray, J. M., Martin, D., de Lonlay, P. *et al.* (1999). Recognition and management of fatty acid oxidation defects: a series of 107 patients. *Journal of Inherited Metabolic Diseases*, **22**, 488–502.

Scaglia, F., Towbin, J. A., Craigen, W. J. *et al.* (2004). Clinical spectrum, morbidity, and mortality in 113 pediatric patients with mitochondrial disease. *Pediatrics*, **114**, 925–31.

Tein, I. (2003). Carnitine transport: pathophysiology and metabolism of known molecular defects. *Journal of Inherited Metabolic Diseases*, **26**, 147–69.

Wolfsdorf, J. I., Holm, I. A. & Weinstein, D. A. (1999). Glycogen storage diseases. Phenotypic, genetic, and biochemical characteristics, and therapy. *Endocrinology and Metabolism Clinics of North America*, **28**, 801–23.

6

Storage syndrome and dysmorphism

Over the years, the distinction between what was conventionally regarded as dysmorphic syndromes and inborn errors of metabolism has become blurred by the recognition that the consequences of many inborn errors of metabolism include physical features, such as facial dysmorphism, that would almost certainly be regarded as developmental defects if the nature of the underlying metabolic defect were not known. In fact, the discovery of a specific metabolic defect in patients with Smith-Lemli-Opitz (SLO) syndrome, a classical dysmorphic syndrome, has led to the suggestion that perhaps all hereditary dysmorphic syndromes should be regarded similarly – as inborn errors of metabolism – in which the specific metabolic defect has not yet been identified. At the other extreme, if the physical features of Hurler disease, resulting directly from abnormal accumulation of the substrate of a defective enzyme, are regarded as 'dysmorphic', then perhaps any inherited metabolic disease showing physical abnormalities should be regarded as dysmorphic syndromes. The issue is raised to underscore the fact that the distinction between the two types of disorders is breaking down, and various biochemical and metabolic studies are being employed increasingly by clinical geneticists in the investigation of dysmorphism, particularly in infants presenting acutely ill early in life. The questions to be addressed in this chapter are:

- Are there characteristics of the dysmorphism that should prompt metabolic investigation?
- What are the types of inherited metabolic diseases in which dysmorphism might be expected to be prominent?
- What sort of metabolic studies are most likely to be diagnostically productive in the investigation of dysmorphism?

General characteristics of the dysmorphism resulting from inborn errors of metabolism

Developmental physical abnormalities have been classified in general as congenital malformations (primary dysmorphogenesis; poor formation), deformations (structural abnormalities resulting from mechanical interference with growth), and disruptions (structural abnormalities resulting from destructive processes). The mechanism of the dysmorphism occurring as a result of inborn errors of metabolism varies from one disorder to another. A few, such as SLO syndrome, clearly involve disturbances of morphogenesis (malformation). In most, the distortion arises primarily as a result of a combination of deformation and disruption. The mucopolysaccharide storage diseases are good examples. Mucopolysaccharide accumulation causes abnormalities of shape, growth, and the physical properties of any tissue normally containing significant amounts of connective tissue ground substance, such as bone, cartilage, ligaments, skin, blood vessels, dura mater, and heart valves (deformation). However, abnormalities of shape and growth also occur as a result of secondary destructive processes (disruption).

With this in mind, some generalizations can be made concerning the characteristics of the dysmorphism in many inherited metabolic diseases:

- The dysmorphic features associated with inborn errors of metabolism are generally disturbances of shape, rather than fusion or cellular migration abnormalities or abnormalities of number, such as polydactyly.
- The dysmorphism tends to become more pronounced with age.
- Microscopic and ultrastructural abnormalities are often prominent.

There are some important exceptions. For example, cellular migration abnormalities are a prominent feature of the cerebral dysmorphogenesis occurring in infants with Zellweger syndrome, glutaric aciduria type II, and pyruvate dehydrogenase (PDH) deficiency. Fusion abnormalities and abnormalities of number (e.g., polydactyly) are major, though not constant, features of SLO syndrome.

In many inherited metabolic disorders, the facies may be recognized to be unusual, though in a relatively nonspecific or very subtle way. Infants with PDH deficiency, for example, are mildly dysmorphic, though not usually in a way that is sufficiently characteristic to suggest the diagnosis. Generally, the peculiarities of the face are matters of proportion, rather than major structural abnormalities. Unrelated patients with the same disorder often look enough alike to appear to be related, but are not regarded as unusual or dysmorphic by themselves. For example, infants with Tay-Sachs disease generally have very attractive, fine, doll-like facial features. The same has been noted about patients with glycogen storage disease, type I, who are often described as resembling 'cupie dolls' because of their chubby cheeks. Children with multiple sulfatase deficiency tend to have fine, attractive facial features. With a few exceptions, the peculiarities of the face in these conditions are not sufficiently striking or specific to be diagnostically helpful. However, the physician may be alerted to the possibility by determining that the child does not resemble any other member of the family very closely, something that is often elicited by asking who the child takes after in the family, or be examining photos of their parents or siblings taken at about the same age.

Table 6.1 Classification of inborn errors with significant dysmorphism

Lysosomal disorders	*Peroxisomal disorders*
Mucopolysaccharidoses	Zellweger syndrome and variants
MPS I (Hurler & Scheie diseases)	Rhizomelic chondrodysplasia punctata
MPS II (Hunter disease)	Adult Refsum disease
MPS III (Sanfilippo disease)	*Mitochondrial disorders*
MPS IV (Morquio disease)	PDH deficiency
MPS VI (Maroteaux-Lamy disease)	Glutaric aciduria, type II
MPS VII (Sly disease)	3-Hydroxyisobutyric aciduria
Glycoproteinoses	Mitochondrial ETC defects
Infantile sialidosis	*Biosynthetic defects*
Galactosialidosis	Mevalonic aciduria
Fucosidosis	SLO syndrome
α-Mannosidosis	CDG syndrome
β-Mannosidosis	Sjögren-Larsson syndrome
Aspartylglucosaminuria	Albinism
Pycnodysostosis	Primary defects in hormone biosynthesis
Sphingolipidoses	Primary disorders of collagen biosynthesis
GM1 gangliosidosis	Homocystinuria*
Farber lipogranulomatosis	Menkes disease*
Gaucher disease, type I	Alkaptonuria*
Combined defects	*Receptor defects*
I-cell disease	Familial hypercholesterolemia
Multiple sulfatase deficiency	Pseudohypoparathyroidism
	Other hormone receptor defects

Abbreviations: MPS, mucopolysaccharidosis; PDH, pyruvate dehydrogenase; ETC, electron transport chain; CDG, carbohydrate-deficient glycoprotein; SLO, Smith-Lemli-Opitz.
*The biosynthetic defect in these conditions is secondary to the metabolic consequences of the primary inborn error of metabolism.

What are the types of inherited metabolic diseases in which dysmorphism might be expected to be prominent?

Most of the inherited metabolic diseases associated with dysmorphism involve defects in organelle metabolism, biosynthetic processes, or receptor defects (Table 6.1). In some cases, serious structural defects, such as major neuronal migration abnormalities, are present at birth. Except for defects of hormone biosynthesis, which represent a special case, the response of all of them to treatment by environmental manipulation is incomplete at best, even when the accumulating substrate of the defective reaction is water-soluble and diffusible (e.g., PDH deficiency).

What follows are brief descriptions of some of the more common inherited metabolic diseases in which dysmorphism is a major feature. They are organized according to the organelle or process involved.

Lysosomal disorders

Except for the uncommon instances in which lysosomal disorders present in the newborn period with non-immune fetal hydrops (see Chapter 7), the dysmorphic features in patients with inborn errors of lysosomal enzyme activity are usually not clinically obvious at birth, even though ultrastructural changes in tissues may be present as early as 20 weeks of gestation. Many of these disorders are characterized by the development, during infancy and early childhood of 'storage syndrome'.

Storage syndrome

Storage syndrome is a constellation of clinical findings suggesting accumulation of macromolecular material in various tissues causing distortion of shape and growth manifested as:
- characteristic facies;
- bone changes (dysostosis multiplex) and short stature;
- organomegaly (megalencephaly, hepatosplenomegaly).

Although affected infants are usually considered normal at birth, a history of large birth weight associated with peripheral edema, sometimes severe enough to cause non-immune fetal hydrops, may be elicited. The onset of symptoms and awareness that something is wrong is usually gradual. Recurrent bouts of otitis media and persistent mucous nasal discharge are common, but rarely are they sufficiently different from what a normal child might experience to generate suspicion of the presence of a storage disorder before the development of other signs of disease.

Affected children may come to attention in a number of ways. The otolaryngologists, consulted because of the recurrent otitis media or persistent nasal discharge, may be the first to notice that the child has unusual facial features suggestive of a genetic disorder. Others come to attention because of abnormalities of growth, either excessively rapid growth of the head, suggesting the possibility of hydrocephalus, or growth retardation causing short stature. The incidental detection of hepatomegaly or hepatosplenomegaly often prompts further investigation. Sometimes the child comes to attention as a result of the investigation of developmental delay or extraordinarily difficult behavior. Occasionally the characteristic skeletal abnormalities are found incidentally on plan radiographs obtained because of suspected lower respiratory tract infections.

The face in patients with storage syndrome shows subtle changes that become more pronounced with age, but at such a slow rate that parents often do not notice them. The changes include relative macrocephaly with prominence of the forehead, prominence of the brow, some puffiness of the eyelids, broadening and flattening of the bridge of the nose, anteverted nares, and thick upper lip. The general impression is one of 'coarse' facial features (Figure 6.1). The hair is usually coarse, and the pinnae of the ears are generally thickened and fleshy. The tongue is enlarged with some exaggeration of the fissuring. The teeth, which generally erupt on schedule,

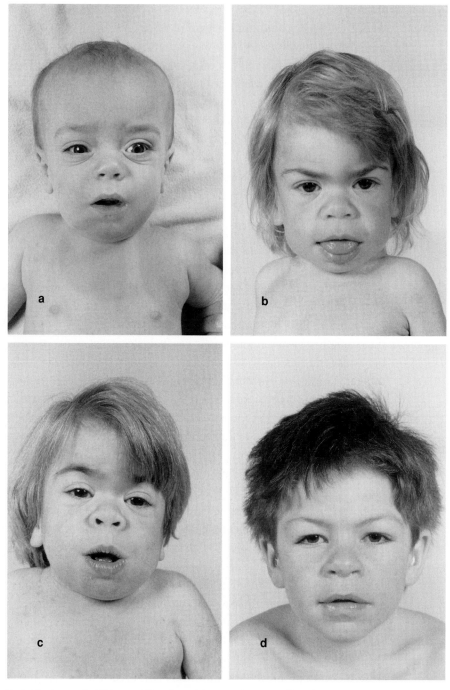

Figure 6.1   Facial features of children with various lysosomal storage disorders.
Panels **a**, Hurler disease (MPS IH) at four months of age; **b**, MPS IH at three years of age;
c, MPS IH at seven years of age; **d**, Hunter disease (MPS IIA) at seven years of age; **e**,
Hunter disease (MPS IIB) at 42 years of age; **f**, seven-month-old infant with I-cell disease;
g, mannosidosis at 5 years of age; **h**, 11-month-old boy with Niemann-Pick disease, type A.

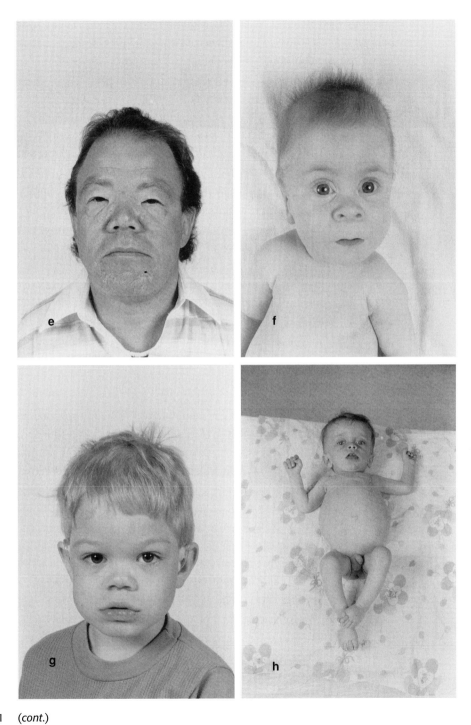

Figure 6.1   (*cont.*)

are often small, widely spaced, and dysplastic. The gums may be thickened. Clouding of the cornea is a feature of many of the inherited metabolic diseases presenting as storage syndrome, though it is generally only clinically obvious in the mucopolysaccharidoses, Hurler disease, Scheie disease, and Maroteaux-Lamy disease.

A prominent feature of virtually all the inherited metabolic diseases presenting with storage syndrome is short stature. Linear growth may actually be accelerated during the first year of life. However, growth during the second year slows suddenly, often arresting completely or showing little further gains after three to five years of age. The axial skeleton is shortened and often shows lumbar kyphosis. In Hurler disease (MPS IH), the kyphosis, caused by wedging of lumbar vertebrae, is often acute, producing the characteristic 'gibbus' deformity of the spine. Careful examination often shows limitation of active and passive movement of various joints, particularly the shoulders, elbows, fingers, and hips. Restriction of elevation of the arm at the gleno-humeral joint often occurs early. Limitation of active and passive movement of the elbows is also early and includes restriction of extension of the joint, as well as supination and pronation. Limitation of extension of the hips results in a characteristic crouched standing posture with flexion at the knees and exaggerated lordosis of the lumbar spine. The fingers generally appear thickened and short, and they gradually become fixed in a partially flexed position over a period of several months or years. Similar changes occur in the toes, producing hammer-toe deformities.

Morquio disease (MPS IV) is a prominent exception to the generalized and severe restriction of joint movement seen in patients with most other mucopolysaccharide storage diseases. In this condition, abnormalities of the skeleton dominate the clinical picture; hepatosplenomegaly is usually mild or absent, and mental retardation is rare. More than any of the other inherited metabolic diseases presenting with storage syndrome, Morquio disease closely resembles a nonmetabolic spondyloepiphyseal dysplasia. In marked contrast to all the other MPS disorders, many of the joints in Morquio disease show abnormally *increased* mobility. The instability caused by hypermobility of joints interferes with efficient muscle action producing an impression of muscle weakness severe enough to suggest a primary myopathy.

Plain radiographs show widespread changes typical of mucopolysaccharide storage diseases in general, but not generally specific for any one in particular (Figure 6.2). The skull is enlarged and thickened, and the sella turcica is enlarged. Late radiographs of the thoraco-lumbar spine show flattening of the vertebrae, beaking of the antero-inferior lip, and often posterior displacement of one of more upper lumbar vertebrae. Radiographs of the hands show shortening and broadening of the metacarpals and phalanges, producing a rounded, bullet-like shape, with generalized under-mineralization and increased coarse trabeculation. The ilia of the pelvis are externally rotated and the acetabula are poorly formed. Radiographs

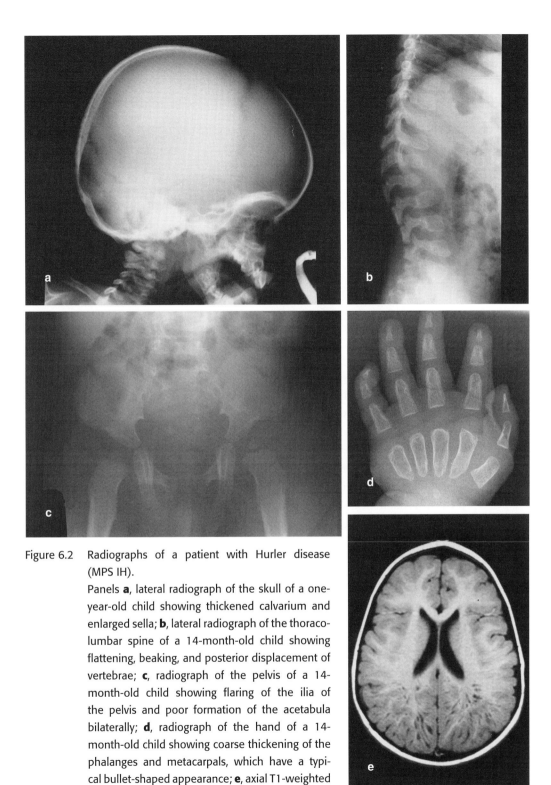

Figure 6.2 Radiographs of a patient with Hurler disease (MPS IH).

Panels **a**, lateral radiograph of the skull of a one-year-old child showing thickened calvarium and enlarged sella; **b**, lateral radiograph of the thoracolumbar spine of a 14-month-old child showing flattening, beaking, and posterior displacement of vertebrae; **c**, radiograph of the pelvis of a 14-month-old child showing flaring of the ilia of the pelvis and poor formation of the acetabula bilaterally; **d**, radiograph of the hand of a 14-month-old child showing coarse thickening of the phalanges and metacarpals, which have a typical bullet-shaped appearance; **e**, axial T1-weighted MRI [TR600/TE15] of the brain of a 4-year-old child showing marked dilatation of Virchow–Robin perivascular spaces, distended by accumulated glycosaminoglycan.

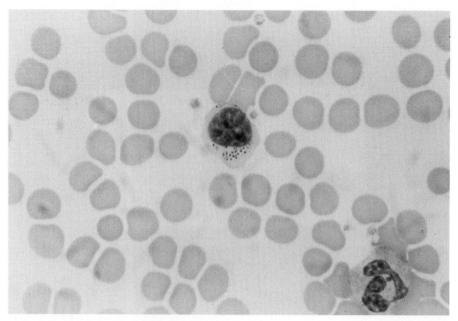

Figure 6.3   Alder-Reilly bodies in peripheral blood lymphocyte from patient with Hurler disease (MPS IH). (Courtesy of Dr. Annette Poon.)

of the upper cervical spine in patients with Morquio disease, type A or type B, show hypoplasia or absence of the odontoid process producing instability of the atlanto-axial joint, which can be appreciated by comparing lateral radiographs of the neck taken in flexion and extension. Radiographic skeletal abnormalites similar to those seen in children with mucopolysaccharide storage diseases are sometimes seen in patients with congenital disorders of glycosylation, type Ia.

In many of the lysosomal disorders presenting as storage syndrome, examination of a routine, Wright-stained peripheral blood smear shows the presence of metachromatic granulation of mononuclear cells called Alder-Reilly bodies (Figure 6.3). However, this sign must be differentiated from the nonspecific granulation occurring in various acquired conditions, such as viral infections, and it is often absent, particularly in the relatively mild MPS variants. Examination of bone marrow aspirates often shows the presence of storage histiocytes even if they are not present in the peripheral blood.

Some of the major clinical features of different lysosomal disorders presenting as storage syndrome are summarized in Table 6.2.

A number of conditions are commonly confused with inherited lysosomal disorders presenting as storage syndrome. Infants with congenital virus infections, such as congenital CMV or rubella, often present with a history of developmental delay, failure to thrive, and hepatosplenomegaly. The presence of generalized

Table 6.2 Some clinical features of lysosomal disorders presenting as 'storage syndrome'

Disorder	Facies	Neurologic	Dysostosis multiplex	Eye findings	Hepatosplenomegaly	Other
Mucopolysaccharidoses						
MPS IH (Hurler)	Coarse	Severe MR	+++	Corneal clouding	+++	Death by age 10 years
MPS IH/S (Hurler–Scheie)	Coarse	± MR	++	Corneal clouding	Intermediate between MPS IH and MPS IS	Short stature, multiple joint contractures
MPS IS (Scheie)	'Normal'	Carpal tunnel syndrome	+	Corneal clouding	+	Short stature
MPS IIA (Hunter)	Coarse	Severe MR	+++	0	++	Death in late teens, often cardiac
MPS IIB (Hunter)	Coarse	0	+ – ++	0	+	Short stature
MPS III (Sanfilippo)	Mild coarsening	Severe MR	±	Corneal opacities	0	Severe behavior abnormalities
MPS IV (Morquio)	Unusual	Cervical compression myelopathy	+++	Corneal opacities	0	Hypoplasia/absence of the odontoid process
MPS VI (Maroteaux–Lamy)	Mild coarsening	± MR	++	Corneal clouding	±	Short stature
MPS VII (Sly)	Mild coarsening	Severe MR	++	?	+	Highly variable phenotype

(*cont.*)

Table 6.2 (*Cont.*)

Disorder	Facies	Neurologic	Dysostosis multiplex	Eye findings	Hepatosplenomegaly	Other
Glycoproteinoses						
Infantile sialidosis (type II)	Coarse	MR	+++	CRS	±	Renal tubular dysfunction
Juvenile sialidosis (type I)	Normal	Myoclonus	0	CRS	0	Angiokeratomata
Galactosialidosis	'Normal'	+ – +++	+ – +++	CRS	±	Angiokeratomata
Fucosidosis, type I	Mild coarsening	MR, seizures	++	0	++	Increased sweat chlorides
Fucosidosis, type II	Mild coarsening	MR	++	Telangiectasia	+	Angiokeratomata
α-Mannosidosis, type I	Coarse	Severe MR	+++	Cataracts, corneal opacities	+++	Early sensorineural hearing loss
α-Mannosidosis, type II	Mild coarsening	MR	++	Cataracts, corneal opacities	++	Early sensorineural hearing loss
Aspartylglucosaminuria	Mild coarsening	MR	+	Mild cataracts	0	Photosensitivity, acne
Pycnodysostosis	Unusual	0	+++	0	0	Osteosclerosis
Sphingolipidoses						
GM1 gangliosidosis (infantile)	Coarse	Severe MR	++	± CRS	++	Early visual failure, hyperacusis
GM1 gangliosidosis (juvenile)	Normal	Moderate MR	±	0	0	Spasticity, ataxia

Abbreviations: MR, mental retardation; CRS, cherry-red spot; +, present; ±, variably present; 0, absent.

lymphadenopathy or chorioretinitis are features that help to differentiate this group of conditions from inborn errors of metabolism presenting as storage syndrome. Appropriate serological and virus isolation studies are generally sufficient to confirm the diagnosis of congenital infection. Disseminated neuroblastoma in young infants is often associated with hepatosplenomegaly. Unusual involuntary eye movements (i.e., opsiclonus) might suggest a metabolic neurodegenerative condition. The true nature of the underlying disease is usually revealed by examination of bone marrow smears showing the presence of neoplastic, not storage, cells. Histiocytosis X is another malignant condition that clinically may initially be confused with a storage disorder. Hepatosplenomegaly, along with pallor, developmental delay, and blindness, is characteristic of osteopetrosis. The skeletal radiographs in that disorder are so characteristic that confusion with one of the lysosomal storage diseases is impossible. Massive hepatosplenomegaly and failure to thrive are characteristics of familial erythrophagocytotic lymphohistiocytosis (FEL), which often suggest storage disease. However, the bone marrow findings are generally typical, showing histiocytosis and marked erythrophagocytosis.

Gaucher disease, type I

Non-neuronopathic Gaucher disease should be considered high on the list of diagnostic possibilities in any patient of any age presenting with asymptomatic splenomegaly or hepatosplenomegaly. It is particularly common among Ashkenazi Jews in whom the prevalence may be as high as 1 in 1000. Gaucher disease is a lysosomal storage disease caused by deficiency of acid glucocerebrosidase, called β-glucosidase when activity is measure using a synthetic substrate. It is characterized by intracellular accumulation of glucocerebroside in macrophages throughout the reticuloendothelial system, especially in the spleen, liver, bone marrow, and lungs. The symptoms of disease are directly related to the tissue distribution of the pathology.

The commonest presentation of the disease is asymptomatic splenomegaly or complications of hypersplenism. Unusual bruising, excessive bleeding during dental surgery, or postpartum hemorrhage may be the first indication of marked thrombocytopenia. Affected individuals usually have a sallow complexion and mild to moderate normocytic, normochromic anemia and mild neutropenia, and they often complain of fatiguability. Discovery of the anemia often prompts treatment with iron, even though bone marrow studies generally show ample, or even excessive, iron stores. The splenomegaly may become massive. Spleen weights in excess of 2 kg are not unusual. Enlargement of the spleen and liver often cause protuberance of the abdomen. Occasionally, patients experience bouts of excruciating abdominal pain related to splenic infarction.

Infiltration of the bone marrow with glucocerebroside-containing storage cells causes expansion of the marrow compartment producing thinning of the cortex and a characteristic widening of the ends of long bones. This produces a typical Erlenmeyer flask shape in the distal ends of the femurs (Figure 6.4). Spontaneous fractures are common as a result of thinning of the cortex of bone throughout the body. One of the most debilitating complications of the disease is 'bone crises' characterized clinically by the sudden onset of very severe, localized pain, swelling, tenderness, heat, and redness, usually in one of the long bones of the lower extremities, usually associated with fever. Clinically, the appearance may be indistinguishable from osteomyelitis or septic arthritis, though cultures are generally negative. The crises usually resolve over a period of a few days. Occasionally, the pain persists, without much evidence of inflammation, for several days, even weeks. Radiologically, there may be nothing to see apart from soft-tissue swelling, until well after the pain has resolved. Sclerosis of bone in the area then follows. The pathophysiology of these episodes is unknown, though the clinical features suggest a vascular mechanism. Avascular necrosis of the head of the femur and humerus is also a common and debilitating complication of the disease. Clinical lung involvement is uncommon.

Bone marrow aspirates generally show the presence of typical Gaucher storage cells (Figure 6.5). The diagnosis is confirmed by demonstrating deficiency of β-glucosidase in peripheral blood leukocytes or cultured fibroblasts. Occasionally, similar storage cells are seen in the marrow of patients with Hodgkin's disease or other lymphomas. The diagnosis is made even more challenging because peripheral blood leukocytes of patients with these lymphomas often have markedly depressed β-glucosidase activity. However, the activity in fibroblasts in patients with tumors is normal, and the β-glucosidase activity in peripheral blood leukocytes characteristically returns to normal levels when the tumor regresses with treatment. Mutation analysis is becoming increasingly applied to the diagnosis of Gaucher disease, particularly among Jews, because a high proportion of the disease is associated with a relatively small number of mutant alleles.

The natural history of severe type 1 Gaucher disease has been dramatically changed by the introduction of enzyme replacement therapy for the disease (see Chapter 10). Biweekly infusions of enzyme invariably produce hematologic improvement within a few months. Reversal of bone lesions takes somewhat longer.

Niemann-Pick disease, type B, caused by deficiency of acid sphingomyelinase, another lysosomal enzyme, is clinically indistinguishable from Gaucher disease, type 1. Marked splenomegaly, with some enlargement of the liver, is typical of both conditions. Bone lesions also occur in both, although they are generally less common in Niemann-Pick disease. The morphology of storage histiocytes found in bone marrow aspirates is different in the two diseases. However, definitive diagnosis

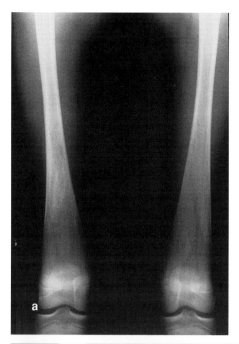

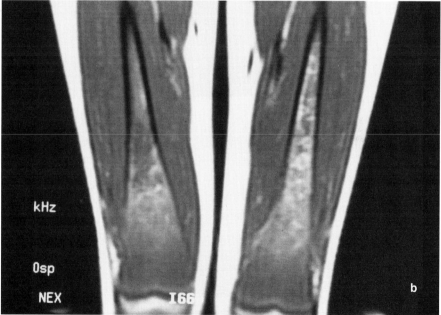

Figure 6.4   Skeletal imaging of the lower extremities in Gaucher disease.
Panels **a**, a plain radiograph showing typical thinning of cortex and expansion of the marrow cavity producing a characteristic Erlenmeyer flask appearance of the distal femurs. **b**, an MRI scan [TR450/TE16] showing mottled signal from the distal femurs. (Courtesy of Dr. Paul Babyn.)

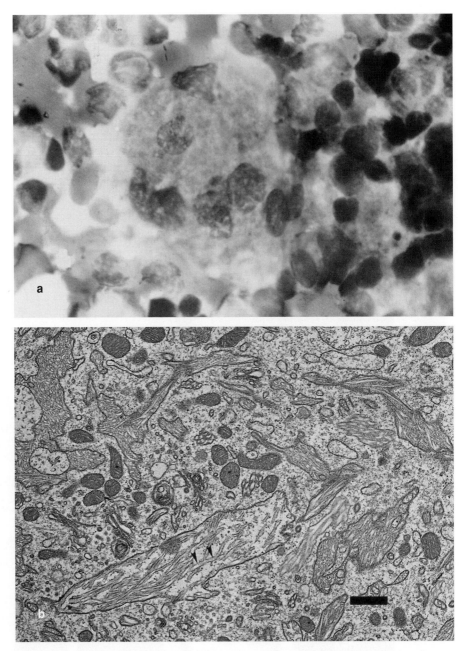

Figure 6.5   Typical storage macrophages in the bone marrow and liver of a patient with Gaucher disease. Panels **a**, a photomicrograph showing the characteristic crinkled tissue paper appearance of Gaucher storage cells. (Courtesy of Dr. Annette Poon.) **b**, an electron photomicrograph showing part of a Kupffer sell. The tubule-like structures (arrowheads) shown within the lysosomes of this cell are diagnostic of Gaucher disease. The bar represents 0.5μm. (Courtesy of Dr. M. J. Phillips.)

requires demonstration of deficiency of one of the two relevant lysosomal enzyme activities, either in leukocytes or cultured skin fibroblasts.

Farber lipogranulomatosis

Classical Farber lipogranulomatosis, an autosomal recessive sphingolipid storage disorder caused by deficiency of the lysosomal enzyme, ceramidase, is characterized by onset in the first few weeks to months of life of painful swelling of joints, particularly of the distal extremities, subcutaneous nodules, a hoarse cry and respiratory distress, failure to thrive, and fever. Lymphadenopathy and moderate hepatomegaly may also occur, but splenomegaly is rare. One of our patients had massive hepatomegaly, evidence of significant hepatocellular dysfunction, and ascites. Affected infants are typically irritable and appear apprehensive, particularly during handling, which causes pain. Most, though not all, show psychomotor retardation; some have seizures. Generalized muscle weakness, atrophy, and hypotonia are associated with decreased or absent deep tendon reflexes. Eye abnormalities are common; an atypical cherry-red spot is seen in many. The course of the disease is relentlessly progressive, with increasing inanition owing to feeding difficulties, the development of joint contractures, increasing pulmonary infiltration and respiratory difficulties, and death, usually within a few months.

Milder variants of the disease are apparently less common than the classical disease and are characterized by long-term survival, many with apparently normal intelligence. Some patients present in the newborn period with very aggressive disease in which hepatosplenomegaly is prominent and death occurs within a few weeks to months. Massive histiocytic infiltration of lungs, liver, spleen, and thymus, often without the typical subcutaneous nodules, in this malignant variant of the disease, may be misdiagnosed as malignant histiocytosis. Rarely, patients with Farber lipogranulomatosis present at one to three years of age with psychomotor regression and rapidly progressive neurodegeneration, prominent macular cherry-red spots, ataxia, quadriparesis, seizures, and death within several months to a few years. The presence of subcutaneous nodules is an important clue to the clinical diagnosis.

Histopathologic studies on tissues affected in Farber disease show accumulation of histiocytes with secondary fibrosis. Some of the lesions progress to form well-organized granulomas with macrophages, lymphocytes, and multinucleated giant cells surrounding a central core of foamy, PAS-positive, storage histiocytes. The diagnosis is confirmed by demonstrating acid ceramidase deficiency in tissues, including peripheral blood leukocytes, or cultured fibroblasts. This is one lysosomal hydrolase that must be measured using the natural substrate of the enzyme; synthetic, fluorogenic substrates do not work. This limits the immediate availability of the test to laboratories providing specialized biochemical diagnostic services.

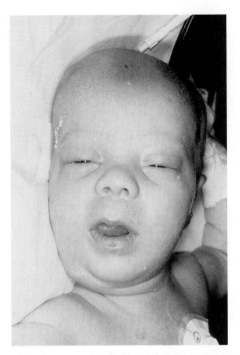

Figure 6.6   Facial features of a newborn infant with classical Zellweger syndrome.

Peroxisomal disorders

Zellweger syndrome

Infants with classical Zellweger syndrome, caused by a defect in peroxisome bio-genesis, display physical features that are so specifically characteristic of the condition that diagnosis is usually possible on inspection alone. The face is typical. It is characterized by a high and prominent forehead, hypoplastic supraorbital ridges, epicanthic folds, and depressed and broad root of the nose (Figure 6.6). Affected infants show typically profound hypotonia and weakness, severe feeding difficulties, very large fontanelles and wide cranial sutures, redundant skin folds of the neck, abnormal external ears, eye abnormalities (nystagmus, corneal clouding, Brushfield spots, glaucoma, cataracts, or pigmentary retinopathy), seizures, single palmar creases, and hepatomegaly.

Abdominal ultrasound examination almost always shows cystic disease of the kidneys, and it often reveals increased echogenicity of the liver. Plain radiographs often show calcific stippling of the patella (Figure 6.7) and synchondrosis of the acetabula. CT and MRI studies of the brain typically show disorganization of the cerebral cortex and white matter abnormalities indicative of severe myelin deficiency and neuronal heterotopias (Figure 6.8).

Electron microscopic examination of liver obtained by biopsy shows absence of peroxisomes. Biochemical studies reveal multiple abnormalities of peroxisomal

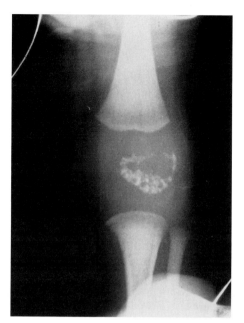

Figure 6.7   Radiograph of the knee in a patient with Zellweger syndrome showing calcific stippling of the patella.

function (see Chapter 9). Measurement of plasma very long-chain fatty acids is generally the most accessible and reliable biochemical test for confirming the diagnosis.

Numerous non-classical variants of Zellweger syndrome have been described, each showing some of the characteristics of the classical disease. On the basis of clinical differences between them, some have been separated off as different diseases, such as neonatal adrenoleukodystrophy (NALD) and infantile Refsum disease (IRD). However, as the number of patients recognized as having peroxisomal defects has increased, the distinction between clinically similar syndromes has become blurred. Moreover, on the basis of complementation studies, many patients with different clinical phenotypes would appear to be genetically indistinguishable. Zellweger syndrome, NALD, and IRD may all represent different positions on a clinical continuum associated with different mutations in the same gene. The results of the same type of complementation studies also indicate that marked genetic heterogeneity exists within distinct clinical phenotypes, such as classical Zellweger syndrome. Many of the disorders have certain characteristics in common that should alert the clinician to the possibility of a peroxisomal disorder. These are features that are prominent in Zellweger syndrome, and collectively they are here called the *severe peroxisomal phenotype*. They include:

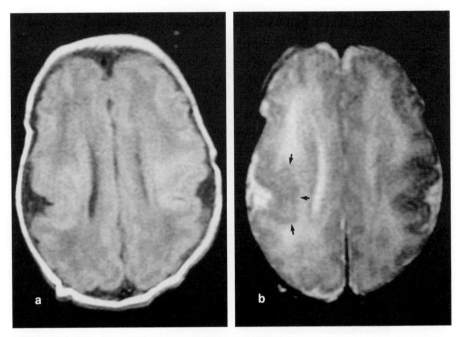

Figure 6.8   MRI scan of the brain in patient with Zellweger syndrome.
Axial MRI scans of the brain show bilateral primitive Sylvian fissures lined by thickened, grossly abnormal cerebral cortex (arrows, Panel b), and poorly formed gyrae throughout. Panels **a**, T1-weighted scan [TR600/TE20]; **b**, T2-weighted scan [TR3000/TE120]. (Courtesy of Dr. Susan Blaser.)

- marked psychomotor retardation;
- profound hypotonia and weakness;
- intractable seizures;
- sudanophilic leukodystrophy;
- variable hepatocellular dysfunction;
- impairment of special senses (visual impairment or sensorineural hearing loss).

Table 6.3 shows a classification of some of the more common peroxisomal disorders based on the nature of the basic defect. It is important not to make too much of the apparent clinical differences between various syndromes, which share so many features in common, associated with the severe peroxisomal phenotype. Ultimately, the group of disorders will be classified according to the biochemical or genetic defect as these become elucidated.

Rhizomelic chondrodysplasia punctata (RCDP)

RCDP is another disorder of peroxisomal function associated with severe and relatively typical dysmorphism. Affected infants show dysmorphic facial features redolent of Zellweger syndrome, moderate to severe psychomotor retardation, profound

Table 6.3 Classification of peroxisomal disorders

Defect	Some distinguishing clinical features
Disorders of peroxisomal biogenesis with multiple functional defects	
Zellweger syndrome	'Severe peroxisomal phenotype' with characteristic facial dysmorphism, disturbances of neuronal migration (polymicrogyria, neuronal heterotopias), corneal clouding, nystagmus, cataracts, congenital heart disease, poor feeding, failure to thrive, death within a few months
Neonatal adrenoleukodystrophy	'Severe peroxisomal phenotype' with more subtle facial dysmorphism, disturbances of neuronal migration (polymicrogyria, neuronal heterotopias), chemical evidence of adrenal insufficiency, poor feeding, failure to thrive, survival for up to a few years
Infantile Refsum disease	'Severe peroxisomal phenotype' with facial dysmorphism, subtle disturbances of neuronal migration (polymicrogyria, neuronal heterotopias), decreased plasma cholesterol, increased plasma phytanate, prominent retinal degeneration and sensorineural hearing impairment, survival for up to a few years
Hyperpipecolic acidemia	'Severe peroxisomal phenotype' with prominent retinal degeneration, cirrhosis, increased plasma and urinary pipecolate, survival for up to many years
Multiple functional defects with peroxisomes present	
Rhizomelic chondrodysplasia punctata (RCDP)	'Severe peroxisomal phenotype' with facial dysmorphism, severe proximal shortening of limbs, chondrodysplasia punctata (stippled epiphyses), skin lesions, cataracts, survival highly variable
Single enzyme defects with 'severe peroxisomal phenotype'	
DHAP acyltransferase deficiency	Identical to classical RCDP
Acyl-CoA oxidase deficiency	'Severe peroxisomal phenotype'
Bifunctional enzyme deficiency	'Severe peroxisomal phenotype' with neuronal heterotopias, polymicrogyria
3-Ketoacyl-CoA thiolase deficiency	'Severe peroxisomal phenotype'; ± facial dysmorphism, renal cysts, neuronal heterotopias, early death
Dihydroxy- & trihydroxycholestanoic acidemia	'Severe peroxisomal phenotype' with subtle facial dysmorphism and liver disease, survival variable
Single enzyme defects with specific phenotype	
X-linked adrenoleukodystrophy	Rapidly progressive X-linked recessive leukodystrophy associated with adrenal insufficiency (see Chapter 2)
Primary hyperoxaluria, type 1	Progressive renal impairment due to renal oxalosis, nephrocalcinosis, and recurrent urolithiasis
Acatalasemia	Predisposition to certain types of bacterial infections, relatively benign

Table 6.4 Inherited metabolic diseases associated with punctate calcification of epiphyses

---

Rhizomelic chondrodysplasia punctata (autosomal recessive, peroxisomal)
Zellweger syndrome
I-cell disease
GM1 gangliosidosis
Sialidosis
Galactosialidosis
Multiple sulfatase deficiency
Mucopolysaccharidoses
Niemann-Pick disease
Vitamin K epoxide reductase deficiency
Metachromatic leukodystrophy
Smith-Lemli-Opitz syndrome

---

hypotonia, cataracts, and ichthyosis. In addition, affected infants show severe shortening of proximal limbs, and the calcific stippling of epiphyses is more generalized than in Zellweger disease. Lateral radiographs of the spine typically show calcific stippling and coronal clefts of vertebral bodies. Rarely, the disease presents somewhat later in infancy or early childhood as psychomotor retardation associated with calcific stippling of epiphyses, but without significant shortening of long bones.

Unlike in Zellweger syndrome and other peroxisomal disorders, plasma very long-chain fatty acid levels are normal in patients with RCDP. However, plasmalogen biosynthesis and phytanic acid oxidation are both impaired. As a result, erythrocyte plasmalogen levels are decreased and phytanic acid levels in plasma are increased in affected infants (see Chapter 9).

Chondrodysplasia punctata (CDP) is a feature of other conditions, such as Conradi-Hünermann syndrome, an autosomal dominant condition in which limb length and intellect are normal. X-linked recessive CDP is associated with cataracts, mental retardation, and erythematous desquamative skin changes in the newborn period evolving within a few months into striated ichthyosiform hyperkeratosis. X-linked dominant CDP, a male-lethal condition, is also associated with congenital erythroderma in heterozygous females, but intellect is normal. CDP may also occur as a feature of some lysosomal storage disorders, congenital infections, coumadin embryopathy, or other disorders (Table 6.4).

Mitochondrial disorders

Subtle facial dysmorphism and moderately severe structural anomalies of the brain, such as congenital absence of the corpus callosum, are seen in many patients with severe variants of PDH deficiency. Facial dysmorphism and associated anomalies are much more prominent and characteristic in patients with the severe, neonatal form of glutaric aciduria type II (GA II).

Glutaric aciduria, type II

The severe hypoglycemia and metabolic acidosis in infants with neonatal GA II are often associated with multiple congenital anomalies, including facial dysmorphism (including high forehead, midface hypoplasia with depressed nasal bridge, hypertelorism, and low-set ears), muscular defects of the anterior abdominal wall, hypospadias, rocker-bottom feet, and enlargement of the kidneys. The liver is also enlarged as a result of massive microvesicular steatosis. Abdominal ultrasound examination shows prominent cystic disease of the kidneys, and neuroimaging studies show evidence of disorganization of the cerebral cortex, a reflection of neuronal migration abnormalities.

The metabolic abnormalities generally dominate the clinical presentation, and investigation of the metabolic acidosis typically reveals massive excretion of glutaric acid and other metabolites as a result of the defect in mitochondrial electron transport flavoprotein (ETF) or ETF dehydrogenase (see Chapter 3). GA II may be difficult to distinguish clinically from severe neonatal CPT II deficiency.

Biosynthetic defects

Menkes disease

Menkes disease is an X-linked recessive disorder of copper transport caused by mutations in a copper-transporting ATPase. The gene has been cloned, and many mutations have been characterized. Many of the characteristic physical abnormalities of the disease are present at birth, but they may be quite subtle and are often overlooked. The face is unusual (Figure 6.9), and the skull shows abnormalities similar to those seen in patients with Zellweger syndrome: long, narrow calvarium, with high forehead and huge fontanelles; small nose, puffy eyes, hyperplastic alveolar ridges, and loose, velvety soft skin. The hair is characteristically brittle and shows pili torti on microscopic examination. Feeding problems, hypotonia, hypothermia, and diarrhea are prominent features of the disease in newborn infants. The clinical course is characterized by continued failure to thrive, profound hypotonia, intractable seizures, persistent mild normochromic normocytic anemia, chronic diarrhea, and severe developmental retardation. Survival of infants with classical severe disease rarely extends beyond two to three years.

Skeletal radiographs show generalized osteopenia and the presence of prominent wormian bones in the skull. Visualization of blood vessels reveals marked tortuosity of the arteries throughout the body. Diverticula of the bladder are common

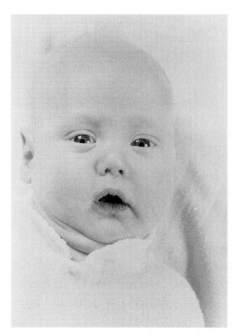

Figure 6.9   Facial features of an infant with Menkes disease.

and give rise to recurrent urinary tract infections. The diagnosis is suggested by finding markedly decreased copper and ceruloplasmin levels in plasma. Copper concentrations in liver are profoundly decreased; the levels in intestinal mucosa are markedly increased above normal. The copper content of cultured fibroblasts and the uptake of radioisotopic copper are greatly increased.

Treatment of the disease by daily injections of copper histidine (about 200–1000 micrograms per day) results in normalization of plasma copper and ceruloplasmin levels. If treatment is begun within the first few days of birth, it appears to alter dramatically the course of the disease, resulting in long-term survival, freedom from seizures, and near-normal psychomotor development.

Mevalonic aciduria

Patients with mevalonic aciduria, an inborn error of cholesterol and nonsterol isoprenoid biosynthesis, present in early infancy or childhood with mildly dysmorphic facial features (Figure 6.10), severe psychomotor retardation, failure to thrive, delayed closure of the cranial sutures and fontanelles, hypotonia and muscle weakness, progressive cerebellar ataxia in about half, anemia, and recurrent attacks of fever, vomiting, diarrhea, arthralgia, edema, and skin rash. In some patients, hepatosplenomegaly, lymphadenopathy, arthralgia, and uveitis during febrile crises, coupled with a dramatic response to corticosteroid treatment, might suggest a

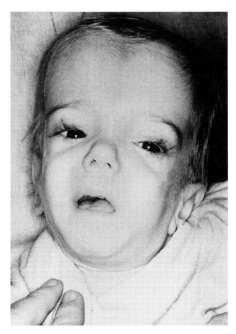

Figure 6.10 Facial features of an infant with mevalonic aciduria. (Courtesy of Prof. Dr. G. Hoffmann.)

collagen vascular disease. Plasma cholesterol levels are usually normal or only slightly decreased. Creatine phosphokinase (CPK) levels are markedly elevated in the majority, particularly during febrile crises. Neuroimaging shows progressive atrophy of the cerebellar hemispheres and vermis. Urinary organic acid analysis shows high concentrations of mevalonic acid. In patients with periodic fevers, plasma IgD levels are elevated (hyper-IgD syndrome). The diagnosis is confirmed by demonstrating deficiency of mevalonate kinase in fibroblasts.

Smith-Lemli-Opitz (SLO) syndrome

The discovery of a specific inborn error of cholesterol metabolism in patients with classical Smith-Lemli-Opitz syndrome challenged the somewhat arbitrary separation of dysmorphic syndromes from inherited metabolic diseases. It is characterized by microcephaly, failure to thrive, hypotonia, unusual facies (high forehead; cataracts; broad, short nose with anteverted nares; ptosis; micrognathia; cleft palate) and limb abnormalities (syndactyly of the toes, polydactyly) (Figure 6.11), in addition to genital anomalies in affected males (hypospadias, ambiguous genitalia, cryptorchidism), endocrine abnormalities, heart and kidney malformations, and psychomotor retardation. Gas chromatographic analysis of sterols shows that cholesterol levels in affected patients are decreased, and the concentration of its immediate precursor, 7-dehydrocholesterol (7-DHC), is increased

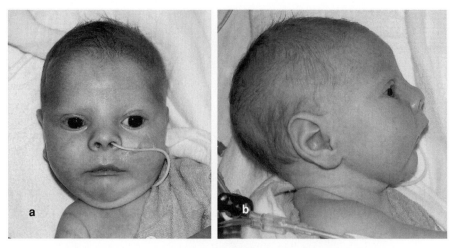

Figure 6.11   Facial features of a 3-week-old infant boy with Smith-Lemli-Opitz syndrome.
Panels **a**, front view; **b**, side view. In addition to facial dysmorphism, the infant had hypospadias and syndactyly of the toes (Courtesy of Dr. Margaret Nowaczyk.)

in plasma, erythrocytes, and cultured skin fibroblasts. Plasma cholesterol levels measure by enzymic-colorimetric analysis using cholesterol oxidase, which does not discriminate between cholesterol and 7-DHC, are not decreased. The diagnosis can usually be confirmed by demonstrating a marked increase in the 7-DHC-to-cholesterol ratio in plasma. However, in some patients, confirmation requires measurement of 7-dehydrocholesterol reductase activity in cultured fibroblasts or mutation analysis.

Besides mevalonic aciduria and Smith-Lemli-Opitz syndrome, a number of other disorders of cholesterol biosynthesis have been described (Table 6.5). All those that have been described to date are associated with failure to thrive, severe developmental delay, congenital skeletal abnormalities and multiple congenital malformations.

Congenital disorders of glycosylation (CDG) [formerly known as 'carbohydrate-deficient glycoprotein syndrome']

CDG are a group of uncommon autosomal recessive multisystem diseases associated with abnormalities in the synthesis of circulating glycoproteins. The frequency of these disorders is estimated to be comparable in northern Europe to the incidence of metachromatic leukodystrophy. Several subtypes of CDG syndrome have been identified, with extraordinary clinical variation among them (Table 6.6). The most common subtype, type Ia, caused by deficiency of phosphomannomutase (PMM), is characterized clinically by onset in early infancy of failure to thrive, marked hypotonia, severe developmental delay, particularly affecting gross motor

Table 6.5 Some inherited disorders of sterol biosynthesis

Disease		Clinical features	Diagnosis
Mevalonic aciduria	AR	Facial dysmorphism, severe phsychomotor retardation, failure to thrive, delayed closure of cranial sutures and fontanelles, hypotonia, progressive cerebellar ataxia, anemia, recurrent episodes of fever, vomiting, diarrhea, arthralgia, edema and skin rash	Increased mevalonic acid in urine on organic acid analysis
Smith–Lemli–Opitz syndrome	AR	Dysmorphic facies (microcephaly, prominent forehead, ptosis, anteverted nares, cleft palate, thick alveolar ridges, micrognathia, ±cataracts), syndactyly, congenital heart defects, genital malformations in males (hypospadias), gastrointestinal anomalies, failure to thrive, developmental retardation	Increased 7-DHC:cholesterol ratio in plasma; deficiency of 7-DHC reductase in fibroblasts; mutation analysis (DHCR7)
Desmosterolosis	AR	Extremely rare, craniofacial malformations (macrocephaly, cleft palate, thick alveolar ridges), congenital heart disease, hypoplastic lungs, renal hypoplasia, ambiguous genitalia, short limbs, osteosclerosis	Marked increases in desmosterol concentration in plasma; mutation analysis (DHCR24)
Chondrodysplasia punctata, type 2 (Conradi-Hunermann-Happle syndrome)	XLD	Generalized congenital ichthyosiform erythroderma, splitting of the nails, cataracts, patchy alopecia, skeletal abnormalities (chondrodysplasia punctata, asymmetrical rhizomelic limb shortening, scoliosis, polydactyly)	Increased 8-dehydrocholesterol and cholesta-8(9)-en-3β-ol in tissues; mutation analysis (EBP)
CHILD syndrome	XLD	Congenital hemidysplasia with ichthyosiform erythroderma, limb defects, which are strikingly asymmetrical in affected females.	Mutation analysis (NSDHL)
Greenberg dysplasia	AR	Lethal combination of facial dysmorphism, hydrops fetalis, cystic hygroma, incomplete lung lobation, pulmonary hypoplasia, extramedullary hematopoiesis, gastrointestinal malformations, polydactyly, limb shortening, abnormal ossification of long bones and calvarium	Increased cholesta-8,14-dien-3β-ol and cholesta-8,14,24-trien-3β-ol in tissues
Antley-Bixler syndrome	AR	Craniosynostosis, brachycephaly, propotosis, midface hypoplasia, dysplastic ears, femoral bowing, multiple joint contractures and fractures, genital anomalies, imperforate anus	Increased lanosterol and dihydrolanosterol in cultured cells

Abbreviations: AR, autosomal recessive; XLD, X-linked dominant; 7-DHC, 7-dehydrocholesterol; CHILD, congenital hemidysplasia with ichthyosiform erythroderma and limb defects

Table 6.6 Classification of subtypes of congenital disorders of glycosylation (CDG)

Subtype	Gene	Enzyme defect	Clinical features
Ia	PMM2	Phosphomannomutase 2	Psychomotor retardation, dysmorphic facies, strabismus, inverted nipples, joint restrictions, abnormal fat pads on hips, pericardial effusion, cardiomyopathy, failure to thrive, stroke-like episodes, cerebellar atrophy, pigmentary retinopathy, peripheral neuropathy, hypogonadism (late)
Ib	PMI1	Phosphomannose isomerase	Protein-losing enteropathy, coagulopathy, hyperinsulinemic hypoglycemia, hepatocellular dysfunction, recurrent vomiting and diarrhea, responsive to treatment with mannose
Ic	ALG6	Dolichol-phosphoglucose:$Man_9GlcNAc_2$-PP-dolichol glucosyltransferase	Similar to type Ia, though milder, without cerebellar atrophy or peripheral neuropathy. Low plasma cholesterol levels.
Id	ALG3	Dolichol-phosphomannose:$Man_5GlcNAc_2$-PP-dolichol mannosyltransferase	Profound psychomotor retardation, infantile spasms with hypsarrhythmia, microcephaly, optic atrophy, iris coloboma
Ie	DPM1	Dolichol-phosphomannose synthase 1	Severe psychomotor retardation, failure to thrive, dysmorphism, severe seizure disorder, recurrent evidence of hepatocellular dysfunction, cortico-subcortical cerebral hypoplasia with normal cerebellum and midbrain
If	MPDU1	Mannose-P-dolichol utilization defect 1	Psychomotor retardation, hypotonia, contractures, seizures, failure to develop speech, failure to thrive, visual impairment with retinitis pigmentosa, (ichthyosis in some)
Ig	ALG12	Dolichol-phosphomannose:$Man_7GlcNAc_2$-PP-dolichol mannosyltransferase	Psychomotor retardation, hypotonia, seizures, microcephaly, supragluteal fat pads, facial dysmorphism (only 1 case described)
Ih	ALG8	Dolichol-phosphoglucose:Glc_1Man_9 $GlcNAc_2$-PP-dolichol α1,3-glucosyltransferase	Severe failure to thrive, inverted nipples, hypotonia, cardiomyopathy, pericardial effusion, recurrent infections, proximal renal tubular dysfunction, protein-losing enteropathy, facial dysmorphism, early death
Ii	ALG2	GDP-Man:$ManGlcNAc_2$-PP-dolichol mannosyltransferase	Severe psychomotor retardation, visual impairment, seizures, delayed myelination

Type	Gene	Enzyme	Clinical features
Ij	*DPAGT1*	UDP-GlcNAc:Dolichol-P-GlcNAc-1 phosphate transferase	Psychomotor retardation, microcephaly, seizures, severe hypotonia, facial dysmorphism, skin dimples on thighs, single palmar creases, 5th finger clinodactyly
Ik	*ALG1*	GDP-mannose:GlcNAc$_2$-PP-dolichol mannosyltransferase	Nonimmune fetal hydrops, facial dysmorphism (large fontanelle, hypertelorism, micragnathia), hepatosplenomegaly, hypogonadism, contractures, absent DTR, dilated cardiomyopathy, early death
Il	*ALG9*	α1,2-mannosyltransferase	Psychomotor retardation, microcephaly, hypotonia, seizures, hepatomegaly
IIa	*MGAT2*	UDP-N-Acetylglucosamine:α-6-D-mannoside-β-1,2-N-acetylglucosaminyltransferase II	Psychomotor retardation, facial dysmorphism, stereotypic behaviors, hypotonia, without peripheral neuropathy or cerebellar atrophy
IIb	*HSAGLUCIE*	α-Glucosidase I	Facial dysmorphism (broad nose, retrognathism, high-arched palate), hypotonia, peripheral neuropathy, hypoventilation and apnea, seizures, hepatomegaly (with steatosis, bile duct proliferation, fibrosis, and multilamellar inclusions), early death (only 1 case described)
IIc	*FUCT1*	GDP-fucose transporter	Psychomotor retardation, short limbs, facial dysmorphism, broad palms, persistent leukocytosis, Bombay blood group, recurrent pyogenic infections
IId	*B4GALT1*	UDP-Gal:GlcNAc β1,4-galactosyltransferase I	Hypotonia, myopathy with increased CK, macrocephaly with Dandy-Walker malformation, hydrocephalus (only 1 case described)
IIe	?	?	Anemia, thrombocytopenia, hypoalbuminemia, proteinuria, dry skin, macrocephaly, hypotonia
IIf	?	CMP-sialic acid transporter	Severe psychomotor retardation, facial dysmorphism, hypotonia, coagulopathy, immunodeficiency, ichthyosis (in some), seizures, failure to thrive,

Abbreviations: DTR, deep tendon reflexes.

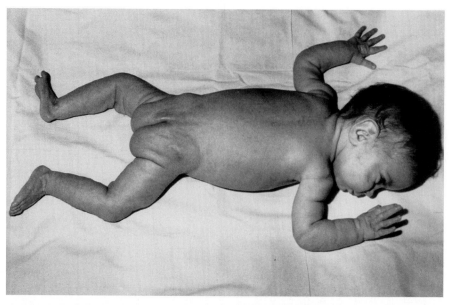

Figure 6.12   Lipodystrophy of the buttocks and thighs of a 6-week-old infant with congenital disorder of glycosylation syndrome, type Ia. (Courtesy of Prof. Dr. Jaak Jaeken.)

skills, and intermittent episodes of hepatocellular dysfunction, recurrent pericardial effusions, acute encephalopathy, or stroke-like episodes. Most show facial dysmorphism with broad nasal bridge, prominent jaw and forehead, large ears, strabismus, and inverted nipples. Unusual fat pads are present over the upper, outer aspects of the buttocks, associated with thickening of the skin on the legs. Alternating areas of lipohyperplasia and lipoatrophy may occur on the thighs (Figure 6.12). The liver is enlarged and liver function tests are abnormal. In addition to marked hypotonia and generalized muscle weakness, deep tendon reflexes are initially depressed, then disappear within two to three years.

Within three to four years, the hepatocellular and cardiac problems resolve, and the principal problems relate to the nervous system. Psychomotor development is severely impaired, and few affected children are able to walk independently. Fine motor skills are not so severely affected, and regression is not a prominent feature of the disease. Ataxia and dyskinesia become more prominent. Virtually all affected children have strabismus and develop progressive retinal degeneration. Stroke-like episodes or acute encephalopathy, seizures, and hemiparesis are particularly common in middle childhood, usually precipitated by intercurrent febrile illnesses. As a rule these neurologic crises are followed by complete recovery.

Adolescence in children with CDG syndrome is characterized by marked weakness and atrophy of the muscles, particularly of the lower extremities, and slowing of nerve conduction velocities, along with continuing cerebellar ataxia and incoordination. Neuroimaging often shows cerebellar and brain stem atrophy. The chest becomes increasingly pigeon-breasted and associated with progressive thoracic kyphoscoliosis. Some patients show hypogonadism. Communication skills are characteristically more advanced than gross motor development, and affected individuals often display an almost euphoric affect. Mobility becomes increasingly compromised by the progression of flexion contractures, particularly affecting the lower extremities.

Liver function tests are generally abnormal early in the disease, but improve with age. Similarly, the CSF protein is usually somewhat elevated early in the disease, becoming normal with age; however, in some patients, the CSF protein increases with age. Affected individuals have subnormal levels of various plasma glycoproteins: thyroxine-binding globulin, haptoglobin, transcortin, apolipoprotein B and low-density lipoprotein (LDL)-cholesterol, and coagulation factors. The most characteristic biochemical finding is a pronounced abnormality of the N-linked oligosaccharides of circulating glycoproteins, especially transferrin. Typically, the terminal trisaccharides of many of the glycoprotein oligosaccharides are missing. Demonstration of the abnormality requires isoelectric focusing analysis of the glycoprotein (Figure 6.13). The levels of transferrin as measured by conventional immunochemical techniques are generally normal.

Infants with CDG type Ib present with a history of failure to thrive, hypotonia, persistent vomiting and diarrhea, protein-losing enteropathy, coagulopathy, hyperinsulinemic hypoglycemia, and hepatocellular dysfunction. In contrast to patients with type Ia disease, the nervous system is spared and psychomotor development is generally normal. This condition is caused by deficiency of phosphomannose isomerase (PMI). Treatment with dietary mannose supplementation often results in rapid resolution of the symptoms of the disease.

Other variants of CDG are very rare. Although the clinical features vary significantly from one variant to another, they do have certain features in common that should suggest the nature of the underlying defect. With only a handful of exceptions, the CDGs are characterized by psychomotor retardation, marked hypotonia, and seizures. The known CDGs in which psychomotor retardation and neurological abnormalities are not prominent, such as CDG type Ib, failure to thrive, with protein-losing enteropathy, renal tubular dysfunction, and immunodeficiency tend to be prominent.

Secondary defects of protein glycosylation, including typical CDG abnormalities in the isoelectric focusing pattern of plasma transferrin, may occur in galactosemia or in hereditary fructose intolerance (HFI). In the case of galactosemia, measurement of galactose-1-phosphate uridyltransferase in red cells is generally

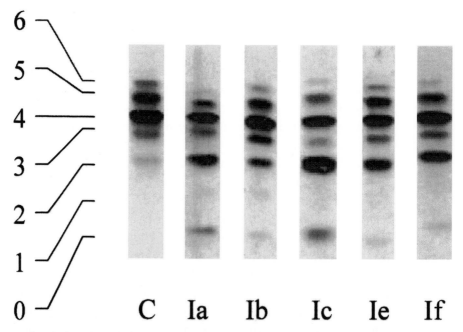

Figure 6.13 Isoelectric focusing of plasma transferrin in congenital disorders of glycosylation (CDG) syndrome.

Plasma transferrin species separated by isoelectric focusing on the basis of the number of sialic acid residues (shown as numbers 0 to 6). Lanes **C**, Control; **Ia**, CDG type Ia; **Ib**, CDG type Ib; **Ic**, CDG type Ic; **Id**, CDG type Id; **Ie**, CDG type Ie; **If**, CDG type If. (Courtesy of Prof. Dr. Jaak Jaeken.)

sufficient to resolve the confusion. In HFI, enzymic diagnosis requires liver biopsy, which is not without risk in a patient with a significant coagulopathy. However, treatment of HFI with a fructose-restricted diet results in rapid clinical improvement, and the plasma transferrin abnormality returns to normal within a few weeks.

Homocystinuria

Marked accumulation of homocystine (a dimer of homocysteine), irrespective of the underlying cause, is associated with certain dysmorphic features arising, in part, as a result of the effects of the amino acid on the levels and cross-linking of various connective tissue elements. Homocysteine is an intermediate in the biosynthesis of methionine and cystathionine (Figure 6.14). Accumulation occurs as a result of defects in any of a number of reactions (Table 6.7), including several involving the metabolism of vitamin B_{12}, an obligatory cofactor for methionine synthase activity (see Figure 3.5). The commonest genetic cause of

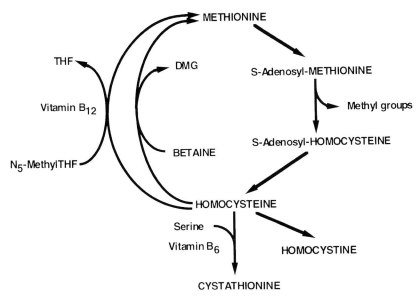

Figure 6.14 Metabolism of homocysteine and methionine.
Abbreviations: N_5-methylTHF, N_5-methyltetrahydrofolate; THF, tetrahydrofolate; DMG, *N,N*-dimethylglycine.

Table 6.7 Genetic and some acquired causes of homocystinuria/ hyperhomocyst(e)inemia

---

Impaired cystathionine β-synthase (CBS) activity
Genetic CBS deficiency
Some drugs (e.g., 6-azauridine triacetate)

Impaired methionine synthase activity
Tetrahydrofolate reductase deficiency
Pernicious anemia (intrinsic factor deficiency)
Failure of vitamin B_{12} absorption (Immerslund syndrome)
Impaired cellular uptake of B_{12} (transcobalamin II deficiency)
Impaired release of B_{12} from lysosomes (*cblF*)
Impaired reduction of cobalamin (*cblC* or *cblD*)
Impaired conversion of B_{12} to adenosylcobalamin (*cblA* or *cblB*)
Impaired conversion of B_{12} to methylcobalamin (*cblE* or *cblG*)
Nutritional B_{12} deficiency
Nutritional folate deficiency

---

homocystinuria/hyperhomocyst(e)inemia, and that associated with the most severe accumulation of the amino acid, is cystathionine β-synthase (CBS) deficiency.

Homocystinuria due to genetic deficiency of CBS is characterized by moderately severe mental retardation, connective tissue abnormalities affecting the skeleton and eyes, vascular abnormalities, and other less prominent physical anomalies. Affected children usually come to initial medical attention in the first one to two years of life as a result of developmental retardation. The psychomotor development of untreated patients varies tremendously; most remain moderately retarded. Seizures may also occur. Psychiatric and behavioral problems are common, but frank psychosis is rare.

One of the most consistent and prominent physical abnormalities in CBS-deficiency homocystinuria is dislocation of the ocular lens. Dislocation is generally downward, as opposed to the upward dislocation of the lens in Marfan syndrome, and it usually occurs between 4 and 12 years of age. Some patients escape this complication until the third decade of life. The parents may be the first to notice the shimmering iridodonesis of the iris, a quivering movement of the membrane usually precipitated by movement of the head. The disease is also associated with the development of marked myopia, and spontaneous retinal detachment is common. Less commonly, it is associated with glaucoma, cataracts, retinal degeneration, and optic atrophy.

Osteoporosis is also a prominent feature of the disease by the late teens, most commonly affecting the spine. It is often associated with the development of thoracic scoliosis. Abnormal lengthening of the long bones (dolichostenomelia) causes affected individuals to be very tall and lean by the time they reach late adolescence. Pectus carinatum, pes cavus, genu valgum, and radiologic abnormalities of the vertebrae are common. Although the body habitus is Marfanoid, affected patients do not have true arachnodactyly, hypermobility of joints, or the cardiac abnormalities of Marfan syndrome.

Thromboembolism is the most frequent cause of death of individuals with CBS-deficiency homocystinuria. The most common site of intravascular thrombosis is a peripheral vein, setting the stage for embolization to the lungs. Cerebrovascular, peripheral arterial, and coronary artery thrombosis also occur. Thromboembolism may occur at any age, even in infants with the disease. However, the likelihood of clinically significant problems increases with age, the cumulative risk reaching 25% by age 15–20 years.

In about half the patients with CBS-deficiency homocystinuria, the biochemical abnormalities are normalized by treatment with large doses (250–500 mg per day) of pyridoxine. In general, the extent and severity of the complications of the disease, including thromboembolism, are greater in patients who are unresponsive to vitamin therapy.

Table 6.8 Initial metabolic investigation of patients presenting with storage syndrome or dysmorphism

Urinary mucopolysaccharides screening test
Urinary oligosaccharides screening test
Urinary organic acid analysis
Plasma lactate and pyruvate
Plasma very long-chain fatty acids
Plasma phytanic acid
Isoelectric focusing of plasma transferrin
Plasma amino acid analysis

What sort of metabolic studies are most likely to be diagnostically productive in the investigation of dysmorphism?

If disorders of organelle metabolism are major contributors to those inherited metabolic diseases associated with dysmorphism, it follows that investigation aimed at assessing organelle function would be particularly important to establishing a diagnosis. In order to be able to concentrate here on general principles, much of the detail relating to the investigation of organelle function is discussed later in Chapter 9.

Morphologic studies are often helpful in the assessment of possible disorders of organelle function. Non-invasive imaging studies (ultrasound examination, plain radiographs, CT scanning, and MRI studies) help to establish the pattern and degree of involvement of various organs and tissues. Sometimes the type and pattern of abnormalities are characteristic enough to suggest a specific diagnosis. More often, the abnormalities may suggest a class of disorders, such as lysosomal storage disease, but are not specific enough to pin down the diagnosis to a specific inborn error of metabolism. For example, finding generalized dysostosis multiplex on plain radiographs is a strong indication of a lysosomal storage disorder. Similarly, the presence of CT or MRI evidence of cerebral cortical disorganization is typical, though not diagnostic, of some peroxisomal disorders. Confirmation of a metabolic diagnosis invariably requires specific biochemical studies.

Unlike disorders of small molecule metabolism, in which histopathologic changes are generally not very helpful, inborn errors of organelle function are commonly associated with histopathologic and ultrastructural abnormalities that are sufficiently characteristic to suggest a short list of diagnostic possibilities. For example, the histopathologic and histochemical characteristics of the storage histiocytes in subcutaneous granulomas in patients with Farber lipogranulomatosis are virtually pathognomonic of the disease. The absence of normal peroxisomes in the liver is characteristic of severe peroxisomal assembly defects, like Zellweger syndrome.

The increased number and abnormal structure of the mitochondria in skeletal or cardiac muscle is highly suggestive of a mitochondrial ETC defect, though which subunit or complex is involved would require further studies.

The types of biochemical studies needed ultimately to arrive at a diagnosis include tests directed primarily at the organelle-classification of a disorder (Table 6.8) and tests for specific defects. If the results of any of these are abnormal, further studies would be needed to identify a specific enzyme defect.

The approach to the identification of dysmorphism arising as a result of defects in biosynthesis, such as CDG syndrome, is not nearly so direct. In fact, the recommendation of any particular test to screen for inborn errors of biosynthesis would obviously omit some of the known and most of the currently unknown defects in biosynthesis presenting with dysmorphic features. Instead, the approach to be encouraged is one of intellectual receptivity. That is to say, the clinician should approach the metabolic investigation of a dysmorphic patient with the commitment to explain every laboratory abnormality that comes to light. This is contrary to the general tendency to ignore or dismiss any information, particularly from the laboratory, that does not fit the presumptive clinical diagnosis. This is a particularly difficult group of diseases to manage: there are no 'screening tests' for inborn errors of biosynthesis.

SUGGESTED READING

Grabowski, G. A., Andria, G., Baldellou, A. *et al.* (2004). Pediatric non-neuronopathic Gaucher disease: presentation, diagnosis and assessment. Consensus statements. *European Journal of Pediatrics*, **163**, 58–66.

Haas, D., Kelley, R. I. & Hoffmann, G. F. (2001). Inherited disorders of cholesterol biosynthesis. *Neuropediatrics*, **32**, 113–22.

Keir, G., Winchester, B. G. & Clayton, P. (1999). Carbohydrate-deficient glycoprotein syndromes: inborn errors of protein glycosylation. *Annals of Clinical Biochemistry*, **36**, 20–36.

Kelley, R. I. & Hennekam, R. C. (2000). The Smith-Lemli-Opitz syndrome. *Journal of Medical Genetics*, **37**, 321–35.

Marklova, E. & Albahri, Z. (2004). Pitfalls and drawbacks in screening of congenital disorders of glycosylation. *Clinical Chemistry and Laboratory Medicine*, **42**, 583–9.

Marquadt, T. & Denecke, J. (2003). Congenital disorders of glycosylation: review of their molecular bases, clinical presentations and specific therapies. *European Journal of Pediatrics*, **162**, 359–79.

Moser, A. B., Rasmussen, M., Naidu, S. *et al.* (1995). Phenotype of patients with peroxisomal disorders subdivided into sixteen complementation groups. *Journal of Pediatrics*, **127**, 13–22.

Muenzer J. (2004). The mucopolysaccharidoses: a heterogeneous group of disorders with variable pediatric presentations. *Journal of Pediatrics*, **144** (5 Suppl), S27–34.

Poggi-Travert, F., Fournier, B., Poll-The, B. T. & Saudubray, J. M. (1995). Clinical approach to inherited peroxisomal disorders. In *Diagnosis of Human Peroxisomal Disorders*, ed. F. Roels, *et al.*, pp. 1–18. Cordrecht: Kluwer Academic Publishers.

Porter, F. D. (2002). Malformation syndromes due to inborn errors of cholesterol synthesis. *Journal of Clinical Investigation*, **110**, 715–24.

Raymond, G. V. (1999). Peroxisomal disorders. *Current Opinions in Pediatrics*, **11**, 572–6.

7

Acute metabolic illness in the newborn

There are few situations in clinical medicine as acutely stressful as the precipitate deterioration of a previously healthy newborn infant, coupled with the recognition that, irrespective of the cause, delay in the initiation of appropriate management often leads to death or irreparable brain damage. Severe illness in the newborn, regardless of the underlying cause, tends to manifest itself in a rather stereotypic way with relatively nonspecific findings, such as poor feeding, drowsiness, lethargy, hypotonia, and failure to thrive. Because inherited metabolic diseases are individually rare, clinicians have a tendency to pursue the possibility only after other more common conditions, such as sepsis, have been excluded. Further delay often occurs because the type of investigation required to make the diagnosis of inherited metabolic disease includes unfamiliar tests, which the clinician may feel uncomfortable interpreting owing to a general lack of confidence regarding metabolic problems.

The need for dispatch requires that inborn errors of metabolism be considered along with and at the same time as common acquired conditions, such as sepsis, hypoxic-ischemic encephalopathy, intraventricular hemorrhage, intoxications, congenital viral infections, and certain types of congenital heart disease. Appropriate laboratory investigation, including some simple bedside tests, such as urine tests for reducing substances and ketones, should be initiated without delay, even done at the bedside if possible. Despite the apparent non-specificity of presenting symptoms in neonates, there are some features that increase the likelihood of an inborn error of metabolism.

Suspicion

A history of acute deterioration after a period of apparent normalcy, which may be as short as a few hours, is a feature of many inherited metabolic diseases presenting in the newborn period. This is particularly true of inborn errors of metabolism in which symptoms are caused by postnatal accumulation of toxic, low molecular

Table 7.1 Circumstances suggesting the possibility of
an inherited metabolic disease

- deterioration after a period of apparent normalcy
- parental consanguinity
- family history of neonatal death
- rapidly progressive encephalopathy of obscure etiology
- severe metabolic acidosis
- hyperammonemia
- peculiar odor

weight metabolites, which had been removed prenatally by diffusion across the placenta and metabolized by the mother. Conditions in which this occurs include some of the amino acidopathies (notably nonketotic hyperglycinemia, maple syrup urine disease (MSUD), and hepatorenal tyrosinemia), urea cycle enzyme defects, many of the organic acidopathies, galactosemia, and hereditary fructose intolerance. Although a period of apparent normalcy is a frequent characteristic of these disorders, its absence does not exclude them from consideration. It may be obscured by coincident neonatal problems, such as birth trauma or complications of prematurity. The danger signals are summarized in Table 7.1.

Along with a history of acute deterioration after a period of apparent normalcy, a family history of a similar illness in a sibling or other blood relative, or a history of parental consanguinity, increases the possibility of an inherited metabolic disease.

Prominent nonspecific signs of diffuse cerebral dysfunction, especially if they are progressive, are a strong indication of inherited metabolic disease. The onset is usually gradual, often no more than poor sucking, drowsiness, and some floppiness. The mother may notice a change in the baby that is often initially dismissed by medical attendants. Vomiting often occurs, and it may be severe enough to suggest mechanical bowel obstruction. Deterioration is marked by increasing somnolence, progressing to stupor and coma, associated with the development of abnormalities of tone (hypotonia or hypertonia) and posturing (fisting, opisthotonus), abnormal movements (tongue-thrusting, lip-smacking, bicycling, tonic elevation of the arms, coarse tremors, myoclonic jerks), and disturbances of breathing (periodic respiration, tachypnea, apneic spells, hiccupping), bradycardia, and hypothermia. Early in the course of the deterioration, the signs of encephalopathy often fluctuate, with periods of what might seem like improvement alternating with periods of obvious progression, or periods of hypotonia punctuated by episodes of hypertonia, tremulousness, posturing, and myoclonus. The EEG generally shows nonspecific encephalopathic changes, often progressing to a burst-suppression pattern indicative of severe diffuse encephalopathy.

Much has been made of the importance of unusual odors in the early recognition of the possibility of an inborn error or metabolism. However, with the exception of MSUD and possibly isovaleric acidemia, these odors are rarely prominent or characteristic enough in newborn infants to be diagnostically useful. In fact, unusual dietary preferences of mothers appear to be a more common cause of abnormal odors in breast-fed infants. Signs specifically attributable to inherited metabolic diseases are sometimes obscured by problems commonly associated with acquired diseases. For example, organic acidopathies presenting in the newborn period are commonly associated with neutropenia, and sepsis often occurs in these patients as a result of the increased susceptibility to bacterial infection. The encephalopathy and metabolic acidosis caused by the metabolic disorder may be wrongly attributed entirely to the septicemia. The recognition of subtle clinical discrepancies between the severity of the apparent sepsis and the degree of acidosis in this situation may make the difference between early diagnosis of an inborn error of organic acid metabolism and missing it completely. There are some apparently acquired conditions in newborns that are particularly common complications of inherited metabolic disease. For example, *Escherichia coli* sepsis is common in infants with classical galactosemia. Primary respiratory alkalosis or pulmonary hemorrhage may be important clinical clues to hyperammonemia caused by a urea cycle enzyme defect (UCED).

Initial laboratory investigation

It is impossible to exaggerate the importance of speed in the investigation and treatment of possible inborn errors of metabolism in the newborn. Metabolic investigations should be initiated as soon as the possibility is considered, not after all other explanations for illness have been eliminated. This is particularly important for those conditions associated with hyperammonemia, such as UCEDs, transient hyperammonemia of the newborn (THAN) and the organic acidopathies. The outcome of treatment of these disorders is directly related to the rapidity with which metabolic problems are suspected and appropriate basic medical management is initiated.

An outline of the initial laboratory investigation of suspected inherited metabolic disease in an acutely ill infant is presented in Table 7.2. Some laboratory studies undertaken in the course of the investigation of other causes of disease are also helpful in the identification of possible inborn errors of metabolism. For example, plasma electrolyte abnormalities, identified in the course of the management of a newborn in shock of obscure etiology may suggest adrenogenital syndrome. The routine urinalysis may be very helpful in the investigation of a newborn infant presenting with acute encephalopathy due to MSUD: the urine often tests strongly for ketones, something in the newborn that should always be considered abnormal

Table 7.2 Initial laboratory investigation of suspected inherited metabolic disease presenting in the newborn period

Blood	Hemoglobin, white blood count, platelets
	Blood gases and plasma electrolytes (calculate anion gap)
	Glucose
	Ammonium
	Lactate
	Galactosemia screening test
	QUANTITATIVE Amino acid analysis
	Carnitine, total and free
	Blood or plasma acylcarnitine analysis (tandem MSMS)
	Calcium and magnesium
	Liver function tests, including albumin and prothrombin and partial thromboplastin times
	Plasma for storage at −20 °C: 2–5 ml
Urine	Ketones (Ames Acetest)
	Reducing substances (Ames Clinitest)
	Ketoacids (DNPH)
	Sulfites (Merck Sulfitest)
	Organic acids (GC-MS)
	Urine for storage at −20 °C: 10–20 ml

Abbreviations: DNPH, dinitrophenylhydrazine; GC-MS, gas chromatography-mass spectrometry; tandem MSMS, tandem mass spectrometry-mass spectrometry (see Chapter 9).

and investigated further. Similarly, the presence of marked neutropenia and thrombocytopenia in a newborn infant with clinical evidence of an encephalopathy and acute metabolic acidosis may signal a diagnosis of methylmalonic acidemia or propionic acidemia. The measurement of blood gases and plasma electrolytes and glucose is so widespread in acute-care pediatrics that a severe persistent metabolic acidosis would not likely be missed in an acutely ill infant. The measurement of blood ammonia should be carried out at the first indication of trouble, at the same time one might consider measuring the blood glucose, gases and electrolytes in a seriously sick newborn.

The importance of the analysis of plasma amino acids and urinary organic acids in the diagnosis of inborn errors of amino acid metabolism is widely accepted. It is imperative that the analysis of plasma amino acids be quantitative and carried out early in the investigation of any acutely ill infant in whom the possibility of an inborn error of metabolism is suspected. While it is somewhat more labor intensive than screening chromatography, quantitative analysis of amino acids in plasma is faster, and it is of critical importance in the diagnosis of specific amino acidopathies and in the differential diagnosis of hyperammonemia. Be contrast, quantitative analysis of amino acids in urine in the newborn period is rarely immediately helpful.

Analysis of urinary organic acids by gas chromatography-mass spectrometry (GC-MS) is critical to the early diagnosis of a number of treatable inborn errors of metabolism, such as methylmalonic acidemia, propionic acidemia, and defects in fatty acid oxidation. The technical issues are discussed in Chapter 9. The results are often diagnostic, even in the absence of any other biochemical abnormality. Analysis of urinary organic acids should, therefore, be considered early in the investigation of a possible inherited metabolic disease. Organic acid analysis, including analysis of organic acid esters, requires only 5–10 ml of urine. If analysis is delayed, the urine should be stored and transported frozen at −20 °C or lower. Under these conditions, most diagnostically important organic acids in urine are stable for several days to weeks.

Analysis of acylcarnitines and selected amino acids, by tandem MSMS, in very small amounts of blood, such as the dried blood spots used for screening for PKU is becoming more widely available as more tertiary-care pediatric institutions adopt this technology. This is a particularly fast and powerful tool for the investigation of a wide range of disorders of organic acid, fatty acid and amino acid metabolism. Tandem MSMS is spreading particularly rapidly in population screening of newborn infants (see Chapter 8).

Although the presence of nonglucose reducing substances in the urine of a sick newborn may suggest galactosemia, their absence does not rule out the possibility. Even short-term galactose restriction is usually sufficient to reverse the galactosuria of the disease. Because the enzyme defect is demonstrable in erythrocytes, but not in plasma, specimens of whole blood should be submitted for galactosemia screening, and the blood must be obtained before the infant receives any transfused blood.

Five clinical 'syndromes'

There are very few pathognomonic clinical signs that permit the immediate clinical diagnosis of inborn errors of metabolism in the newborn period. However, like inherited metabolic diseases presenting later in life, those with onset in the newborn period commonly describe one of five 'syndromes':
- encephalopathy without metabolic acidosis;
- encephalopathy with metabolic acidosis;
- hepatic syndrome;
- cardiac syndrome; or
- non-immune fetal hydrops.

Some of these disorders are associated with dysmorphic features that are discussed in Chapter 6.

Table 7.3 Inherited metabolic diseases presenting in the newborn period with acute encephalopathy without metabolic acidosis

Disease	Distinguishing features
Maple syrup urine disease	Plasma ammonium normal; urine positive for ketones; urinary DNPH test positive; marked elevation of plasma branched chain amino acids
Urea cycle enzyme defects	Plasma ammonium >250 μmol/L in absence of metabolic acidosis; normal liver function tests
Nonketotic hyperglycinemia	Elevated CSF glycine; no acidosis; no hyperammonemia; no hypoglycemia
Pyridoxine-dependent seizures	Therapeutic trial of vitamin B_6: immediate cessation of seizures and EEG abnormalities
Peroxisomal disorders (Zellweger syndrome)	Dysmorphism (see Chapter 6); elevated plasma very long-chain fatty acids
Molybdenum cofactor defect	Sulfites increased in urine; plasma urate levels low; increased S-sulfocysteine in urine

Abbreviations: DNPH, dinitrophenylhydrazine; CSF, cerebrospinal fluid.

Encephalopathy without metabolic acidosis

Encephalopathy without metabolic acidosis is a common problem in neonatology, most often the result of an hypoxic-ischemic insult to the brain occurring at or shortly after birth. A history of a period of apparent normalcy, or the absence of a history of birth trauma in keeping with the degree of encephalopathy, should be treated as indicators of the possibility of an inborn error of metabolism. There are six inherited metabolic diseases that characteristically present in the newborn period in this way (Table 7.3).

Maple syrup urine disease (MSUD)

MSUD is caused by a defect in branched-chain amino acid metabolism character-ized by deficiency of the enzyme, 2-ketoacyl-CoA decarboxylase, which catalyzes the second step in the oxidative metabolism of leucine, isoleucine, and valine. The defect causes accumulation of the respective 2-ketoacids and the branched-chain amino acids. Affected infants commonly present in the second or third week of life, though we have seen infants who presented with encephalopathy as early as the first 24 hours of life. The clinical findings are of a progressive, nonspecific, acute encephalopathy. The diagnosis can sometimes be made at the bedside because of the peculiar odor associated with the disease and the positive test for ketones in the urine. Although the disease received its name from the alleged resemblance of the smell to that of maple syrup, the odor actually more closely resembles that of burnt sugar, which should be a relief to clinicians who do not have access to the

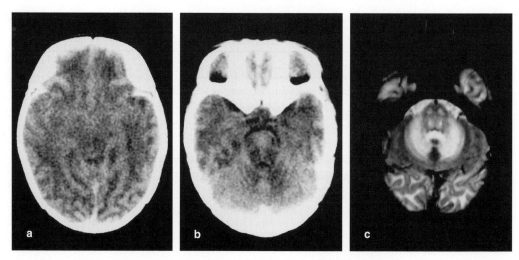

Figure 7.1   Imaging of the brain of an infant with maple syrup urine disease.
Panels **a**, Unenhanced axial CT scan at 10 days of age showing extensive acute supra-
and infra-tentorial edema; and **b**, prominence of brainstem swelling, which contrasts with
the usual sparing of the brainstem in infants with hypoxic-ischemic encephalopathy; **c**, T2-
weighted MRI [TR3000/TE120] at 2 weeks of age showing persistent edema and increased
signal in all visualized white matter with marked involvement of cerebellum.

syrup, a product almost exclusively of eastern Canada and northeastern U.S. Brain
swelling is a characteristic feature of the disease (Figure 7.1). Severe, intractable cerebral edema causing massive intracrainal hypertension, with bulging fontanelle and
diastasis of the sutures, develops relatively early and is invariably an indication of a
poor prognosis. Although hypoglycemia has been reported in newborn infants with
MSUD, this is a rare phenomenon in our experience. Although severe abnormalities of tone (hypotonia and hypertonia), posturing, and abnormal neurovegetative
movements are prominent in infants with advanced leucine encephalopathy, frank
seizures only occur later in the disorder.

   Although the urine of infants with MSUD generally tests strongly positive for
ketones, metabolic acidosis is not a prominent finding until later in the course of
the disease. This is important. The encephalopathy of MSUD is apparently caused
by accumulation of leucine, not by accumulation of the 2-ketoacids. The diagnosis
is confirmed by quantitative analysis of plasma amino acids. Analysis of urinary
organic acids as oxime derivatives (Chapter 9) shows the presence of branched-
chain 2-ketoacids and 2-hydroxyacids. Modest elevations of plasma branched-
chain amino acids are commonly seen in infants and children after short-term
starvation; the levels in MSUD presenting in the newborn period are several times
higher.

Treatment requires aggressive measures to lower plasma leucine levels, invariably including some form of efficient dialysis, such as hemodialysis or continuous venous-venous hemofiltration-dialysis (CVVHD). Intravenous lipid, along with high concentrations of glucose, is administered in an effort to decrease endogenous protein breakdown. Insulin is sometimes given, along with sufficient glucose to prevent hypoglycemia, in an attempt to increase endogenous protein biosynthesis. The clinical effectiveness of insulin in this situation is still not proven. The administration of mannitol, or other measures to control the cerebral edema, is not generally effective.

Urea cycle enzyme defects (UCED)

The metabolism of ammonium is reviewed in some detail in Chapter 2. Some of the defects presenting as hyperammonemic encephalopathy in older children or adults do not cause symptomatic hyperammonemia in the newborn period. The differential diagnosis of neonatal hyperammonemic encephalopathy lends itself well to an algorithmic approach (Figure 7.2), initially proposed by Saul Brusilow and his colleagues at Johns Hopkins Medical Center.

The onset and early course of the acute encephalopathy in infants with UCED are similar to that in MSUD, though hypotonia is more prominent and severe, and breathing may be abnormally rapid producing respiratory alkalosis as a result of central stimulation of ventilation by ammonium. Having determined the presence of significant hyperammonemia (>250 μmol/L; often as high as 2000 μmol/L), measurement of blood gases and plasma electrolytes shows whether ammonium accumulation is likely due to a UCED or is secondary to an organic acidopathy. The degree of the hyperammonemia is of no help in this regard: infants with organic acidopathies or with THAN will often have plasma ammonium levels at presentation in the same range as infants with untreated UCED.

The UCEDs presenting in the newborn period are clinically indistinguishable from each other. Differential diagnosis rests critically on quantitative analysis of plasma amino acids. The citrulline levels is particularly important, though normal levels in newborn infants are so low that some laboratories do not calculate the concentration unless specifically requested. Very high citrulline levels indicate the UCED is citrullinemia caused by deficiency of argininosuccinic acid (ASA) synthetase. Abnormally low citrulline levels suggest a defect in citrulline production, as a result of deficiency of either ornithine transcarbamoylase (OTC) or carbamoylphosphate synthetase I (CPS I). OTC deficiency is the most common of the UCEDs, and it is the only one transmitted as an X-linked recessive disorder. Although heterozygous females often present with subacute or acute encephalopathy later in infancy or childhood, they almost never present with hyperammonemic encephalopathy in the newborn period. OTC deficiency is

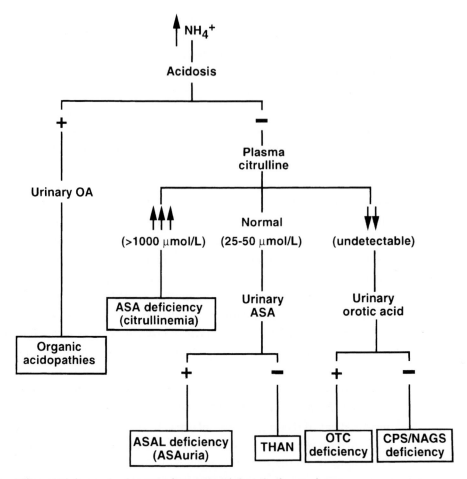

Figure 7.2   Differential diagnosis of urea cycle enzyme defects in the newborn.
Abbreviations: OA, organic acids; ASA, argininosuccinic acid; ASAL, argininosuccinic acid lyase; THAN, transient hyperammonemia of the newborn; OTC, ornithine transcarbamoylase; CPS, carbamoylphosphate synthetase I; NAGS, N-acetylglutamate synthetase.

characterized by accumulation of carbamoylphosphate, an intermediate in cytosolic pyrimidine biosynthesis. Diffusion of the compound from mitochondria into the cytosol stimulates pyrimidine biosynthesis causing accumulation of orotic acid. The presence of increased concentrations of orotic acid in the urine distinguishes OTC deficiency from CPS deficiency.

Normal or only modestly elevated plasma citrulline levels are seen in ASA lyase deficiency and in infants with THAN, which is often clinically indistinguishable from ASA lyase deficiency and other UCEDs. THAN is not an inherited metabolic disease; it is a condition of unknown etiology, generally affecting premature infants, usually with a history of low birth weight and respiratory distress. It also usually presents within the first 24 hours of life, unlike the UCED, which commonly present on or after the third day of life. The presence of ASA and its anhydrides in plasma, which are seen on the same quantitative amino acid analysis used to measure citrulline, confirms the diagnosis of ASA lyase deficiency. This is therapeutically important. The hyperammonemia in infants with ASA lyase deficiency is caused by inadequacy of the supply of intramitochondrial ornithine, derived from arginine, to combine with the carbamoylphosphate produced from condensation of ammonium and bicarbonate. Treatment of affected infants with intravenous arginine produces dramatic resolution of the hyperammonemia over a period of only a few hours, a response that is so typical it is diagnostic of the disease.

Another group of disorders that closely mimic UCEDs in the newborn period are some of the inherited defects of fatty acid oxidation, especially carnitine-acylcarnitine translocase. This condition is characterized by acute encephalopathy, associated with hyperammonemia, evidence of hepatocellular dysfunction, and usually with intractable cardiac dysrrhythmias, such as ventricular tachycardia. In these cases, the encephalopathy is often more severe than can be accounted for by hyperammonemia alone. The response of the hyperammonemia to peritoneal dialysis is particularly brisk, with virtually complete resolution occurring within a few hours. Clinical recovery is typically much slower, and many infants die, usually of the complications of cardiac rhythm defects.

The successful treatment of hyperammonemic encephalopathy caused by UCED demands early and very aggressive measures to control ammonium production and to facilitate its elimination. Intravenous glucose and lipid minimize ammonium production from endogenous protein breakdown. The administration of arginine is recommended even before the specific UCED has been identified because short-term administration of the amino acid is dramatically beneficial in patients with ASA lyase deficiency, at least modestly beneficial in the others, except perhaps in ASA synthetase deficiency, and harmful in none. The intravenous administration of sodium benzoate and sodium phenylacetate (or sodium phenylbutyrate, which is converted to phenylacetate in the body) is used extensively in the treatment of neonatal hyperammonemia, including that associated with UCED. These compounds lower ammonium levels by facilitating waste nitrogen excretion by alternative pathways (see Chapter 10). Specifically, sodium benzoate condenses with glycine to form hippuric acid, which is cleared from the circulation very efficiently by the kidney. Each molecule of benzoate metabolized in this fashion causes excretion of one atom of nitrogen. Sodium phenylacetate condenses with glutamine to form phenylacetylglutamine, which is also excreted in the urine taking with it two atoms of nitrogen per molecule. Since both glycine and glutamine are nonessential amino acids, they perform in this therapeutic strategy as a waste nitrogen 'metabolic sponge'.

Except in infants with ASA lyase deficiency, who respond so well to intravenous arginine, ammonium levels during acute hyperammonemia cannot be controlled adequately by medical measures alone. Restoration of normal plasma ammonium levels requires some form of aggressive dialysis, either hemodialysis or CVVHD. Regrettably, although the prognosis for infants with THAN who are identified and treated early and aggressively is excellent, the mortality associated with the disorder is over 50% in most centers owing primarily to delayed diagnosis.

Nonketotic hyperglycinemia (NKHG)

NKHG, due to deficiency of the hepatic glycine cleavage reaction, is characterized by early onset, rapidly progressive encephalopathy with virtually no secondary biochemical abnormalities to provide a clue to the underlying defect. In fact, it is the lack of acidosis, ketosis, hypoglycemia, hyperammonemia, hepatocellular dysfunction, cardiac, renal, or hematologic abnormalities, in the face of clinical evidence of very severe diffuse cerebral dysfunction that suggests the diagnosis. The encephalopathy characteristically progresses quickly to respiratory arrest, and many affected infants become intubated and ventilated before the diagnosis is confirmed.

Analysis of plasma amino acids usually shows elevation of glycine concentrations. However, plasma concentrations may be only modestly elevated, and sometimes they are normal, presumably because glycine reabsorption by the kidney is not mature at birth. Renal clearances of the amino acid are high, and urinary glycine levels are almost always elevated. Since elevations of plasma glycine are a common manifestation of various disorders of organic acid metabolism, hyperglycinemia by itself is not sufficient to make the diagnosis. The elevation of glycine levels in the CSF is sufficiently consistent and specific to be considered diagnostic of the disease.

Treatment of NKHG is unsatisfactory. Aggressive treatment with intravenous fluids, glucose, and sodium benzoate will restore plasma glycine levels to normal or even much lower. However, it has little effect on CSF glycine levels. Attempts have been made to treat the condition with neuromodulators, such as diazepam, strychnine, and dextromethorphan. Only dextromethorphan appears to have any beneficial effect, and the effect is incomplete. Curiously, after several days of ventilatory support, infants with NKHG often appear to improve and can be safely extubated. However, almost all will have suffered very severe, irreparable brain damage. A small number of cases have been reported in which the defect in glycine metabolism appears to be severe, but transient. Most of the patients with this rare, transient variant are currently alive and apparently well.

Pyridoxine-dependent seizures

Pyridoxine-dependent seizures is one of the few inherited metabolic diseases in which seizures are particularly prominent and severe in the absence of any other significant clinical abnormality (see Chapter 2). Affected infants characteristically present very early, in the first few hours or days of life, with intractable, generalized, tonic-clonic seizures and associated EEG abnormalities. On direct questioning, the mother of the infant will often report that she was aware of paroxysms of fetal movement later in the course of the pregnancy. These have been interpreted to be intrauterine convulsions. Apart from the seizures, affected infants appear normal, though failure to control the convulsions results ultimately in the development of moderately severe mental retardation. The most remarkable feature of this condition, which may be the result of a defect in glutamic acid decarboxylase, is its dramatic response to administration of vitamin B_6 (pyridoxine). The intravenous administration of 100 mg of the vitamin results in prompt cessation of the seizures and normalization of the EEG abnormalities.

Peroxisomal disorders (Zellweger syndrome)

Infants with Zellweger syndrome are often acutely symptomatic within a few hours of birth. They characteristically show profound hypotonia, typical abnormalities of the face and skull, nystagmus, seizures, jaundice, hepatomegaly, and other anomalies that are described in more detail in Chapter 6. Plain radiographs of the long bones show the presence of abnormal punctate calcifications in the epiphyses of the knees and other joints; ultrasound examination of the abdomen shows enlargement of the liver and kidneys with cystic changes in both organs; and CT scans of the head show cerebral dysgenesis with subcortical cystic changes. Routine laboratory studies show evidence of hepatocellular dysfunction with elevations of bilirubin and transaminases, hypoalbuminemia, and prolonged prothrombin and partial thromboplastin times. Confirmatory biochemical abnormalities specific to the disease include elevation of plasma levels of very long-chain fatty acids (C26:0 and C26:1), decreased erythrocyte plasmalogens, and the presence of pipecolic acid and bile acid intermediates in plasma. Liver biopsy shows evidence of bile stasis, cystic changes, and fibrosis; electron microscopic examination reveals the absence of peroxisomes.

Molybdenum cofactor deficiency (sulfite oxidase/xanthine oxidase deficiency

The development, within the first week or two of birth, of intractable tonic-clonic seizures in an encephalopathic infant without hypoglycemia, hypocalcemia, hyperammonemia, or significant metabolic acidosis, is suggestive of molybdenum cofactor deficiency, or the rare disorder, isolated sulfite oxidase deficiency. Imaging studies may show early cerebral edema followed rapidly by marked cerebral and cerebellar atrophy, hydrocephalus *ex vacuo*, and signs of hypomyelination of white matter. The presence of evidence of cerebral dysgenesis suggests that considerable damage occurs before birth.

Molybdenum cofactor deficiency is associated with combined deficiency of the two molybdenum-dependent enzymes, xanthine oxidase and sulfite oxidase. The clinical and pathologic abnormalities in isolated sulfite oxidase deficiency are indistinguishable from the changes in molybdenum cofactor deficiency. The deficiency of xanthine oxidase causes marked depression of plasma uric acid levels, an important and easily accessible clue to the underlying disorder. Urine amino acid analysis shows the presence of increased levels of S-sulfocysteine. However, the diagnosis can often be made at the bedside by tests of the urine for the presence of sulfite using commercially available dipsticks (Merckoquant 10013 Sulfit Test). The urine must be fresh because sulfite is oxidized rapidly in air at room temperature. The disease is almost always associated with severe brain damage and death in early childhood. Survival beyond two years of age is often, though not always, associated with the development of dislocation of the ocular lens.

Encephalopathy with metabolic acidosis

In infants with inherited metabolic diseases characterized by encephalopathy associated with metabolic acidosis, the tachypnea caused by the acidosis may be severe enough to suggest a diagnosis of primary pulmonary disease. Typically, the infant is apparently well until three to five days of age when feeding difficulties and other nonspecific signs of encephalopathy develop, accompanied by a significant increase in respiratory rate and effort. Chest radiographs typically show nothing more sinister than some hyperinflation, and the measurement of blood gases confirms the presence of a primary metabolic acidosis.

The diagnostic workup is similar to that described in more detail in Chapter 3. Metabolic acidosis due to renal tubular bicarbonate losses, severe enough to be clinically obvious, is rare in newborn infants; by comparison, metabolic acidosis caused by accumulation of organic acids is relatively common. The anion gap in these patients is usually increased (>25 mmol/L), and measurement of lactate, 3-hydroxybutyrate, and acetoacetate usually account for only part of the increase. *Identification of the unmeasured anion by urinary organic acid analysis is an important lead to making a diagnosis.*

Organic acidurias

Although many of the disorders of organic acid metabolism presenting later in infancy or childhood (Chapter 3) may present in the newborn period, some are relatively common and are particularly likely to present in the first few weeks of life, rather than later (Table 7.4).

Table 7.4 Organic acidopathies presenting as acute illness in the newborn period

Disease	Defect	Urinary organic acids	Distinguishing clinical features
Propionic acidemia	Propionyl-CoA carboxylase	Propionate, 3-hydroxypropionate, propionylglycine, methylcitrate, tiglylglycine, 3-hydroxybutyrate, acetoacetate	Severe metabolic acidosis, hyperammonemia, neutropenia, thrombocytopenia
Methylmalonic acidemia	Methylmalonyl-CoA mutase; *Cbl* defects, especially *A* and *B*	Methylmalonate, methylcitrate, 3-hydroxybutyrate, acetoacetate	Severe metabolic acidosis, hyperammonemia, neutropenia, thrombocytopenia
Isovaleric acidemia	Isovaleryl-CoA dehydrogenase	Isovalerylglycine, 3-hydroxyisovalerate, lactate, 3-hydroxybutyrate, acetoacetate	Severe metabolic acidosis, hyperammonemia, neutropenia, thrombocytopenia, odor of sweaty feet
Holocarboxylase synthetase deficiency	Holocarboxylase synthetase	Lactate, 3-hydroxybutyrate and acetoacetate (due to PC deficiency); 3-methylcrotonate, 3-methylcrotonylglycine, 3-hydroxyisovalerate (due to 3-MCC deficiency); and propionate, 3-hydroxypropionate, methylcitrate, tiglylglycine (due to PCC deficiency)	Severe metabolic acidosis, hyperammonemia, thrombocytopenia, seizures
HMG-CoA lyase deficiency	HMG-CoA lyase	3-Hydroxy-3-methylglutarate, 3-methylglutaconate, 3-methylglutarate, 3-hydroxyisovalerate	Severe metabolic acidosis without ketosis, hyperammonemia, hypoglycemia, macrocephaly
Glutaric aciduria, type II (multiple acyl-CoA dehydrogenase deficiency)	Electron transfer flavoprotein (ETF) or ETF dehydrogenase deficiency	Glutarate, 2-hydroxyglutarate, ethylmalonate, adipate, suberate, sebacate, dodecanedioate, isovalerylglycine, hexanoylglycine	Facial dysmorphism, cerebral dysgenesis, cystic kidneys
3-Hydroxyisobutyric aciduria	3-Hydroxyisobutyryl-CoA dehydrogenase	3-Hydroxyisobutyrate, lactate	Facial dysmorphism, cerebral dysgenesis, hypotonia, failure to thrive, episodes of acidosis
5-Oxoprolinuria (pyroglutamic aciduria)	Glutathione synthetase	5-Oxoproline (pyroglutamate)	Severe, persistent metabolic acidosis, hemolytic anemia, neutropenia
D-2-Hydroxyglutaric aciduria	D-2-Hydroxyglutaric acid transhydrogenase	D-2-Hydroxyglutarate	Seizures, infantile spasms (with hypsarrhythmia), choreoathetosis

Abbreviations: HMG-CoA, 3-hydroxy-3-methylglutaryl-CoA; ETF, electron transfer flavoprotein; 3-MCC, 3-methylcrotonyl-CoA; PCC, propionyl-CoA carboxylase; PC, pyruvate carboxylase.

Propionic acidemia, methylmalonic acidemia, and isovaleric acidemia are almost clinically indistinguishable from each other when they present as acute illness in the newborn period. In each, metabolic decompensation is heralded by signs of encephalopathy accompanied by marked metabolic acidosis. In isovaleric acidemia, it is often associated with a peculiar odor. Hyperammonemia is common, and it is often severe ($NH_4^+ > 1000$ μmol/L). Neutropenia and thrombocytopenia also occur, predisposing affected infants to bacterial infection and bleeding. Plasma carnitine levels are decreased, and the proportion of esterified carnitine, relative to total carnitine (normally approximately 0.25), is generally markedly increased. Plasma amino acid analysis shows marked increases in glycine concentrations. Tests for ketones in the urine are often positive. Urinary organic acid analysis shows changes typical of the various disorders. In some centers rapid and specific diagnosis is possible by tandem MSMS analysis of plasma acylcarnitines (see Chapter 9). Confirmation of the diagnosis requires analysis of the relevant enzyme activities in cultured skin fibroblasts, coupled in some cases with specific mutation analysis.

Infants with severe, neonatal-onset holocarboxylase synthetase deficiency present with many of the same clinical features as infants with propionic acidemia (Table 7.4), presumably because propionyl-CoA carboxylase is one of the enzymes affected by the defect in biotin metabolism. The urinary organic acid pattern, which shows high concentrations of the immediate substrate of each of the three catalytic carboxylases affected, is diagnostic of the disease. Treatment with pharmacologic doses of biotin reverses the metabolic abnormalities.

Infants with severe variants of 3-hydroxy-3-methylglutaryl-CoA (HMG-CoA) lyase deficiency commonly present with rapidly progressing encephalopathy associated with severe metabolic acidosis, hypoketotic hypoglycemia, and hyperammonemia. Some biochemical evidence of hepatocellular dysfunction, with elevated bilirubin and transaminases, is also generally present. Urinary organic acid analysis shows large amounts of 3-hydroxy-3-methylglutarate, 3-methylglutaconate, 3-methylglutarate, and 3-hydroxyisovalerate. Diagnosis is confirmed by analysis of enzyme activity in cultured skin fibroblasts.

Severe encephalopathy, metabolic acidosis, hyperammonemia, along with facial dysmorphism, cerebral dysgenesis, and other anomalies, are features of severe multiple acyl-CoA dehydrogenase deficiency (glutaric aciduria, type II or GA II) and 3-hydroxyisobutyric aciduria (see Chapter 6). Congenital visceral anomalies, such as renal cystic dysplasia, and hypoglycemia are characteristic of GA II and severe neonatal CPT II deficiency. All are rare conditions, particularly 3-hydroxyisobutyric aciduria. And all are generally rapidly fatal when they present in the newborn period. The diagnosis in each case is suggested by the results of urinary organic acid analysis and is confirmed by specific enzyme analysis in cultured skin fibroblasts.

Congenital lactic acidosis

The differentiation between the encephalopathy associated with congenital lactic acidosis, resulting either from primary defects of pyruvate metabolism or mitochondrial electron transport defects, and hypoxic-ischemic encephalopathy (HIE) may be difficult. Intractable seizures are commonly prominent in both. However, the clinical abnormalities and degree and duration of the lactic acidosis in newborns with defects in mitochondrial energy metabolism are usually out of proportion to the apparent severity of any hypoxic-ischemic insult experienced by the infant.

Signs that are particularly suggestive of severe primary congenital lactic acidosis include:

- small size for gestational age (SGA);
- subtle facial dysmorphism;
- structural malformations of the brain;
- multisystem disease (brain, kidney, liver, heart, eyes).

Simultaneous measurement of plasma lactate and pyruvate levels and calculations of the lactate/pyruvate (L/P) ratio is useful to distinguish pyruvate dehydrogenase (PDH) deficiency, in which the ratio is normal (15–20), from the severe neonatal form of pyruvate carboxylase deficiency (type B) and mitochondrial electron transport defects, in which the ratio is invariably >25. The L/P ratio is also normal in inborn errors of gluconeogenesis, such as glycogen storage disease, type I (GSD I) and fructose-1,6-diphosphatase (FDP) deficiency, which may sometimes present in the newborn period. However, they are associated with prominent hepatomegaly, hypoglycemia, and ketosis (in FDP deficiency), and encephalopathy is not present unless it is the result of severe, uncontrolled hypoglycemia (see section 'Hypoglycemia').

Many infants with severe PDH deficiency have facial dysmorphism suggestive of fetal alcohol syndrome: narrow skull with high, bossed forehead, broad nasal bridge, small nose with anteverted nares, and large ears. In many cases imaging studies of the brain show cerebral and cerebellar atrophy and cystic changes in the cerebrum and basal ganglia, and often agenesis or partial agenesis of the corpus callosum. The lactic acidosis in infants with PDH deficiency is often aggravated by high glucose intakes and ameliorated to some extent by high fat intakes. The diagnosis is confirmed by measurement of enzyme activity in leukocytes or cultured fibroblasts.

Unlike in older infants presenting with milder variants of the disease (see Chapter 3), the L/P ratio in neonates with the pyruvate carboxylase deficiency, type B, is elevated (>25). Postprandial ketoacidosis is a feature of this disorder, but the ratio of 3-hydroxybutyrate to acetoacetate is paradoxically decreased. Other prominent features are hyperammonemia and elevations of the plasma concentrations of the amino acids, citrulline, lysine, and proline, in addition to hyperalaninemia. The diagnosis is confirmed by enzyme assay in leukocytes or cultured skin fibroblasts.

Multisystem involvement is very suggestive of mitochondrial electron transport chain (ETC) defects, most commonly mitochondrial ETC complex I or complex IV (cytochrome c oxidase). One or more of skeletal myopathy, hypertrophic cardiomy-opathy, hepatocellular dysfunction, renal tubular dysfunction, or cataracts are char-acteristic features of the neonatal variants of this class of diseases. The L/P ratio in these disorders is always elevated (>25). Imaging studies show that the brain is small with spongiform degenerative changes in the cerebrum and attenuation of white matter. Muscle biopsy in infants presenting this early does not show the ragged red fibers that are so typical of mitochondrial ETC defects presenting later in life (see Chapters 2 and 9). The diagnosis requires specialized studies on cultured fibroblasts or muscle (see Chapter 9). Most neonatal variants of the mitochondrial ETC defects are invariably and rapidly fatal. However, in a few patients, cytochrome c oxidase (complex IV) deficiency causing severe congenital lactic acidosis reverses spontaneously without serious permanent neurologic deficits.

Dicarboxylic aciduria

Pathologic dicarboxylic aciduria occurs most often as a manifestation of disorders of fatty acid oxidation (see Chapter 4). The clinical features of neonates presenting with fatty acid oxidation defects may be dominated by signs of any combination of encephalopathy, hepatocellular dysfunction, skeletal myopathy, or cardiomyopa-thy. Clinical generalizations about this group of inborn errors of metabolism must be regarded as provisional because the numbers of cases, particularly of patients presenting in the first few days or weeks of life, are small. However, marked hypo-tonia and lethargy seem to be a feature of them all, and hepatomegaly is often prominent. Hypoketotic hypoglycemia, another characteristic feature of this class of disorders presenting in older infants, is common in affected neonates, and it is often accompanied by lactic acidosis, though this is not usually severe. Mild to mod-erately severe hyperammonemia is common. Plasma carnitine levels are decreased, and the esterified fraction is increased markedly. The urinary organic acid abnor-malities, summarized in Table 7.4, are usually characteristic of the diseases.

Medium-chain acyl-CoA dehydrogenase (MCAD) deficiency, the most common of the hereditary fatty acid oxidation defects in older infants (see Chapter 4), is a very rare cause of severe illness in the newborn. It may be heralded by little more than marked hypotonia and mild lactic acidosis and hyperammonemia, without hypoglycemia or significant hepatomegaly. Urinary organic acid analysis shows the presence of large amounts of the medium-chain dicarboxylic acids (adipate, suber-ate, and sebacate) with very low levels of 3-hydroxybutyrate. Short-chain acyl-CoA dehydrogenase (SCAD) deficiency is characterized by nonspecific encephalopathy with poor feeding, failure to thrive, hypotonia, episodes of hypertonia and seizure-like activity, progressive muscle weakness and cardiomyopathy. Urinary organic acid analysis shows large amounts of ethylmalonic acid, methylsuccinate, glutarate, butyrylglycine, and hexanoylglycine. The organic acid pattern is similar to that found in infants with GA II, or with cytochrome c oxidase deficiency.

Long-chain acyl-CoA dehydrogenase (LCAD) deficiency and long-chain hydroxyacyl-CoA dehydrogenase (LCHAD) deficiency, presenting in the newborn period, show encephalopathy, hepatocellular dysfunction, metabolic acidosis, hypoketotic hypoglycemia, and marked hypotonia. However, the prominence and severity of the cardiomyopathy, particularly in infants with LCHAD deficiency, sets this group apart from MCAD and SCAD deficiency. Urinary organic acid analysis shows large amounts of long-chain dicarboxylic and monocarboxylic acids in addition to medium-chain dicarboxylics. In the case of LCHAD deficiency, the 12-carbon and 14 carbon 3-hydroxydicarboxylic and monocarboxylic acids are particularly characteristic, though small amounts may sometimes be seen in infants with neonatal hepatitis.

Neonatal hepatic syndrome

The pattern of clinical abnormalities in patients with inherited metabolic disorders presenting with acute liver disease in the newborn period may be dominated by:
• jaundice;
• severe hepatocellular dysfunction (jaundice, hypoglycemia, hyperammonemia, elevated transaminases, ascites and anasarca, and coagulopathy);
• hypoglycemia with little evidence of generalized hepatocellular dysfunction.

Jaundice

Jaundice is the principal, if not the only, sign of inborn errors of bilirubin metabolism, such as Gilbert syndrome, Lucey-Driscoll syndrome, Crigler-Najjar syndrome, and Dubin-Johnson syndrome (see Chapter 4). All are benign except for the type I variant of Crigler-Najjar syndrome, caused by total deficiency of hepatic uridine diphosphate (UDP)-glucuronosyltransferase. Infants with this defect develop severe intractable unconjugated hyperbilirubinemia within 24–48 hours of birth and invariably develop kernicterus.

In all other inherited metabolic conditions in which neonatal jaundice may be prominent, the hyperbilirubinemia is generally conjugated and is associated with other evidence of generalized hepatocellular dysfunction. Infants with classical galactosemia commonly present with a history of persistent hyperbilirubinemia. The bilirubin is often unconjugated in the early stages of the disease, later becoming predominantly conjugated. The liver is enlarged and firm, and some evidence of hepatocellular dysfunction, sometimes severe, is invariably present, including hypoglycemia, elevated transaminases, mild to moderate coagulopathy, and mild hypoalbuminemia. Ascites is often seen, even in the absence of portal hypertension or hypoalbuminemia. Hyperchloremic metabolic acidosis, hypophosphatemia, and generalized amino aciduria indicate the presence of some renal tubular damage. Slit-lam examination of the eyes often shows the presence of punctate lens opacities, even very early in the disease. These early cataracts generally resolve on treatment. Some infants with galactosemia present with severe cerebral edema and signs of intracranial hypertension. For reasons that are not well understood, infants with galactosemia are particularly susceptible to fulminant *Escherichia coli* sepsis. In fact any infant with *E. coli* sepsis should be considered possibly to have the disease and be investigated accordingly.

The presence of nonglucose reducing substances in the urine in an infant with these findings is strong presumptive evidence of classical galactosemia. The galactosuria in infants with the disease is evanescent: if the infant has been off galactose-containing formula for more than a few hours, tests for reducing substances are likely to be normal. Testing for reducing substances, using Clinitest tablets (Ames), can and should be done at the bedside at the earliest opportunity. Most hospitals caring for sick infants make available a galactosemia screening test, a semi-quantitative measurement of galactose-1-phosphate uridyltransferase (GALT) in red blood cells. Blood must be taken for this test before the infant receives any blood transfusions. The test is done on dried blood spots collected on filter paper, similar to the spots used for screening for PKU (see Chapter 8). It relies on the presence of glucose-6-phosphate dehydrogenase (G6PD) activity in the sample, and the screening test may, therefore, be falsely positive in infants with G6PD deficiency. Confirmation of the diagnosis is by quantitative analysis of GALT in red cells.

Galactosemia caused by generalized deficiency of UDPgalactose 4-epimerase is extremely rare and clinically indistinguishable from classical galactosemia. In patients with 4-epimerase deficiency, galactosemia screening tests based on analysis of red cell galactose-1-phosphate may be positive, while those based on measurement of GALT activity are negative. The diagnosis is suggested by strong clinical evidence for galactosemia, including galactosuria, with normal GALT activity, and it is confirmed by measurement of 4-epimerase activity in cultured skin fibroblasts.

Neonatal hepatitis, with intrahepatic cholestasis, multiple amino acidemia (citrulline, threonine, methionine, and tyrosine), hypoproteinemia, galactosemia, hypoglycemia, and mild elevation of transaminases, is characteristic of citrin deficiency (citrullinemia, type II; CTLN2). Elevations of plasma galactose concentrations may be sufficient to cause cataracts. Newborn screening tests based on measurement of plasma galactose levels may be positive, but measurements of GALT and UDP-galactose 4-epimerase activities are typically normal. The condition often resolves with nothing more than supportive therapy only to re-emerge, several years later, as hyperammonemic encephalopathy (see Chapter 2). The diagnosis is confirmed by demonstration of mutations in the *SLC25A13* gene, a gene coding for a calcium-binding mitochondrial aspartate-glutamate carrier. A significant number of patients with CTLN2 develop hepatomas at relatively young ages. Almost all reported cases have been Japanese.

Infants with alpha-1-antitrypsin deficiency may present with persistent neonatal jaundice, predominantly conjugated and accompanied by other evidence of cholestasis. The jaundice commonly resolves spontaneously over a period of 6–10 weeks, and affected children often remain well until some months later when they present with cirrhosis with portal hypertension (see Chapter 4). The diagnosis may be suspected on the basis of the presence of typical inclusions in liver obtained by biopsy. Confirmation is based on demonstration of the presence of homozygosity for the protease inhibitor PI type ZZ phenotype, or by mutation analysis.

Severe hepatocellular dysfunction

Severe hepatocellular dysfunction due to inborn errors of metabolism presenting in early infancy is characterized by hypoglycemia, ascites, anasarca, hypoalbuminemia, hyperammonemia, hyperbilirubinemia (often only mild), and coagulopathy. The manifestations of liver disease are relatively nonspecific. Identification of the underlying defect is often based on recognition of specific secondary metabolic abnormalities (Table 7.5).

Hepatorenal tyrosinemia (hereditary tyrosinemia, type I), caused by deficiency of fumarylacetoacetase (FAH), may present in the newborn period, though it more commonly presents later in infancy (see Chapter 4). Presentation in the first few weeks of life is characterized by evidence of massive, acute hepatocellular dysfunction, along with evidence of renal tubular dysfunction (hyperchloremic metabolic acidosis, hypophosphatemia, glucosuria, and generalized amino aciduria). The liver is enlarged, hard, and irregular in shape, a reflection of the degree of fibrosis already present at birth. Cardiomyopathy, sometimes severe enough to cause congestive heart failure, is common.

Analysis of plasma amino acids shows increased levels of tyrosine, phenylalanine, and methionine, though the levels may not be significantly higher than in infants with other types of severe hepatocellular disease. Other biochemical abnormalities supporting the diagnosis include depressed plasma cysteine levels and marked elevation of plasma α-fetoprotein levels. The coagulopathy of hepatorenal tyrosinemia is characterized by dysfibrinogenemia, which is reflected in disproportionate prolongation of the reptilase time compared with the thrombin time. Urinary organic acid analysis usually shows the presence of succinylacetone, which is a specific characteristic of the disease. The absence of succinylacetone in the urine

Table 7.5 Inherited metabolic diseases presenting with severe hepatocellular dysfunction in the newborn period

Disease	Associated findings	Distinguishing features
Amino acidopathies		
Hepatorenal tyrosinemia	Renal tubular dysfunction	Massive elevation of plasma α-fetoprotein; presence of succinylacetone in urine
Disorders of carbohydrate metabolism		
Hereditary fructose intolerance	Renal tubular dysfunction; lactic acidosis, hyperuricemia, hypoglycemia	History of exposure to fructose in the diet; deficiency of fructose-1-phosphate aldolase in liver
Glycogen storage disease, type IV	Hypoglycemia, severe coagulopathy	Severe generalized hepatocellular dysfunction; deficiency of hepatic glycogen brancher enzyme activity in liver
Fatty acid oxidation defects		
MCAD deficiency	Hypoketotic hypoglycemia, encephalopathy	Medium-chain dicarboxylic aciduria
LCAD deficiency	Hypoketotic hypoglycemia, cardiomyopathy, encephalopathy	Long-chain monocarboxylic aciduria
LCHAD	Encephalopathy, cardiomyopathy	Long-chain 3-hydroxymono- and dicarboxylic aciduria
CPT II deficiency	Hypoketotic hypoglycemia, cardiomyopathy, encephalopathy, dysmorphic features, cystic kidneys, cardiac arrhythmias	Deficiency of CPT II in cultured fibroblasts
CACT deficiency	Encephalopathy, metabolic acidosis, hyperammonemia, myopathy, cardiac arrhythmias	Marked elevation of plasma and urine long-chain acylcarnitines
Disorders of mitochondrial energy metabolism		
Cytochrome c oxidase deficiency	Encephalopathy, myopathy, lactic acidosis, retinitis pigmentosa, sensorineural hearing impairment	Paradoxical increase in plasma ketones after meals; deficiency of cytochrome c oxidase in liver and muscle
Mitochondrial DNA depletion syndrome	Myopathy, lactic acidosis, ketosis, renal tubular dysfunction	Marked depletion of mtDNA in muscle, brain, ± liver
Lysosomal storage diseases		
Niemann-Pick disease	Neonatal hepatitis	Storage histiocytes in bone marrow; deficiency of acid sphingomyelinase in type A variant; deficiency of cholesterol esterification in type C

Abbreviations: MCAD, medium-chain acyl-CoA dehydrogenase; LCAD, long-chain acyl-CoA dehydrogenase; LCHAD, long-chain 3-hydroxyacyl-CoA dehydrogenase; CPT carnitine palmitoyltransferase; CACT, carnitine-acylcarnitine translocase.

does not exclude the diagnosis of hepatorenal tyrosinemia. If the clinical suspicion is high, urinary organic acid analysis should be repeated at least three times and fumarylacetoacetase activity should be measured in leukocytes or fresh liver tissue.

The association of encephalopathy with evidence of moderately severe hepato-cellular dysfunction and cardiomyopathy are features of fatty acid oxidation defects (FAOD), which may make them difficult to distinguish from hepatorenal tyrosine-mia. Generalized hypotonia, the result of involvement of skeletal muscle, may be profound in both. However, biosynthetic defects (hypoalbuminemia and coagu-lopathy) are not generally as prominent FAOD, and the cardiomyopathy is generally much more severe, except in MCAD deficiency, sometimes progressing rapidly to intractable congestive heart failure, fatal cardiac arrhythmias, and death. Plasma α-fetoprotein levels are not elevated, and renal tubular function is not disturbed. Urinary organic acid analysis shows the presence of aromatic tyrosine metabolites and fatty acid oxidation intermediates, similar to those seen in older children with FAOD (see Chapter 4), but succinylacetone is not found, regardless of the sever-ity of the liver disease. The organic acid abnormalities in infants with FAOD are notoriously evanescent. They may clear early, making the presumptive diagnosis on the basis of urinary organic acid analysis difficult. In these situations, analysis of plasma acylcarnitines by tandem MSMS is particularly helpful. The diagnosis and classification of the FAOD is generally confirmed by analysis of fatty acid oxidation in cultured skin fibroblasts by laboratories with special expertise in this area (see Chapter 9).

The clinical features of acute, neonatal hepatorenal tyrosinemia and early-onset variants of the hereditary fatty acid oxidation defects may be difficult to distinguish from neonatal hemochromatosis or neonatal hepatitis. In both these acquired con-ditions, plasma α-fetoprotein levels may be very high, though not usually as high as in tyrosinemia. In neonatal hemochromatosis, plasma ferritin concentrations are typically extremely high. Urinary organic acid analysis will show the presence of the same mixture of aromatic tyrosine metabolites that occurs in tyrosinemia as a result of severe hepatocellular dysfunction, but the presence of succinylacetone is specific for hepatorenal tyrosinemia. The histopathologic appearances of tissue obtained by liver biopsy are also different in the three diseases.

The association of acute hepatocellular dysfunction (hypoglycemia, hepato-megaly, elevated transaminases), severe lactic acidosis, hyperuricemia, hypophos-phatemia, and hyperchloremic metabolic acidosis with the ingestion of fructose is characteristic of hereditary fructose intolerance (HFI) presenting in the newborn period. This most commonly occurs when feeding problems prompt the use of soy protein-based formulas in which the carbohydrate is supplied as sucrose. However, it may also occur when sugar-water, prepared with cane sugar, is given in efforts to sooth a fussy baby. The hypoglycemia and lactic acidosis may be severe enough to be life-threatening. Presentation of HFI in the newborn period has become less common now that neonates requiring supplementation are given oral glucose solution, rather than sugar-water. Enzymic confirmation of the diagnosis is difficult because the deficient enzyme (fructose-1-phosphate aldolase) is expressed only in liver. Fructose loading tests are dangerous and should not be done. Mutation analysis, testing for the common mutations associated with HFI, is safe and often diagnostic.

Defects in the acylcarnitine synthesis-translocation-hydrolysis process (see Chapter 4), such as carnitine palmitoyltransferase I (CPT I) deficiency, CPT II deficiency, or carnitine-acylcarnitine translocase deficiency (CACT), generally present with hepatomegaly and severe hepatocellular dysfunction, along with encephalopathy, hyperammonemia, metabolic acidosis, and hypotonia. Cardiac arrhythmias appear to be a prominent feature of CACT deficiency. Unlike the other inherited defects of fatty acid oxidation, the urinary organic acids are usually completely normal, or show only nonspecific abnormalities. In CPT I deficiency, the plasma carnitine concentrations are often elevated, and the acylcarnitines are generally not remarkable. However, in CACT deficiency, plasma carnitine levels are often profoundly depressed, and tandem MSMS analysis shows accumulation of long-chain acylcarnitines in plasma. Mitochondrial DNA depletion syndrome may present with similar clinical findings. However, affected infants are usually severely ketotic.

We have managed two infants presenting with severe cirrhosis in the first week of life because of glycogen storage disease, type IV (GSD IV) caused by brancher enzyme deficiency. The total failure of biosynthetic functions was particularly remarkable. Disease presenting this early is invariably rapidly fatal, and diagnosis is generally confirmed by the typical histopathologic findings in the liver and biochemical studies done at autopsy. We have also seen a few infants with Woman disease (lysosomal acid lipase deficiency) presenting in early infancy with marked failure to thrive, massive hepatomegaly, and hepatocellular dysfunction. The diagnosis is supported by demonstrating calcification of the adrenal glands, and it is confirmed by analysis of acid lipase in peripheral blood leukocytes.

Many infants who present later in infancy or childhood with neurologic or hepatic abnormalities of Niemann-Pick disease, irrespective of the variant of the disease, have a history of persistent neonatal jaundice. The histopathologic changes in liver obtained by biopsy are often indistinguishable from giant cell hepatitis. The jaundice and associated hepatomegaly generally resolve spontaneously over a period of days of a few weeks.

Hypoglycemia

Hypoglycemia is a frequent, nonspecific complication of almost any severe illness in the newborn. Prematurity, intrauterine growth retardation, maternal diabetes mellitus, sepsis, and asphyxia are just a few of the common conditions associated with symptomatic hypoglycemia. The underlying disorder is generally obvious, and the blood glucose is relatively easy to control. Hypoglycemia may also be prominent, though generally not difficult to control, in infants with adrenal insufficiency or growth hormone deficiency. The hypoglycemia occurring as a result of hyperinsulinism caused by nesidioblastosis is typically much more difficult to correct, requiring iv glucose infusion rates exceeding 12 mg/kg body weight/minute, or administration of glucagon, to control. Infusion of glucose at rates exceeding 12 mg/kg/minute often produces lactic acidosis, which may cause diagnostic confusion unless the relationship with the rapid infusion of glucose is noted.

In many of the inherited metabolic diseases that may be associated with neonatal hypoglycemia, instability of the blood glucose is a relatively trivial matter compared with other problems, such as metabolic acidosis and hyperammonemia or severe hepatocellular dysfunction. However, hypoglycemia is often the only sign of disease in infants with primary disorders of gluconeogenesis presenting in the first week or two of life. The hypoglycemia is clearly related to fasting, and, although it may be severe, it is typically relatively easy to control with nothing more that regular feeds at intervals of three to four hours.

GSD I may present in the newborn period with hypoglycemia associated with lactic acidosis. The hypoglycemia is usually easy to control by intravenous administration of relatively small amounts of glucose (6–7 mg/kg/minute), or frequent feeds. Typically, the hypoglycemia does not respond to glucagon. The underlying diagnosis is often missed at this stage. As soon as an infant with GSD I is able to tolerate full feeds, symptomatic hypoglycemia generally resolves only to reappear at three to four months of age when attempts are made to extend the interval between feeds. The liver of infants with the disease may be normal or only slightly enlarged during the first few days of life. However, by one week of age, often after the hypoglycemia occurring in the first few days of life has been controlled, the liver becomes markedly enlarged. The diagnosis is suggested by the association of hypoglycemia with lactic acidosis and hyperuricemia. In GSD, type Ib, the neutropenia characteristic of the disease develops within the first few days of life, though increased susceptibility to infection may not become a problem until some months later. The diagnosis of GSD I is supported by failure of the hypoglycemia to respond to injections of glucagon. Confirmation requires liver biopsy and measurement of glucose-6-phosphatase in fresh tissue or histochemically, bearing in mind that special studies are necessary to make the diagnosis of GSD Ib or Ic (see Chapter 4).

Hypoglycemia resulting from other defects in gluconeogenesis, such as fructose-1,6-diphosphatase (FDP) deficiency, is less common, but may be clinically indistinguishable from GSD, type Ia. Massive hepatomegaly, marked intolerance of fasting, lactic acidosis, hyperuricemia, and ketosis are features of both; however, ketosis is generally much more prominent in FDP deficiency.

Cardiac syndrome

Structural congenital heart disease is an uncommon manifestation of inborn errors of metabolism, with one important exception: maternal PKU embryopathy. As many as 40% of infants born to women with unrecognized or poorly controlled classical PKU have congenital structural heart disease, most commonly, tetralogy of Fallot. The infants are also small for gestational age and have congenital microcephaly. If the PKU screening test is done within the first 24–48 hours of birth, it will also generally be positive as a result of maternal hyperphenylalaninemia, even if the infant itself is not affected with the disease. A screening test done on the mother will be positive, of course. Recognition of the cause of the congenital anomalies is important in the prevention of the problem recurring in future infants.

Severe, life-threatening heart disease caused by inherited metabolic diseases in the newborn period may be dominated by:
- intractable cardiac arrhythmias
- cardiomyopathy

Intractable cardiac arrhythmias

Neonates affected with severe fatty acid oxidation defects, especially with carnitine-acylcarnitine translocase (CACT) deficiency, often present with severe, intractable cardiac arrhythmias. The origin of the arrhythmia may be supraventricular, but it is often ventricular and is characteristically resistant to conventional anti-arrhythmia medication. In fact, treatment with amiodarone may exacerbate the rhythm disturbance. Myocardial function is generally impaired, which often prompts debate about which came first, the arrhythmia or the cardiomyopathy. Some evidence of hepatocellular dysfunction is almost always present, including moderately severe hyperammonemia. Metabolic acidosis is generally not prominent, in the absence of obvious cardiac decompensation.

Analyses of urinary organic acids or plasma acylcarnitines may reveal the presence of the dicarboxylic acid intermediates of fatty acid oxidation. In CACT, systemic carnitine deficiency, and neonatal carnitine-palmitoyltransferase II deficiency (CPT II) deficiency, these may not be abnormal. However, the plasma carnitine concentrations are profoundly decreased, an important clue to the underlying disorder. Confirmation of the diagnosis requires studies on cultured skin fibroblasts or specific mutation analysis. Treatment with carnitine and the substitution of medium-chain triglyceride fats for the usual long-chain triglyceride dietary fats results in significant, though generally transient, improvement.

Cardiomyopathy

Impaired myocardial function is a prominent feature in many neonates with inherited disorders of energy metabolism. These have been classified as disorders of substrate availability (fatty acid transport defects), disorders of substrate utilization (fatty acid oxidation defects and disorders of glycogen mobilization and gluconeogenesis), and defects in energy generation (mitochondrial ETC defects). These conditions are reviewed in Chapters 2, 4, 5, and 9. The investigation of the newborn with possible metabolic cardiomyopathy is not significantly different from the investigation of older infants and children with cardiomyopathy (see Figure 5.1). Persistent severe lactic acidosis, initially with or without evidence of hepatic or brain involvement, is typical of cytochrome *c* oxidase deficiency in which the cardiomyopathy is often severe and rapidly fatal.

Nonimmune fetal hydrops

The list of conditions associated with nonimmune fetal hydrops is long and includes a wide range of genetic disorders, in addition to severe anemia, congenital heart disease, and congenital infection. In a significant proportion of cases, an underlying explanation for it is never found. A small proportion is the result of inherited metabolic diseases (Table 7.6). The hydrops associated with inborn errors of red blood cell energy metabolism is undoubtedly the result of heart failure precipitated by severe anemia. The relationship between fluid accumulation, heart failure, and anemia is obvious, and investigation of the hematologic disorder generally identifies the underlying defect.

The birth weight of infants with lysosomal storage diseases, particularly the mucopolysaccharidoses, is sometimes excessive and associated with some noticeable swelling of the extremities. Marked weight loss often occurs during the first several days of life as accumulated subcutaneous fluid is resorbed and excreted. Why some newborn infants with lysosomal storage diseases are born with massive generalized edema and ascites is not clear. Severely affected infants usually go on to die as a result of respiratory embarrassment, circulatory failure, or coagulopathies. In a few milder cases, the fluid accumulation resolves spontaneously. The presence of dysostosis multiplex, marked hepatosplenomegaly, vacuolated mononuclear cells in the peripheral smear, and storage histiocytes in bone marrow or other tissues are strongly suggestive of a lysosomal storage disease. However definitive diagnosis invariably requires enzyme analyses of cultured skin fibroblasts or tissues.

Initial management

Early and aggressive management of many inherited metabolic diseases is often life saving. The principles of initial management are summarized in Table 7.7.

Eliminate dietary or other intake of the precursors of possibly toxic metabolites. This applies most often to suspected inborn errors of amino acid or organic acid metabolism. In both cases, dietary or parenteral intake of protein and amino acids should be eliminated immediately an inborn error of metabolism is suspected.

Table 7.6 Inherited metabolic diseases presenting as nonimmune fetal hydrops

Disease	Metabolic abnormality
Hematologic disorders	
G6PD deficiency	Glucose-6-phosphate dehydrogenase deficiency
Pyruvate kinase deficiency	Pyruvate kinase deficiency
Glucosephosphate isomerase deficiency	Glucose-6-phosphate isomerase deficiency
Disorders of steroid biosynthesis	
Smith-Lemli-Opitz syndrome	7-Dehydrocholesterol reductase
Mevalonic aciduria	Mevalonate kinase
Lysosomal storage diseases	
Mucopolysaccharidoses	
Hurler disease (MPS IH)	α-L-Iduronidase
Morquio disease (MPS IVA)	*N*-Acetylgalactosamine-6-sulfatase deficiency
Sly disease (MPS VII)	β-Glucuronidase deficiency
Mucolipidoses	
GM1 gangliosidosis	β-Galactosidase deficiency
Galactosialidosis	Protective protein deficiency
Sialidosis	α-Neuraminidase (sialidase) deficiency
I-Cell disease (mucolipidosis, type II)	*N*-Acetylglucosamine-1-phosphotransferase deficiency
Infantile sialic acid storage disease	Defective lysosomal transport of sialic acid
Sphingolipidoses	
Farber lipogranulomatosis	Acid ceramidase deficiency
Gaucher disease, type 2	Glucocerebrosidase (β-glucosidase) deficiency
Niemann-Pick disease, type C	NPC1 protein deficiency
Miscellaneous	
Zellweger disease	Various defects in peroxisomal biogenesis
CDG syndrome	Various
Glycogen storage disease, type IV	Glycogen brancher enzyme
Congenital lactic acidosis	Various mitochondrial ETC defects

Abbreviations: G6PD, Glucose-6-phosphate dehydrogenase; CDG, congenital disorders of glycosylation; ETC, electron transport chain.

Because inherited disorders of fatty acid oxidation may not initially be easily distinguished from the amino acidopathies, dietary and intravenous fat intake should also be eliminated, at least initially.

Administer a metabolically simple source of **calories**, i.e., glucose, at a rate sufficient to suppress mobilization of endogenous sources of the metabolites, especially protein. In acute, metabolically decompensated MSUD, the goal should be to provide 100 cal/kg/day intravenously. This is achieved by the intravenous administration of 10% dextrose supplemented by Intralipid. Intravenous lipid is specifically

Table 7.7 Initial management of possible inherited metabolic diseases presenting in the newborn period

Principle	Specific initiative
Minimize intake and endogenous production of toxic metabolites	Eliminate protein and fat from the diet
	Administer high-calorie, high-carbohydrate intravenous fluids: 10% dextrose in 0.2% NaCl at 1.5 times calculated maintenance, and add KCl when urinary output is established
Correct acidosis	Administer intravenous sodium bicarbonate CAUTIOUSLY if plasma bicarbonate is <10 mmol/L
Treat intercurrent illness	
In the presence of intractable seizures without hyperammonemia or metabolic acidosis	Pyridoxine, 100–200 mg iv
Accelerate elimination of toxic metabolites	Hemodialysis
In the presence of suspected urea cycle enzyme defect	Continuous venous-venous hemofiltration
	Administer arginine hydrochloride, 2–4 mmol/kg, iv over one hour followed by 2–4 mmol/kg/24 hours in 4 divided doses*
	Administer sodium benzoate, 250 mg/kg iv immediately followed by 250 mg/kg/24 hours in 4 divided doses
	Administer sodium phenylacetate, 250 mg/kg, iv immediately followed by 250 mg/kg/24 hours in 4 divided doses

Note: *Arginine hydrochloride, which is generally readily available in most hospital pharmacies, should be replaced by arginine free base as soon as possible to avoid hydrochloride-induced metabolic acidosis.

contraindicated in children with suspected defects in fatty acid oxidation, although some of these patients may turn out to have defects (such as systemic carnitine deficiency) responsive to replacement of usual dietary fat by medium-chain triglyceride (MCT) oil. In cases of congenital lactic acidosis resulting from PDH deficiency or mitochondrial ETC defects, the administration of large amounts of glucose often drive plasma lactate levels even higher. Blood gases and plasma lactate levels should be monitored and appropriate adjustments made in these cases.

Administer greater than maintenance amounts of **fluids** to promote diuresis and accelerate excretion of water-soluble, toxic metabolites. Care must be taken to avoid fluid over-load in children with acute, encephalopathic MSUD or UCED.

Treat shock, hypoglycemia, metabolic acidosis, electrolyte imbalances, infections, and coagulopathies by conventional methods. Metabolic acidosis should be treated cautiously. Bicarbonate is generally not indicated unless the plasma bicarbonate is <10 mmol/L; deficits should be only half corrected.

In cases involving potentially vitamin responsive enzymopathies, administer pharmacologic doses of the relevant vitamin. This is most important in the treatment of suspected pyridoxine dependency seizures of the newborn. As a general rule, vitamin-responsive enzymopathies are clinically less severe than non-responsive variants. A trial of therapy with vitamins would be indicated nevertheless in any acutely ill patient in whom a strong presumptive diagnosis of a specific, potentially vitamin-responsive, inborn error of metabolism is made.

Administer pharmacologic agents known to detoxify or accelerate the excretion of toxic metabolites. The efficacy of nontoxic drugs, such as sodium benzoate and sodium phenylacetate, that accelerate nitrogen excretion in patients with UCED by forming innocuous, rapidly cleared amino acid conjugates (hippuric acid and phenylacetylglutamine, respectively) is well established.

Consider dialysis for treatment of resistant, life-threatening metabolic acidosis, rapidly progressive encephalopathy, or treatment-induced electrolyte disturbances, e.g., hypernatremia. Patients with UCED presenting in the newborn period with severe hyperammonemia usually require hemodialysis or CVVH to control ammonium levels. Peritoneal dialysis is too slow. Exchange transfusion brings the plasma ammonium down quickly, but rebound hyperammonemia occurs just as quickly. It may be useful in some circumstances as an adjunct to hemodialysis.

Summary comments

Treatable inherited metabolic diseases often present in early infancy or childhood as acute, life-threatening illness. Diagnosis is often delayed, however, because the conditions are individually rare, the presenting signs and symptoms are often non-specific, and diagnosis usually rests on biochemical testing that may not be readily available. This chapter presents an approach to the problem that stresses those clinical signs or situations suggesting the strong possibility of disease due to inborn errors of metabolism, the initial investigation, and the initial management of infants with suspected inherited metabolic diseases. The approach is based on experience that suggests diagnosis is often unnecessarily delayed because premonitory signs are misinterpreted, that a clinically useful presumptive diagnosis can often be made with the aid of relatively easily accessible laboratory facilities, and that effective initial management, while often relatively nonspecific, allows time for more definitive investigation and specific, long-term treatment.

SUGGESTED READING

Burton, B. K. (1998). Inborn errors of metabolism in infancy: a guide to diagnosis. *Pediatrics,* **102**, E69.

Cornblath, M. & Ichord, R. (2000). Hypoglycemia in the neonate. *Seminars in Perinatology*, **24**, 136–49.

Ellaway, C. J., Wilcken, B. & Christodoulou, J. (2002). Clinical approach to inborn errors of metabolism presenting in the newborn period. *Journal of Paediatrics and Child Health*, **38**, 511–517.

Leonard, J. V. & Morris, A. A. (2000). Inborn errors of metabolism around the time of birth. *Lancet*, **356**, 583–7.

Ogier de Baulny, H. (2002). Management and emergency treatments of neonates with a suspicion of inborn errors of metabolism. *Seminars in Neonatology*, **7**, 17–26.

Rinaldo, P., Yoon, H.-R., Yu, C., Raymond, K., Tiozzo, C. & Giordano, G. (1999). Sudden and unexpected neonatal death: a protocol for the postmortem diagnosis of fatty acid oxidation disorders. *Seminars in Perinatology*, **23**, 204–10.

Saudubray, J. M., Nassogne, M. C., de Lonlay, P. & Touati, G. (2002). Clinical approach to inherited metabolic disorders in neonates: an overview. *Seminars in Neonatology*, **7**, 3–15.

Stone, D. L. & Sidransky, E. (1999). Hydrops fetalis: lysosomal storage disorders *in extremis*. *Advances in Pediatrics*, **46**, 409–40.

Sue, C. M., Hirano, M., DiMauro, S. & De Vivo, D. C. (1999). Neonatal presentations of mitochondrial metabolic disorders. *Seminars in Perinatology*, **23**, 113–24.

Tein, I. (1999). Neonatal metabolic myopathies. *Seminars in Perinatology*, **23**, 125–51.

8

Newborn screening

Large-scale screening is a well-established way to identify members of a population, such as newborn infants, affected by a specific disease before the development of clinical signs of the condition, with the objective of initiating treatment that would prevent serious disability or even death. The initiative for most population-based screening programs rests with the state, rather than with the subject to be tested, who may not even be aware that testing is being done. In most cases, consent for testing is considered to be implied unless the individual or parent specifically objects. Therefore, the state assumes responsibility for ensuring that the facilities and resources are available to provide appropriate follow-up investigation and treatment of individuals identified by the screening program.

Screening newborn infants for PKU was the first, large-scale genetic screening initiative to be widely adopted in a direct attempt to ameliorate the impact of genetic disease. The principles that have evolved since its introduction have served as a model for the development of numerous subsequent newborn screening programs. For many years, the principles originally articulated by Wilson and Jungner[1] for screening in general and later modified and expanded by Pollitt et al.[2] with specific reference to newborn screening have been accepted as the criteria for neonatal screening. They are:

1. The condition sought should be an important health problem. This is viewed as a combination of the incidence of the condition and the consequence for the affected individual.
2. There should be an accepted treatment for patients with recognised disease. What is meant by this is treatment of the disease at an earlier stage than normal affects the course and ultimate outcome for the affected individual. The lack of effective treatment is not considered by many to be an absolute contraindication

[1] Wilson, J. M. G. & Jungner, G. (1968). *Principles of screening for disease*. Geneva: World Health Organization, 26–39.
[2] Pollitt, R. J., Green, A., McCabe, C. J. *et al.* (1997). Neonatal screening for inborn errors of metabolism: cost, yield and outcome. *Health Technology Assessment*, 1, 1–202.

to screening; however, the evidence that it has significant benefit in spite of the absence of an effective therapeutic intervention needs to be strong.

3. Screening for medical intervention should be carried out as part of an integrated program with the facilities, resources, and personnel to provide
   - the necessary education and counselling for the population and participating health professions,
   - the screening test,
   - retrieval of individuals with positive screening tests,
   - diagnostic confirmation,
   - treatment, and
   - evaluation of out-come.

4. There should be a recognisable presymptomatic or early symptomatic stage when detection and therapeutic intervention would materially alter the out-come of treatment of affected individuals.

5. There should be a suitable test or examination that is technically simple and inexpensive, with high sensitivity (the proportion of affected infants with a positive test), specificity (the proportion of unaffected infants with a negative test), and predictive value of a positive test (the ratio of true-positive to false-positive tests).

6. The test must be acceptable to the population. In the past, acceptability has often been defined as the absence of denial. However, the pressure is mounting, on ethical grounds, to demonstrate that the population being screened, or the parents in the case of newborn screening, understands the process. Whether this requires formal informed consent is still being debated.

7. The natural history of the condition, including development from presymptomatic to symptomatic disease, needs to be adequately understood.

8. An agreed policy must exist for whom to treat as patients.

9. The costs of identifying and treating infants affected with a specific disease should be weighed against the healthcare benefits of the intervention, not merely the costs avoided as a result of the intervention. Economic evaluations of newborn screening programs have historically focused on comparing the costs of screening and treating identified patients with the costs of managing patients who present symptomatically, i.e., the costs avoided by early detection and intervention. Pollitt and his colleagues felt that this approach to economic evaluation was too limited, and it is also inconsistent with the approach taken to the evaluation of other healthcare interventions. They recommended that newborn screening be evaluated according to the more conventional approach, weighing the costs of intervention against the healthcare benefits derived.

10. Screening should be understood to be a continuous process, not a "once and for all" project.

Screening for medical intervention

When the goal of the screening project is medical intervention, to alter the natural history of a disease by early detection and treatment, the condition for which screening is contemplated should be medically significant, in terms of individual suffering and overall disease burden, in the population under consideration. Affected individuals should benefit significantly as a result of any medical intervention initiated on the basis of the screening procedure. To prove that treatment initiated early as a result of screening, rather than later when symptomatic, has a significant impact on the health and long-term well-being of the patient is sometimes difficult. Individuals should be informed of the goals, operation, and implications of the screening program, and they should have the right to refuse testing without prejudice. The outcome and impact of any screening program, regardless of the rationale for undertaking it in the first place, should be evaluated and the program modified, if necessary, based on the results of the evaluation.

The prototype of this type of screening is newborn screening for PKU and congenital hypothyroidism. In many jurisdictions, screening programs have expanded to include testing for galactosemia, the organic acidurias, fatty acid oxidation defects, and other inherited metabolic conditions, although few have been subjected to thorough cost-utility analysis to evaluate the overall merit of the undertaking.

Screening for reproductive planning

The goal of screening for reproductive planning is to identify individuals at particularly high risk for conceiving offspring affected with a particular inherited disorder *before* pregnancy occurs, in order for them to make optimum reproductive choices for themselves. The knowledge of a high risk for having offspring with a certain disease is used to make decisions about what measures they may take to decrease or eliminate the risk. In some cases, this might even determine whether a couple marries or not. In most, it involves consideration of various options, including adoption, artificial insemination by donor, egg donation and *in vitro* fertilization, or prenatal diagnosis.

In order for testing to be effective as a guide to prenatal diagnosis, identification of high-risk pregnancies must be done early enough to allow time for appropriate counselling, decision-making, carrying out chorionic villus sampling (CVS) or amniocentesis, and whatever laboratory procedures that may be necessary to determine the status of the fetus. All this must be done in time to allow the woman to undergo termination of the pregnancy safely with a minimum of stress if the fetus is found to be affected with the disease under investigation.

Screening for carriers of Tay-Sachs disease has been particularly successful as an approach to preventing the disease. The development in the late 1960s of a biochemical test for carriers of the disease gene, prompted the organization of a number of large-scale community screening clinics in the United States and elsewhere directed at identifying couples at risk for having offspring with the disease. Before the advent of carrier screening, the frequency of Tay-Sachs disease among Ashkenazi Jews was one hundred times higher than among most other ethnic groups. Since the introduction of carrier screening, many of us have seen more Tay-Sachs disease among non-Jews than among the offspring of the high-risk Ashkenazi Jewish community.

Screening newborn infants has been introduced in some places for the purposes of reproductive planning by using the birth of an infant affected with a genetic condition, such as Duchenne muscular dystrophy or nonketotic hyperglycinemia, to identify parents who are at particularly high risk for having more children affected with the same disease. The ethics of this type of screening has been challenged because the infant undergoing testing does not benefit directly from the procedure.

Screening to answer epidemiological questions

Screening has been undertaken from time to time to determine the frequency of specific disease-associated biochemical phenotypes in certain populations. This type of screening is usually done in an effort to determine the true incidence of a disease and whether or not a population-based screening program would be cost-effective. Studies of this type are considered research, and the ethical constraints applying to all research projects must be observed. A rich source of material for this type of project has been the dried blood spots collected and stored from newborn infants during the course of screening for PKU. Many centers store the unused portion of the filter-paper requisition for many years, making retrospective, anonymous surveillance studies relatively easy. As long as the anonymity of the infants being tested is assured, and the period under study is far enough in the past that medical intervention as a result of a positive test alone would be unlikely to be necessary, the general requirement for informed consent might be foregone. PKU blood spots have been used in this way to estimate the frequency of medium-chain acyl-CoA dehydrogenase (MCAD) deficiency, usually by testing for the presence of abnormal concentrations of acylcarnitines or for a single mutation, K329E, that accounts for 98% of the disease-associated mutant alleles in Caucasian populations in which it has been studied. Prospective surveillance studies are somewhat more difficult because they cannot be undertaken without the explicit, informed consent of the parents of the infants, adding significantly to the cost of the study.

Case-finding

Case-finding is the term David Sackett (1975) applied to a process, often called 'screening', by which a health care professional carries out certain tests on selected individuals presenting to them for care, regardless of the problem that generated the consultation. The goal is the same as for population screening: it is to identify the risk of disease at an early stage when specific intervention might be expected to alter the natural history by treatment or prevent the disease altogether. In case-finding, however, the process is initiated by the patient presenting to her physician, generally with some completely unrelated problem. The nature of the contract between the individual and the physician is different. The parties to the contract are the patient or parent and the physician. Although the physician may be held responsible for failing to provide what might be regarded as good general medical care as a result of having failed to test the patient for some high-incidence, preventable or treatable condition, the state is generally not involved. The responsibility for following up on the results of testing rest with the individual and the physician, and the state would not normally be held responsible for ensuring that the resources are available to provide further investigation or treatment.

Case-finding has worked demonstrably well in identifying individuals at high risk for certain hereditary conditions in various groups of patients. In many centers, for example, limited population screening for Tay-Sachs disease carriers has been replaced by a case-finding approach by which the physicians of Ashkenazi Jewish patients offer carrier testing for this and other 'Jewish diseases' as a routine part of their medical care. The experience of centers that have made this shift, from population screening to case-finding, has shown, however, that a large proportion of general physicians, as well as many of their patients, regard carrier detection by case-finding as an aspect of reproductive *care*, rather than part of reproductive *planning*. As a result, women are often pregnant before carrier testing is undertaken, and their husbands generally do not present for testing at all, unless the woman is found to be a carrier. The inevitable delays that result often mean that prenatal diagnosis testing is not even considered until the middle of the second trimester of pregnancy.

Problems created by false positive screening tests

The price of maximum sensitivity in newborn screening programs is often a large number of false positive tests. For example, in some PKU screening programs, the number of false positive tests outnumbers positive tests in infants with PKU or benign hyperphenylalaninemia by 10 to 1 or more, making the predictive value of a positive test less than 10%. Although most of these are recognized and eliminated from further consideration simply by re-testing the same blood sample, or by analysis of tyrosine levels on the same sample, the number of infants requiring retrieval and more detailed investigation is substantial. The situation with congenital hypothyroidism is the same. The cost of follow-up investigation of these infants and counselling of their parents is a major direct cost of newborn screening. Some investigators have also shown that parents of infants with false positive screening tests tend to regard these children as unusually vulnerable. Their utilization of health care resources is greater than their healthy siblings. The magnitude of this indirect cost of screening is unknown.

Screening technology

The earliest form of newborn screening for inherited metabolic diseases involved the use of color reagents for the detection of abnormal metabolites in urine. The ferric chloride test for the presence of phenylpyruvic acid, for the detection of PKU, and the Benedict's test for reducing substances, for the detection of galactosemia, were two such tests that were widely used in the early 1960s. About the same time, Scriver and Efron developed a simple paper chromatographic technique for screening urine for a wide range of amino acid abnormalities. This technique was also adopted by several jurisdictions for newborn screening, some of which continue to employ the method.

Colorimetric tests are cumbersome because they require the collection of urine from newborn infants or a wet diaper uncontaminated by stool. The tests are not particularly sensitive, and the results of testing are often confounded by the presence of drugs, drug metabolites and harmless endogenous metabolites that produce false positive tests. Chromatography is more sensitive and generates fewer false positives. However, it is also cumbersome owing to the need to salvage fresh, uncontaminated urine from the infant.

Bacterial inhibition assays – the 'Guthrie test'

One of the most important breakthroughs in newborn screening for inherited metabolic diseases was the development of the 'Guthrie test', a bacterial inhibition assay of the phenylalanine concentration in blood named after the late Robert Guthrie, the American physician-microbiologist who invented it. This is the most commonly used screening test for PKU in the world. Only a few drops of blood, soaked into a piece of filter paper and allowed to dry in air, are needed for the test. At the screening laboratory, small circles of blood-soaked filter paper are applied to the surface of agar plates containing a strain of *Bacillus subtilis* that requires phenylalanine for growth. The agar is impregnated with β-2-thienylalanine, a phenylalanine analogue that inhibits the utilization of phenylalanine by the organism. The amount of growth around the blood-soaked filter paper disks is proportional to the phenylalanine concentration in the blood. The capital and operating costs of

Table 8.1 Classification of inherited disorders of phenylalanine metabolism

Disorder	Characteristics
Classical phenylketonuria (PKU)	Plasma phenylalanine levels >1200 μmol/L on unrestricted diet
Atypical (mild) PKU	Plasma phenylalanine levels 600–1200 μmol/L on unrestricted diet
Persistent benign hyperphenylalaninemia	Plasma phenylalanine levels <600 μmol/L on unrestricted diet
Transient hyperphenylalaninemia	Early dietary phenylalanine intolerance becoming normal within a few weeks or months
Dihydropteridine reductase deficiency	Plasma phenylalanine levels 800–1200 μmol/L on unrestricted diet; requires treatment with diet and neurotransmitter precursors (dopa, Carbidopa, 5-HTP)
BH4 biosynthesis defects	Plasma phenylalanine levels 800–1200 μmol/L on unrestricted diet; requires treatment with BH4 and neurotransmitter precursors (dopa, Carbidopa, 5-HTP)
Maternal PKU	Low birth-weight, microcephaly, mental retardation, congenital heart defects, and subtle facial dysmorphism in the offspring of women with PKU

Abbreviations: BH4, tetrahydrobiopterin; 5-HTP, 5-hydroxytryptophan; dopa, dihydroxyphenylalanine.

screening based on this test are relatively low. However, quantitation of blood phenylalanine by this test is unreliable when concentrations of the amino acid are less than 200 or above 1500 μmol/L.

Like most biological assays, the Guthrie test requires careful standardization and the inclusion of suitable controls with each plate. Substances in the blood, such as antimicrobials, may interfere with bacterial growth, producing spuriously low phenylalanine concentrations. The test is highly sensitive for the detection of PKU in infants more than 3 days old. However, tests done in the first day of life, before plasma phenylalanine levels have risen into the pathological range, may be falsely negative.

Because of the relative insensitivity of the Guthrie test, an increasing number of screening laboratories began to switch to semi-automated chemical or enzymic methods for the measurement of blood phenylalanine levels. The most common is a spectrofluorometric method, which is relatively inexpensive and yields more reliable results than the Guthrie test, particularly at very low and at very high phenylalanine concentrations.

Table 8.2 Investigation of neonatal hyperphenylalaninemia

Quantitative analysis of plasma amino acids
To determine accurately the plasma phenylalanine concentration and the concentration of tyrosine in order to distinguish hyperphenylalaninemia caused by transient or hereditary defects in tyrosine metabolism

Blood DHPR assay
For the diagnosis of DHPR deficiency. This can be done on dried blood spots.

Urinary biopterin/neopterin ratio and percentage BH4
To identify defects in biopterin biosynthesis. Must be done before BH4 loading test.

BH4 loading test
Another approach to the identification of defects in BH4 biosynthesis. Serial measurements of plasma phenylalanine are done immediately before and at 4-hour intervals after oral administration of BH4, 20 mg per kg body weight.

PAH mutation analysis
Rarely needed for diagnosis of PKU. However, it is necessary for prenatal diagnosis of the condition in future pregnancies.

Abbreviations: BH4, tetrahydrobiopterin; 5-HTP, 5-hydroxytryptophan; DHPR, dihydropteridine reductase.

The inherited disorders of phenylalanine metabolism that often present with a positive PKU screening test are summarized in Table 8.1. An outline of the investigation of neonatal hyperphenylalaninemia is shown in Table 8.2.

Tandem MSMS

The introduction of tandem MSMS for newborn screening represents a technological breakthrough of the same magnitude as the Guthrie test. The sample collection is identical to that currently used throughout the world for screening for PKU and congenital hypothyroidism: blood obtained by heel-stick is applied to a filter-paper requisition to fill 4–6 circles approximately 1 cm in diameter, allowed to dry in air, and sent to a central screening laboratory for analysis. Small circles of dried blood-soaked filter paper are punched out and metabolites extracted with organic solvents. Aliquots of deuterated internal standards of the metabolites of interest are added, and the samples are derivatized, usually by formation of the butyl esters, prior to injection into the tandem MSMS for analysis (see Chapter 9).

The sensitivity of tandem MSMS testing in screening for PKU is greater than the sensitivity of any bacterial inhibition or biochemical method for measuring blood phenylalanine levels. However, one of the greatest benefits it provides is greatly enhanced predictive value of a positive test, with far fewer false positive tests. The false positive rate in one major PKU screening program in the United States showed a 75% decrease with the introduction of tandem MSMS testing. This is achieved in part by measuring phenylalanine and tyrosine simultaneously and calculating the phenylalanine-to-tyrosine ratio.

The power of newborn screening by tandem MSMS is enormously enhanced by the ability to analyze several metabolites simultaneously in the same blood specimen. Newborn screening programs have tended to focus on three groups of metabolites: amino acids, fatty acid oxidation intermediates, and short-chain organic acids (Table 8.3). Although the instrument and methodology is capable of analyzing many more compounds, routine screening is generally confined to the detection of disorders that are reliably detectable by this technology and are treatable. Analysis takes only a few minutes per sample. A laboratory with a single instrument fitted with an automatic sample-injector and appropriate computer programming and software is capable of analyzing and reporting on the concentrations of a number of metabolites in 300 or more samples per day.

The post-analysis follow-up of infants tested in a program using tandem MSMS is identical in principle to that used in screening programs for PKU and congenital hypothyroidism. Based on estimates of the incidence of various disorders of amino acid, urea, fatty acid, and organic acid metabolism, some have predicted that one out of 4000 newborns would be identified pre-symptomatically with a treatable inherited metabolic disease. The cost of the tandem MSMS instrument and accessories is high, a potent disincentive for cost-conscious government agencies involved in newborn screening. However, analyses of the incremental costs and potential benefits of the technology have shown that the payoff in lives saved and morbidity avoided is substantial. The number of jurisdictions employing tandem MSMS for newborn screening is growing rapidly throughout the Western world, especially in the United States.

One of the most vexing problems created by the wide-spread use of tandem MSMS for newborn screening is the identification of apparently healthy individuals with acylcarnitine abnormalities which have been generally associated with severe clinical disease. For example, for years, physician-investigators have debated whether short-chain acyl-CoA dehydrogenase (SCAD) deficiency causes disease. The discovery, by newborn screening, of an increasing number of healthy infants with biochemical abnormalities characteristic of SCAD deficiency has created doubt about the significance of this inborn error of metabolism. Some patients are clearly symptomatic, while others, who appear to have the same biochemical defect, are apparently healthy. Close follow-up clinical and biochemical monitoring are needed to determine the significance of the abnormality in any individual infant.

Another relatively frequently encountered abnormality is elevated 3-hydroxy-isovalerylcarnitine (C5OH), accumulating in plasma, along with 3-methylcrotonyl-glycine (3MCG) in urine, as a result of 3-methylcrotonyl-CoA carboxylase

Table 8.3 Inherited metabolic disorders detectable in the newborn period by tandem MSMS testing of blood spots

Disorder	Primary metabolic indicator
Amino acidopathies	
Phenylketonuria (PKU)	Phe
Maple syrup urine disease (MSUD)	Leu/Ile, Val
Homocystinuria (cystathionine β-synthase deficiency)	Met
Hypermethioninemia	Met
Citullinemia	Cit
Argininosuccinic aciduria	Cit
Hepatorenal tyrosinemia (tyrosinemia, type I)	Tyr
Fatty acid oxidation defects	
Medium-chain acyl-CoA dehydrogenase (MCAD) deficiency	C8, C10, C10:1, C6
Very long-chain acyl-CoA dehydrogenase (VLCAD) deficiency	C14:1, C14, C16
Short-chain acyl-CoA dehydrogenase (SCAD) deficiency	C4
Multiple acyl-CoA dehydrogenase deficiency (GA II)	C4, C5, C8:1, C8, C12, C14, C16, C5DC
Carnitine palmitoyl transferase (CPT) deficiency	C16, C18:1, C18
Carnitine-acylcarnitine translocase (CACT) deficiency	C16, C18:1, C18
Long-chain 3-hydroxyacyl-CoA dehydrogenase (LCHAD) deficiency	C16OH, C18:1OH, C18OH
Trifunctional protein deficiency	C16OH, C18:1OH, C18OH
Organic acidopathies	
Glutaric aciduria, type I	C5DC
Propionic acidemia	C3
Methylmalonic acidemia	C3
Isovaleric acidemia	C5
3-Hydroxy-3-methylglutaryl-CoA lyase deficiency	C5OH
3-Methylcrotonyl-CoA carboxylase deficiency	C5OH

Abbreviations: Phe, phenylalanine; Tyr, tyrosine; Leu, leucine; Ile, isoleucine; Val, valine; Cit, citrulline; Met, methionine. The abbreviations for fatty acid oxidation products and organic acid intermediates, such as C5, C16OH, C18:1, etc., refer to carnitine esters of aliphatic, monocarboxylic acids with chain length indicated by the number adjacent to C, and the number of double bonds indicated by the number after the colon. For example, C18:1, refers to an aliphatic, monocarboxylic acid with 18 carbon atoms and a single double bond. C5DC refers to a 5-carbon, aliphatic, dicarboxylic acid.

Source: CDC Morbidity and Mortality Weekly Report, Using tandem mass spectrometry for metabolic disease screening among newborns (2001).

(3MCC) deficiency. However, in this case, a high proportion of newborns with high levels of C5OH in blood tested in the course of newborn screening have turned out to be the offspring of mothers with 3MCC deficiency, but unaffected themselves with the enzyme defect. The affected mothers have generally been clinically healthy, and the C5OH in their unaffected infants cleared rapidly and was unaccompanied by high levels of 3MCG in the urine. Some infants affected with 3MCC deficiency suffer recurrent episodes of moderately severe metabolic acidosis during metabolic decompensations requiring aggressive treatment. The majority would appear to require either no special treatment or only modest dietary manipulation, i.e., avoidance of high protein foods, and supplementation with carnitine, though whether this is really necessary is not at all clear.

Experience with SCAD and 3MCC underscores the need for well-designed studies to elucidate the mechanism and natural history of abnormalities discovered incidently in the course of newborn screening with high-power technologies, such as tandem MSMS. On the basis of the well-known work of Sir Harry Harris on biochemical polymorphisms, we should not be surprised to encounter more 'abnormalities' resulting from enzyme polymorphisms in the population. The need to retrieve and investigate infants with these 'abnormalities' is one of the inevitable costs of a screening technology that generates such adventitious information requiring exploration and explanation.

Radioimmunoassay

Radioimmunoassay for the measurement of hormones, such as thyroid stimulating hormone (TSH) or 17-hydroxyprogesterone, is widely used in newborn screening programs for congenital hypothyroidism and congenital adrenal hyperplasia (CAH), respectively. Testing is done on the same types of dried blood spots used for screening for PKU, making sample collection particularly easy. The sensitivity of this type of testing for congenital hypothyroidism is high, but the proportion of false positives requiring further investigation is also high, especially in infants less than 24 hours old. Despite the problems caused by false positive tests, screening for congenital hypothyroidism by this technique is deeply entrenched and is unlikely to be replaced in the foreseeable future. Although the sensitivity of testing for severe, salt-losing variants of CAH is high, the proportion of false positives is also as high as 200 times the true incidence of the disease. Yet milder variants of the disease are often missed when testing is done in the first few days of life.

Enzyme assay

Screening for a number of conditions, notably galactosemia and biotinidase deficiency, is based on measurement of the enzyme reponsible for the disease. In the case of galactosemia screening, measurement of galactose-1-phosphate uridyltransferase activity is supplemented by measurement of galactose-1-phosphate or galactose levels in blood.

With the advent of treatment of lysosomal storage diseases (LSD) by enzyme replacement therapy (ERT), interest is growing in screening for these disorders in the newborn period. The discovery that many of the lysosomal enzymes associated with storage diseases are robust and retain activity even after drying on filter-paper and storage at room temperature prompted Chamoles in Argentina to develop methods for measuring these enzymes on the same dried blood spots used for screening for PKU and congenital hypothyroidism. Another group extended the technique by coupling it with tandem MSMS to permit multiplex testing for several disorders in one reaction. Like screening for LSD by measurement of lysosome-associated membrane proteins (LAMP1 and LAMP2) in dried blood spots, these enzyme-based screening tests are still under investigation.

Specific mutation testing

The recognition that the number of mutant alleles responsible for some inherited metabolic diseases, especially within certain ethnically defined communities, may be very small has prompted interest in using molecular genetic testing for newborn screening. For example, one allele, K329E, accounts for over 95% of the mutant alleles associated with medium-chain acyl-CoA dehydrogenase (MCAD) deficiency among Caucasians. However, this approach to large-scale newborn screening is still prohibitively expensive, and the technology is reserved, in general, for follow-up investigation of infants with positive or suspicious biochemical or immunological screening tests and for carrier detection within high-risk groups.

SUGGESTED READING

Bok, L. A., Vreken, P., Wijburg, F. A. *et al.* (2003). Short-chain Acyl-CoA dehydrogenase deficiency: studies in a large family adding to the complexity of the disorder. *Pediatrics*, **112**, 1152–5.

Centers for Disease Control and Prevention. (2001). Using tandem mass spectrometry for metabolic disease screening among newborns: a report of a work group. *Morbidity and Mortality Weekly Report*, **50**, 1–34.

Chace, D. H., Hillman, S. L., Van Hove, J. L. K. & Naylor, E. W. (1997). Rapid diagnosis of MCAD deficiency: quantitative analysis of octanoylcarnitine and other acylcarnitines in newborn blood spots by tandem mass spectrometry. *Clinical Chemistry*, **43**, 2106–13.

Chace, D. H., Sherwin, J. E., Hillman, S. L., Lorey F. & Cunningham, G. C. (1998). Use of phenylalanine-to-tyrosine ratio determined by tandem mass spectrometry to improve newborn screening for phenylketonuria of early discharge specimens collected in the first 24 hours. *Clinical Chemisty*, **44**, 2405–9.

Chamoles, N. A., Blanco, M. B., Gaggioli, D. & Casentini, C. (2001). Hurler-like phenotype: enzymatic diagnosis in dried blood spots on filter paper. *Clinical Chemistry*, **47**, 2098–102.

Clague, A. & Thomas, A. (2002). Neonatal biochemical screening for disease. *Clinica Chimica Acta*, **315**, 99–110.

Council of Regional Networks for Genetic Services (CORN). (2000). U. S. newborn screening system guidelines II: follow-up of children, diagnosis, management, and evaluation. *Journal of Pediatrics*, **137** (Supplement), S1–S46.

Koeberl, D. D., Millington, D. S., Smith, W. E. *et al.* (2003). Evaluation of 3-methylcrotonyl-CoA carboxylase deficiency detected by tandem mass spectrometry newborn screening. *Journal of Inherited Metabolic Disease*, **26**, 25–35.

Li, Y., Scott, C. R., Chamoles, N. A. *et al.* (2004). Direct multiplex assay of lysosomal enzymes in dried blood spots for newborn screening. *Clinical Chemistry*, **50**, 1785–96.

Meikle, P. J., Ranieri, E., Simonsen, H. *et al.* (2004). Newborn screening for lysosomal storage disorders: clinical evaluation of a two-tier strategy. *Pediatrics*, **114**, 909–16.

National Academy of Sciences (National Research Council). (1975). *Genetic Screening: Programs, Principles, and Research.* Washington: National Academy of Sciences.

Newborn Screening Task Force. Serving the family from birth to the medical home. Newborn screening: a blueprint for the future. (2000). *Pediatrics*, **106** (Supplement):380–427.

Pandor, A., Eastham, J., Beverley, C., Chilcott, J. & Paisley, S. (2004). Clinical effectiveness and cost-effectiveness of neonatal screening for inborn errors of metabolism using tandem mass spectrometry: a systematic review. *Health Technology Assessment*, **8**, 1–121.

Pollitt, R. J., Green, A., McCabe, C. J. *et al.* (1997). Neonatal screening for inborn errors of metabolism: cost, yield and outcome. *Health Technology Assessment*, **1**, 1–202.

Sackett, D. L. & Holland, W. W. (1975). Controversy in the detection of disease. *Lancet*, **2**, 357–9.

Thomason, M. J., Lord, J., Bain, M. D. *et al.* (1998). A systematic review of evidence for the appropriateness of neonatal screening programmes for inborn errors of metabolism. *Journal of Public Health Medicine*, **20**, 331–43.

Wilcken, B., Wiley, V., Hammond, J. & Carpenter, K. (2003). Screening newborns for inborn errors of metabolism by tandem mass spectrometry. *New England Journal of Medicine*, **348**, 2304–12.

9

Laboratory investigation

It is impossible to exaggerate the importance of the diagnostic clinical chemistry laboratory in the investigation of inherited metabolic diseases. Access to comprehensive routine laboratory testing is indispensable to the establishment of the diagnosis of any suspected inherited metabolic condition, and the clinical biochemist is an extremely important collaborator whose allegiance should be cultivated carefully. In this chapter, I present information relating to the laboratory investigation of inherited metabolic diseases to help the clinician understand some of the technical principles involved, to give enough detail about certain tests to provide a feel for the interpretation of test results, and some of the more common sources of error. It is not intended to be a detailed technical treatise on clinical chemistry. However, I have found that the initial laboratory investigation of patients with possible inborn errors of metabolism is generally more appropriate when the clinician has some understanding of laboratory issues. Treating some of the diagnostic laboratory information in a separate chapter like this does create its own problems. Specifically, it is difficult at times to decide whether a particular point should be included here, or if it would not be more logically placed alongside of the presentation of the clinical aspects of a particular disease. This has been resolved in most cases by a compromise. If the laboratory aspects of, for example, amino acid analysis, are relevant to more than one major clinical presentation, such as chronic encephalopathy (covered in Chapter 2), metabolic acidosis (Chapter 3), and hepatocellular dysfunction (Chapter 4), it seemed more appropriate to place it in a separate chapter. However, the physiologic rationale for some laboratory studies seemed more appropriate in the chapter in which presentation of the information would be helpful in grasping the pathophysiology of a particular disease.

Laboratory chemists supervise the technical aspects of specific testing. They not only provide information regarding the availability and appropriateness of specific tests, the limitations of the investigation, and the interpretation of the results, they can often influence the scheduling of testing so that results that are needed urgently are obtained with a minimum of delay. When certain specialized testing is not available locally, the clinical chemist is often the one who knows where it can be obtained and will facilitate referral to an appropriate reference laboratory.

The goal of various laboratory studies, including biochemical testing, may be to:

- determine the extent and severity of organ or tissue involvement;
- classify a presumed inherited metabolic problem according to the aspect of metabolism involved; or
- establish a specific diagnosis.

The types of tests that might be undertaken to determine what organs of tissues are involved in a disease process, and the severity of the involvement, include the wide range of biochemical, hematologic, electrophysiologic, imaging, and histopathologic studies that are useful for the assessment of any disorder, inherited or acquired. They include routine biochemical tests like measurements of arterial blood gases, plasma electrolytes, glucose, urea, creatinine, liver function tests, routine hematologic tests, and various endocrinologic tests, such as thyroxine, triiodothyronine, thyroid stimulating hormone. They also include somewhat more specialized electrophysiologic studies, such as EEG, evoked potentials, EMG, and nerve conduction studies, as well as ECG. Imaging studies that are particularly helpful, though not specific to the investigation of inherited metabolic disorders, include routine skeletal radiography, echocardiography, CT scanning, and magnetic resonance imaging. The advent of magnetic resonance spectroscopy (MRS), though not yet widely available, adds a new and powerful dimension to the noninvasive investigation of complex metabolic disorders. For example, the accumulation of lactic acid in the brain, identifiable by MRS, may be the only disease-specific metabolic abnormality in some children with Leigh disease who do not show consistent peripheral lactic acidosis or elevation of CSF lactate levels. Histopathologic, histochemical, and ultrastructural studies are particularly useful in the investigation of inherited disorders of organelle function (see Chapter 6).

A number of somewhat less readily available biochemical tests are used to identify metabolic abnormalities and classify them according to the general area or pathway of metabolism involved. The tests are generally not specific enough to differentiate primary from secondary metabolic abnormalities, though the pattern of abnormalities may be suggestive of a specific diagnosis. Studies in this category include measurements of lactate, pyruvate, amino acids, 3-hydroxybutyrate, acetoacetate, and free fatty acids in plasma; analyses of urinary organic and amino acids; tests for mucopolysacchariduria and oligosacchariduria; and measurements of certain trace elements, such as copper.

The ultimate specific diagnosis of inherited metabolic disease generally requires the demonstration of a primary biochemical abnormality, such as a specific enzyme deficiency, or mutations that have been shown to cause disease. These tests are

Table 9.1 Clinical differentiation of organelle disease and small molecule diseases

Feature	Organelle disease	Small molecule disease
Onset	Gradual	Often sudden, even catastrophic
Course	Slowly progressive	Characterized by relapses and remissions
Physical findings	Characteristic features	Nonspecific
Histopathology	Often reveals characteristic changes	Generally nonspecific changes
Response to supportive therapy	Poor	Brisk

generally available only in large metropolitan teaching hospitals or university medical centers.

A useful first step in helping to focus the laboratory investigation of possible inherited metabolic diseases is to try to determine whether the disease is due to a defect in the metabolism of water-soluble intermediates, such as amino acids, organic acids, or other low molecular weight compounds, or is likely due to an inherited defect of organelle metabolism, such as lysosomal, mitochondrial, or peroxisomal metabolism. Table 9.1 summarizes some features that are helpful in differentiating the two classes of disorders.

The *onset of signs of disease* is an important, though not infallible, clue to the nature of the underlying disorder. Diseases presenting with a sudden or catastrophic onset are generally more likely to be attributable to inherited defects of small molecule metabolism. Catastrophic deterioration on a background of chronic disease is also more likely to be due to small molecule disorders, particularly if the clinical history is one of recurrent exacerbations and remissions separated by periods of relatively good health. However, the interpretation of the diagnostic significance of sudden deterioration requires some care. The disease process in patients with organelle disease may erode the general health of the patient, or the function of some specific organ or tissue, to the extent that intercurrent infections or otherwise trivial illnesses cause generalized organelle dysfunction or severe organ failure. An example is acute deterioration of patients with mitochondrial disorders occurring as a result of sudden metabolic decompensation in the face of an otherwise trivial viral illness. An acute-on-chronic presentation is not, therefore, invariably an indication that the underlying defect is in small molecule metabolism.

Similarly, although a gradual onset of symptoms is characteristic of many organelle disorders, like lysosomal storage disease and peroxisomal disorders, it is also a feature of some of the small molecule diseases, especially some of the

Table 9.2 Some general clinical characteristics of defects of organelle metabolism

Lysosomal	Peroxisomal	Mitochondrial
Disease limited to nervous system ± RES	Multisystem disease	Multisystem disease
Chronic course	Failure to thrive	Failure to thrive
Hepatosplenomegaly, variable	Profound hypotonia	Cerebral dysgenesis
Leukodystrophy, often severe	Cerebral dysgenesis	Sensorineural hearing loss
Cerebellar atrophy, marked	Hepatocellular dysfunction	Peripheral neuropathy
Skin lesions (angiokeratomata)	Sensorineural hearing loss	Myopathy
'Cherry-red' macular spot	Neuropathy	Extraocular ophthalmoplegia
Behavior/psychiatric problems	Cystic disease of kidneys	Cardiomyopathy
Seizures, late	Seizures, early and intractable	Retinitis pigmentosa
		Seizures, variable

Note: Abbreviations: RES, reticuloendothelial system.

amino acidopathies, like phenylketonuria (PKU) and homocystinuria. In this case, the course of the disease must be considered in the light of other clinical findings, such as the presence or absence of what might be characterized as particular physical findings or dysmorphic features.

The presence of *specific physical findings or dysmorphic features* suggests in general that the underlying defect is in organelle metabolism. While the generalization may hold most of the time, there are also some important exceptions. Urinary organic acid analysis would usually be regarded as a 'small molecule' test. However, some of the inherited metabolic diseases associated with diagnostic organic aciduria, such as mevalonic aciduria and glutaric aciduria type II, often present with severe dysmorphism. Among the various inherited disorders of organelle metabolism, the type and extent of tissue and organ involvement often provides a clue to which organelle might be implicated (Table 9.2). Here again, the summary information presented in Table 9.2 is intended to serve only as a guide; there are many exceptions to these generalizations. For example, hypertrophic cardiomyopathy is a common manifestation of mitochondrial cytopathies. However, it is often the presenting sign of GSD II, a lysosomal storage disorder.

Specific histopathologic or ultrastructural abnormalities may be sufficiently characteristic to permit a strong presumptive diagnosis in many of the organelle diseases. Often microscopic examination of tissues or organs not obviously involved with the disease provides invaluable diagnostic information in these cases. For example, the clinical abnormalities in neuronal ceroid lipofuscinosis are confined to the central nervous system (CNS). However, electron microscopic examination of conjunctival mucosa, skin, peripheral blood lymphocytes, or rectal mucosa, generally shows the presence of the typical lysosomal inclusions that are diagnostic of the disease. Some 35 lysosomal storage disorders are associated with characteristic ultrastructural abnormalities in skin biopsies, making electron microscopic examination of the tissue an effective tool for screening for these disorders (Figure 9.7). Bone marrow examination generally provides histopathologic information specific enough to make a strong presumptive diagnosis of Gaucher disease (see Figure 6.5) or Niemann-Pick disease. Histopathologic and ultrastructural abnormalities may be present in patients with small molecule disorders, but as a rule they are not sufficiently specific to provide a diagnosis.

The *response to aggressive supportive measures*, or 'first-aid', is also different between the organelle diseases and the small molecule disorders. The administration of intravenous fluids, glucose, maintenance electrolytes, and correction of metabolic acidosis, often results in significant early, if not dramatic, improvement of patients with small molecule disease who may be acutely ill as a result of metabolic decompensation. In contrast, patients with organelle disease generally respond slowly and incompletely to supportive measures unless deterioration is sudden and the cause is immediately obvious and correctable, such as acute airway obstruction.

Studies on the extent and severity of pathology

Studies directed at determining the extent and severity of organ or tissue failure are generally nonspecific, although the pattern or distribution of abnormalities may be suggestive of a specific disease. Most imaging studies, such as radiographs, MRI, CT scans, and ultrasound examinations, are in this category. Electrophysiologic studies are also relatively nonspecific, showing that a system is affected by disease, but not usually shedding much light on the basic defect. Routine biochemical studies are also generally nonspecific, though they are often helpful in classifying metabolic defects.

Studies directed at the classification of disease processes (the 'metabolic screen')

In the interests of simplifying the investigation of the possibility of inborn errors of metabolism, many laboratories and hospitals have developed customized batteries of screening tests that are grouped together as a 'metabolic screen'. What is included in the battery of tests varies from one laboratory to another, creating the potential for confusion. One of the main problems with so-called metabolic screens is the potentially false sense of security they may produce in the minds of physicians who may not appreciate the limitations of the screening battery. Metabolic screens are probably here to stay, and it is important to determine for each laboratory what tests are included in the test battery and how to interpret the results in each case.

Tests in this category include analysis of plasma ammonium, plasma lactate, pyruvate, 3-hydroxybutyrate, and free fatty acids, quantitative or semi-quantitative analysis of plasma and urine amino acids, urinary or plasma organic acid analysis urinary mucopolysaccharides (MPS) and oligosaccharides screening tests, and galactosemia screening tests. Definitive diagnosis generally requires further *in vitro* metabolic studies, usually specific enzyme assay. The principles involved in the various analytic techniques are described here, along with some indications of the interpretation of test results and major sources of error.

Investigation of 'small molecule disease'

Plasma ammonium

The measurement of plasma ammonium in most laboratories is now done enzymatically with the aid of an autoanalyzer, eliminating the delays and inherent inaccuracies associated with older spectrophotometric methods. However, the determination of plasma ammonium levels is still subject to significant errors arising from environmental contamination, poor venipuncture technique, and careless sample handling. Blood samples should be drawn from a free flowing vein directly into an anticoagulated tube, placed immediately on ice, and the plasma separated and analysis performed within 15 minutes of the blood being drawn. Normal plasma ammonium concentrations vary somewhat with age, being slightly higher in newborn infants.

Plasma lactate and pyruvate

Plasma lactate and pyruvate levels are generally analyzed enzymatically. The same precautions required for accurate measurement of plasma ammonium apply to measurements of plasma lactate. The use of a tourniquet and delayed sample handling are common causes of spurious elevations of plasma lactate. Levels in arterial blood and cerebrospinal fluid (CSF) are generally more reliable than venous plasma lactates. The measurement of pyruvate is cumbersome, and the results are seriously prone to error. Pyruvate levels in blood are always at least an order of magnitude lower that lactate levels, and pyruvate in blood is unstable. Lactate to pyruvate ratios in plasma should, therefore, be interpreted with care, especially if the lactate concentration is not elevated.

Plasma ketones and free fatty acids

Plasma ketones (3-hydroxybutyrate and acetoacetate) are measured enzymatically. 3-Hydroxybutyrate in plasma is relatively stable stored frozen at $-20\ {}^{\circ}C$.

However, acetoacetate is unstable, and quantitative analysis is technically more difficult than measurement of 3-hydroxybutyrate. Because of the technical difficulties associated with acetoacetate measurements, and the finding that pathologic increases in plasma ketone levels characteristically affect 3-hydroxybutyrate more than acetoacetate, many laboratories offer quantitative measurements only of the former. Semi-quantitative methods for estimating blood ketone levels, with the use of Acetest tablets or Ketostix (Ames), measure acetoacetate only; 3-hydroxybutyrate, the principal ketone in blood, does not react.

Free fatty acids in plasma can be measured in many ways. However, most manual methods are cumbersome and are being replaced by semi-automated assays based on colorimetric measurement of cupric ion binding. This method is *not appropriate* for the analysis of very long-chain fatty acids in the investigation of inherited defects of peroxisomal metabolism.

Amino acid analysis

The capability to detect amino acid abnormalities in various physiologic fluids, like plasma, urine and CSF, is central to the investigation of possible inherited metabolic diseases. The detection of abnormalities may be by:

- some relatively nonspecific chemical reactions producing colored reactions products;
- paper or thin-layer chromatography coupled with staining with ninhydrin and other reagents producing colored products upon reaction with specific amino acids;
- ion-exchange chromatography, the basis of most automated amino acid analyzers used for the amino acid quantitation of physiologic fluids;
- high-performance liquid chromatography (HPLC), beginning to replace automated ion-exchange chromatography as the standard method for amino acid quantitation;
- gas chromatography-mass spectrometry (GC-MS);
- tandem mass spectrometry-mass spectrometry (MSMS).

Many metabolic screens include a selection of relatively nonspecific chemical tests for the presence of compounds containing certain functional groups, such as disulfides. In some laboratories, these are combined with, or replaced by, thin-layer or paper chromatography of urine, plasma, or blood to screen for amino acid abnormalities in low-risk patients or as an adjunct to quantitative amino acid analysis. HPLC analysis of amino acids is rapid, accurate, and relatively inexpensive. However the presence of large amounts of interfering substances sometimes makes application of the method to the analysis of free amino acids in physiologic fluids unreliable. Most clinical laboratories formerly doing amino acid quantitation by automated ion-exchange chromatography are changing over to HPLC as the principal analytic methodology.

High-resolution tandem MSMS is rapid, accurate, and requires only small samples of blood. A significant advantage of this technology is the wide range of chemically unrelated compounds and metabolites that can be analyzed simultaneously in extremely small samples of the relevant physiologic fluid, such as dried blood spots. The potential capacity of this methodology, coupled with low operating costs and rapid turnaround times, makes this a powerful tool for centralized state screening laboratories (see Chapter 8). One significant disadvantage of this technique is the inability to separate structural isomers, such as leucine and isoleucine without special upstream chromatographic separation.

Chemical screening tests for amino aciduria

A number of tests have evolved for rapid detection of specific classes of amino acids or amino acid metabolites in urine (Table 9.3). They are inexpensive, require only small amounts of urine, and are technically simple to perform. They are even adaptable to use at home, in certain circumstances, for monitoring therapy. In general, they are relatively insensitive and nonspecific, being affected by the presence of any of a wide range of compounds, such as drug metabolites. They provide useful initial screening tests, but the results must be interpreted with care.

Paper or thin-layer chromatography

Paper or thin-layer chromatographic separation of amino acids in blood, plasma, or urine, and visualization by treatment with ninhydrin is an excellent technique for detecting *excesses* of single amino acids, such as phenylalanine or tyrosine, or small groups of structurally related amino acids, such as the branched-chain amino acids. It is next to useless for the detection of *deficiencies* of amino acids, a feature that seriously compromises the usefulness of this type of analysis in the investigation of possible urea cycle enzyme defects. Artifacts are common, but generally they are readily recognizable.

Quantitative amino acid analysis

Quantitative amino acid analysis, by semi-automated ion-exchange chromatography, HPLC, or tandem MSMS, is an indispensable component of any diagnostic service involved with the management of inherited metabolic diseases. It meets four important needs:
- It provides for the confirmation of the identity and concentration of abnormal ninhydrin-positive compounds that might have been detected by any of the screening tests discussed above.

Table 9.3 Chemical screening tests for amino acids and amino acid metabolites in urine

Screening test	Compound	Interpretation
Ferric chloride or Phenistix	Phenylpyruvic acid	Typical stable green color occurs in untreated PKU. Other conditions or the presence of a wide range of interfering metabolites (e.g., p-hydroxyphenylpyruvic acid, branched-chain ketoacids, imidazolepyruvic acid, homogentisic acid) or drugs (e.g., acetaminophen, salicylates, phenothiazines, isoniazid) produce different colors.
Dinitrophenylhydrazine	α-Ketoacids	Typical yellow precipitate occurs in MSUD, PKU, or ketoacidosis.
Cyanide nitroprusside	Disulfide bonds	Rapid development of red-purple color occurs in cystinuria, homocystinuria, or β-mercaptolactate-cysteine disulfiduria. The ingestion of certain drugs, notably N-acetylcysteine (Mucomyst), penicillamine, captopril, or synthetic penicillins, also produces a positive reaction. Atypical color reactions occur in ketoacidosis.
Nitrosonaphthol	p-Hydroxylated phenolic acids and 5-hydroxyindoles	Orange-red color occurs in tyrosinemia. Typical or atypical positive reactions are seen in patients with severe hepatocellular dysfunction, intestinal malabsorption or short gut syndrome, neuroblastoma, or carcinoid tumor, and in patients receiving parenteral nutrition containing N-acetyltyrosine.
Merckoquant Sulfite test	Sulfite	A pink color on the reagent strip occurs in sulfite oxidase deficiency or molybdendum cofactor defect. The reaction is inhibited by large amounts of ascorbic acid. The presence of excessive amounts of other inorganic anions and some cations produces atypical positive reactions.
Benedict's reagent (Clinitest)	Reducing substances	Green to orange colors occur in glycosuria (e.g., glucose, galactose, fructose, lactose, mannose, sialic acid or xylose, but not sucrose). Homogentisic acid also produces a positive reaction. The presence of large amounts of ascorbic acid or ampicillin may interfere with the test.
Acetest	Acetoacetate or acetone	Purple color indicates the presence of acetoacetate.
p-Nitroaniline-nitrite reagent	Methylmalonic acid	An emerald green color indicates increased methylmalonic acid. Malonic and ethylmalonic acids, and some drugs used in pediatrics also produce positive reactions.

Note: Abbreviations: MSUD, maple syrup urine disease; PKU, phenylketonuria.

- When it is readily accessible, it ends up being faster than paper or thin-layer chromatographic analysis.
- It provides accurate quantitative information on the levels of amino acids that may be present in subnormal concentrations, in addition to those that are present in excess.
- It is the only way to quantitate reliably the concentrations of amino acids in physiologic fluids, like CSF, in which the levels of all amino acids are normally very low.

Secondary abnormalities of amino acid concentrations in plasma and urine are very common. Severe hepatocellular disease, renal tubular disease, catabolic states, pregnancy, vitamin deficiencies, malnutrition, neoplasia, infection, burns, and injuries are all associated with disturbances of amino acid concentrations in plasma or urine or both. Sorting out whether a particular abnormality is due to an inborn error of metabolism or secondary to some common, acquired disorder is sometimes difficult. In many cases, the matter is resolvable by eliciting a history of injury, stress, or disease. However, in some, the distinction between abnormalities attributable to primary metabolic disease and secondary metabolic responses to acquired disease requires further investigation. This is especially true when a particular inherited disorder of amino acid metabolism, such as hepatorenal tyrosinemia, causes severe generalized or organ-specific tissue damage. In other instances, primary inherited disorders of fat, organic acid, or carbohydrate metabolism are associated with secondary disturbances of amino acid metabolism. The amino acid abnormality in plasma or urine may be wrongly interpreted as evidence that the underlying disease is a primary disorder of amino acid metabolism. The hyperglycinemia occurring in propionic acidemia and methylmalonic acidemia is a signal example of this type of confusion.

A reasonable approach to the interpretation of plasma or urinary amino acid abnormalities might consist in addressing the following questions:

- Is the amino acid abnormality sufficiently characteristic that, along with the clinical findings, the diagnosis of a specific inborn error of metabolism can be made? This applies particularly to inborn errors of specific amino acids in which marked increases in plasma and urine levels are observed (Table 9.4).
- Is the abnormality attributable to an inherited amino acid transport defect? Amino acid transport abnormalities in general are characterized by markedly increased levels in urine, because of defective reabsorption of the amino acids, along with normal or subnormal levels in plasma. The urinary amino acid pattern may be specific enough to suggest the diagnosis (Table 9.5).
- To what extent might the abnormalities be due to inherited metabolic diseases in which the disturbances in amino acid concentrations are secondary (Table 9.6)?

Table 9.4 Plasma amino acid abnormalities in various primary disorders of amino acid metabolism

Amino acid abnormality	Disease (defect)	Associated clinical features
Aspartylglucosamine	Aspartylglucosaminuria	Progressive psychomotor retardation with 'storage syndrome' (see Chapter 6)
Alanine	Nonspecific manifestation of lactic acidosis	
β-Alanine, taurine, GABA	Hyper-β-alaninemia, Carnosinemia	Severe, early-onset neurologic syndrome with intractable seizures
α-Aminoadipic acid (2-ketoadipic acid, 2-hydroxyadipic acid)	α-Aminoadipic aciduria	Hypotonia, intermittent metabolic acidosis, developmental delay in some patients
β-Aminoisobutyric acid	β-Aminoisobutyric aciduria	Benign polymorphism, also occurs secondary to massive tissue destruction (e.g., burns, malignancy, etc.)
Anserine (β-alanyl-1-methylhistidine)	Carnosinemia	Psychomotor retardation, myoclonic seizures
Arginine	Hyperargininemia	Psychomotor retardation, spasticity resembling cerebral palsy
Argininosuccinic acid	Argininosuccinic aciduria	Hyperammonemic encephalopathy (Chapter 2)
Carnosine (β-alanylhistidine)	Carnosinemia	Psychomotor retardation, myoclonic seizures
Citrulline	Citrullinemia	Hyperammonemic encephalopathy (Chapter 2)
Cystathionine	Cystathioninemia (γ-cystathionase deficiency)	Uncertain, may be benign
Cysteine-homocysteine disulfide	Homocystinuria	See below
Glutamine	Nonspecific manifestation of hyperammonemia	
Glycine	Nonketotic hyperglycinemia (glycine cleavage deficiency)	Severe, early-onset acute encephalopathy, seizures, profound mental retardation (Chapter 7). Glycine is also markedly increased in patients with organic acidemias, e.g., MMA, PA, IVA
Histidine	Histidinemia (histidase deficiency)	Probably benign
Homocysteine	Homocystinuria (cystathionine β-synthetase deficiency)	Psychomotor retardation, Marfanoid habitus, ectopia lentis, intravascular thrombosis (Chapter 6)
	Homocystinuria (cobalamin defects)	Megaloblastic anemia, methylmalonic acidemia, psychomotor retardation
Hydroxylysine	Hydroxylysinemia	Possible mental retardation
Hydroxyproline	Hydroxyprolinemia (hydroxyproline oxidase deficiency)	Psychomotor retardation

(cont.)

Table 9.4 (*cont.*)

Amino acid abnormality	Disease (defect)	Associated clinical features
Leucine, isoleucine, valine	MSUD	Acute encephalopathy (Chapter 2)
Lysine	Persistent hyperlysinemia (α-aminoadipic semialdehyde synthetase deficiency)	Psychomotor retardation, seizures
Methionine	Homocystinuria (cystathionine β-synthetase deficiency)	See above
Ornithine	HHH syndrome	Recurrent hyperammonemic encephalopathy
	Hyperornithinemia with gyrate atrophy (ornithine aminotransferase deficiency)	Progressive visual impairment
Phenylalanine	Phenylketonuria	Progressive psychomotor retardation
Phosphoethanolamine	Hypophosphatasia	Skeletal dysplasia
Proline	Hyperprolinemia, type I (proline oxidase deficiency)	Benign
	Hyperprolinemia, type II (Δ^1-pyrroline-5-carboxylate dehydrogenase deficiency)	Seizures, relatively benign
Sarcosine (*N*-methylglycine)	Hypersarcosinemia	Probably benign
S-sulfocysteine	Sulfite oxidase deficiency, Molybdenum cofactor deficiency	Severe, neurologic syndrome with seizures, psychomotor retardation, ectopia lentis
Tyrosine	Hepatorenal tyrosinemia (hereditary tyrosinemia, type I; fumarylacetoacetase deficiency)	Severe, progressive hepatocellular dysfunction, renal tubular dysfunction, porphyric crises (Chapter 4)
	Hereditary tyrosinemia, type II (oculocutaneous tyrosinemia; tyrosine aminotransferases deficiency)	Painful hyperkeratosis of palms and soles, painful inflammation of the eyes, corneal opacities, variable psychomotor retardation
	Hereditary tyrosinemia, type III (*p*-hydroxyphenylpyruvate dioxygenase deficiency)	Probably benign

Note: Abbreviations: GABA, γ-aminobutyric acid; MMA, methylmalonic acid; PA, propionic acidemia; IVA, Isovaleric acidemia; MSUD, maple syrup urine disease; HHH, hyperornithinemia-hyperammonemia-homocitrullinemia.

Table 9.5 Primary inherited disorders of amino acid transport

Amino acid abnormality	Disease (defect)	Associated clinical features
Increased cystine, arginine, lysine, ornithine, glutamine in urine	Cystinuria (defect in dibasic amino acid and cystine transport in kidney and gut)	Kidney stones, recurrent renal colic
Increased urine concentrations and decreased plasma levels of ornithine, lysine, arginine, glutamine	Lysinuric protein intolerance (generalized defect in diamino acid transport)	Dietary protein intolerance, recurrent hyperammonemia, hematologic abnormalities, pulmonary and renal disease
Increased plasma levels of ornithine, homocitrulline	HHH syndrome (defect in intramitochondrial ornithine transport)	Recurrent hyperammonemic encephalopathy (Chapter 2)
Increased urine concentrations and decreased plasma levels of neutral amino acids	Hartnup disease (defect in neutral amino acid transport in kidney and gut)	Pellagra-like skin lesions (Chapter 2)
Increased urine concentrations of glycine, proline, hydroxyproline	Iminoglycinuria (defect in renal transport)	Benign

Note: Abbreviations: HHH, hyperornithinemia-hyperammonemia-homocitrullinemia.

In most of the primary inherited disorders of amino acid metabolism or transport, the plasma and urinary amino acid abnormalities are not subtle. Nonessential amino acid abnormalities are often secondary to other metabolic disorders or acquired conditions. Abnormalities involving more than one amino acid are more likely to be due to primary inherited metabolic disorders if the amino acids are structurally or metabolically related, such as the dibasic amino acids or neutral amino acids. Increased amino acid levels in the urine in the absence of corresponding increases in plasma levels are generally due to inherited or acquired renal transport defects.

Neurotransmitters

The investigation of neurological disorders, especially those characterized by movement disorders, seizures, or autonomic disturbances (Chapter 2), has been greatly advanced by the development of protocols for analysis of neurotransmitters and related metabolites in CSF. A handful of reference laboratories are now providing analyses of tetrahydrobiopterin (BH4), 7,8-dihydrobiopterin (BH2), neopterin, homovanillic acid (HVA), 5-hydroxyindoleacetic acid (5HIAA), and 3-*O*-methyldopa (3OMD) on a service basis. Accurate interpretation of the findings is critically dependent on the care taken with the collection of CSF by lumbar

Table 9.6 Some common secondary abnormalities of plasma or urinary amino acids

Amino acid	Underlying condition or disease
Increased plasma alanine	Lactic acidosis, irrespective of the cause
β-Aminoisobutyric aciduria	Marked tissue destruction (burns, leukemia, surgery, etc.)
Generalized amino aciduria	Proximal renal tubular dysfunction
1-Methylhistidinuria, carnosine	Derived from dietary poultry
Increased plasma methionine, tyrosine, and phenylalanine	Commonly associated with hepatocellular disease, irrespective of the cause
Methioninuria	Resulting from ingestion of D-methionine in semi-synthetic infant formulae supplemented with DL-methionine
Glycylprolinuria or prolylhydroxyprolinuria	Active bone disease
Increased plasma threonine	Ingestion of infant formulas with high whey to casein ratio
Increased plasma cystathionine	Vitamin B_6 deficiency

puncture and the handling of the specimen between the time it is obtained and analysis. Keith Hyland has emphasized that:

- the reference laboratory should be contacted in advance for instructions on collection of samples of CSF and shipping,
- all neurotransmitters and metabolites should be analyzed on the same sample of CSF,
- the CSF should be frozen immediately and stored on dry ice, or collected into a suitable antioxidant, prior to shipping, and
- any contaminating red cells should be removed immediately by centrifugation prior to freezing of the CSF.

Some of the abnormalities found in various disorders of neurotransmitter metabolism are shown in (Table 9.7).

Organic acid analysis

Organic acid analysis, by gas-liquid chromatography with or without mass spectrometry, has become available in most major pediatric hospitals. Although diagnostically important organic acid changes occur in a variety of physiologic fluids, urine is the most easily obtained, the most commonly analyzed, and the fluid for which the most information is available with respect to the identification of pathologic abnormalities. With the spread of the application of tandem MSMS technology to the investigation of inherited metabolic diseases, the analysis of organic acids in blood, as acylcarnitines, will become more accessible. Tandem MSMS offers numerous advantages over conventional amino acid and organic acid analyses; however, the instrumentation is very expensive.

Most of the diagnostically important organic acids occurring in urine are chemically quite stable. The results of analysis are not materially affected by storage

Table 9.7 Cerebrospinal fluid abnormalities in some disorders of neurotransmitter metabolism

Disorder	Levels in CSF					
	BH4	BH2	Neop	HVA	5HIAA	3OMD
GTP-CH deficiency	↓	N	↓	↓	↓	N
Septiapterin reductase deficiency	±↓	↑	N	↓	↓	N
Tyrosine hydroxylase deficiency	N	N	N	↓	N	N
AADC deficiency	N	N	N	↓	↓	↑

Abbreviations: CSF, cerebrospinal fluid; BH4, tetrahydrobiopterin; BH2, 7,8-dihydrobiopterin; Neop, neopterin; HVA, homovanillic acid; 5HIAA, 5-hydroxyindoleacetic acid; 3OMD, 3-O-methyldopa; GTP-CH, GTP cyclohydrolase; AADC, aromatic L-amino acid decarboxylase. *Source:* Table adapted from Hyland (2003).

for periods of months at $-20\ °C$. The addition of chemical preservatives, such as thymol, is not generally necessary so long as the urine is kept frozen. Preparation for analysis includes extraction of the organic acids from the urine into an organic solvent. After extraction, the organic acids all require derivatization to lower the temperature at which they vaporize and to prevent them undergoing thermal decomposition in the heated inlet of the gas chromatograph.

A typical organic acid analysis would involve preliminary measurement of the creatinine concentration and dilution of a volume of urine containing 2.5 μmol to 1.0 ml with distilled water. After acidification and extraction into ethylacetate, the solvent is evaporated off, and trimethylsilyl derivatives of the organic acids are formed immediately prior to injection into the GC-MS. The gas chromatograph is made up of three parts: a heated inlet, a glass or steel column containing a finely ground solid support coated with a microscopic film of nonvolatile liquid phase, and a detector. The detector is often a mass spectrometer. The sample, dissolved in an appropriate solvent, is injected into the inlet where it is vaporized by heating. The vapor is carried through the column by a stream of inert gas. The compounds in the sample are separated from each other on the basis of their relative solubilities in the stationary liquid phase. Preliminary identification of organic acids is based on retention time, that is the time taken for the compound to pass through the column.

The mass spectrometer part of the system also consists of three components: a system for ionizing the compounds to be analyzed, a system for separating them on the basis of the ratio of mass to charge (m/z), and a detector. Most instruments used for clinical purposes are designed to receive the effluent from a gas chromatograph. The compounds in the effluent are ionized, commonly by bombardment by a stream of electrons, which also causes orderly fragmentation of the compounds into derivative ions of specific m/z. They are then propelled into the separating system by application of high voltage. The separating system consists of a magnetic field, most commonly produced by an array of electrodes (quadripole) or a large magnet (magnetic sector), and the intensity of the field is varied electronically so that at any given instant only ions with a specific m/z ratio reach the detector. The detector simply records the impact of positively charged ions as they emerge from the separator and reports the relative abundance of the ions and the m/z ratio. Compounds are identified, with the aid of computer-assisted data analysis, on the basis of a combination of retention time (gas chromatograph) and m/z and fragmentation pattern (mass spectrometer). Some typical pathological urinary organic acid patterns are shown in Figure 9.1.

Primary disorders of organic acid metabolism are reviewed in more detail in Chapter 3. Chemical and biological artifacts are common in the analysis of urinary organic acids. The plasticizers in plastic containers may leach out, in the presence of urine, and produce spurious signals identified as unusual fatty acids, such as azelaic and pimelic acids. Age, drugs, and diet also affect urinary organic acid profiles. Gut bacteria produce large amounts of organic acids, particularly in the very young. Some of the more common causes of urinary organic acid artifacts are shown in Table 3.6.

Acylcarnitines and acylglycines

Urine

Analysis of carnitine and glycine esters in urine has become an important part of the investigation of organic acidopathies. Sample preparation is much easier, and the results obtained, using fast-atom bombardment (FAB) and high-resolution mass spectrometry, are more powerful than conventional GC-MS. However, the capital cost of the required instrumentation puts this out of range of most diagnostic laboratories. The sensitivity of acylcarnitine analysis for the detection of inborn errors of organic acid metabolism is increased when it is combined with carnitine loading. The patient is given an oral dose of 100 mg L-carnitine per kg body weight. Urine is then collected for 8–12 hours and submitted for acylcarnitine analysis. This is sometimes necessary because carnitine levels in patients with organic acidopathies may become so depleted that there is not enough available to form diagnostic carnitine esters.

Analysis of acylglycines is performed with the same apparatus used for acylcarnitine analysis. Some feel that acylglycine analysis is more sensitive that acylcarnitine analysis, especially for the detection of fatty acid oxidation defects. Both analytic

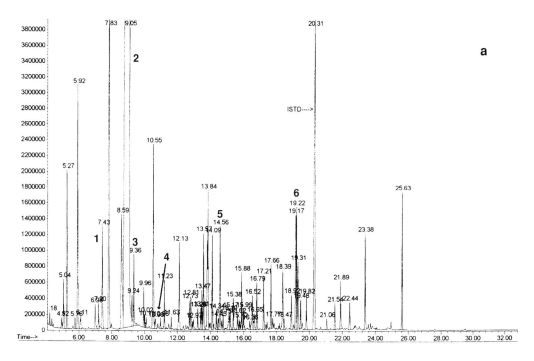

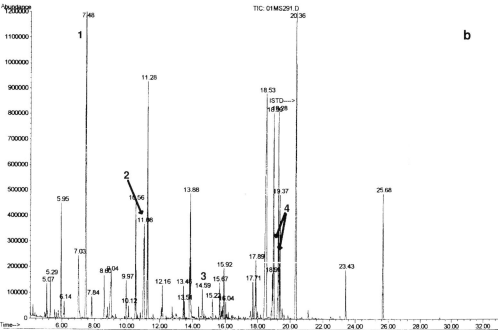

Figure 9.1 Some typical pathological urinary organic acid patterns. The figures show the total ion-current recorded by the mass spectrometer, representing the pattern of organic acids as they pass through the gas chromatograph. Panels **a**, Methylmalonic acidemia (**1**, 3-hydroxy-propionate; **2**, methylmalonate; **3**, 3-hydroxyvalerate; **4**, propionylglycine; **5**, tiglylglycine; **6**, methylcitrate); **b**, Propionic acidemia (**1**, 3-hydroxypropionate; **2**, propionylglycine; **3**, tiglylglycine; **4**, methylcitrate); **c**, Multiple carboxylase deficiency (**1a** and **1b**, 3-hydroxy-isovalerate; **2**, isovalerylglycine; **3**, 3-methylcrotonylglycine); **d**, Medium-chain acyl-CoA dehydrogenase deficiency (**1**, hexanoylglycine; **2**, phenylpropionylglycine; **3**, suberylglycine).

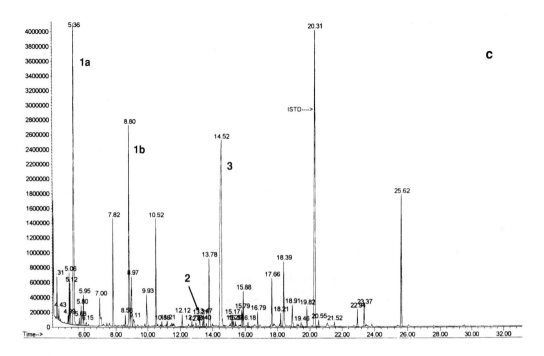

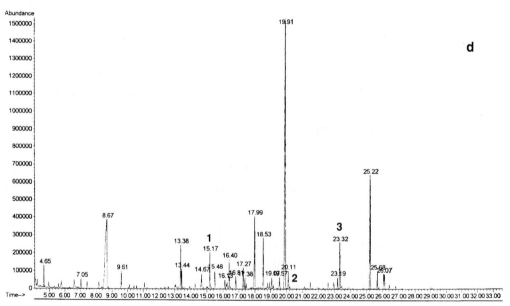

Figure 9.1 (cont.)

techniques are likely to be replaced as diagnostic tools by tandem MSMS analysis of acylcarnitines in blood.

Blood

One of the most important advances in the application of diagnostic laboratory technology for the management of inherited metabolic diseases has been the introduction of tandem MSMS. It has already been introduced in several jurisdictions for newborn screening for a variety of inborn errors of metabolism (see Chapter 8). The analysis of acylcarnitines, amino acids, and other metabolic intermediates in blood is generally performed on compounds eluted from dried blood spots identical to those used throughout the world for newborn screening for PKU. The metabolites in the sample are derivatized by the formation of butyl esters and injected directly into the ionization chamber of the tandem MSMS.

Instead of using gas-liquid chromatography for preliminary separation of metabolites in a physiological mixture, tandem MSMS makes use of a second mass spectrometer. After injection of the sample, the solvent is evaporated and the metabolites become positively charged by a process of electrospray ionization. The positively charged molecular ions are accelerated through the first quadripole, i.e., the first mass spectrometer, where they are separated according to the mass-to-charge (m/z) ratio. The charged molecular ions emerging from the first quadripole enter a collision chamber where collision with an inert gas, such as argon, causes fragmentation of the compounds, producing a series of daughter ions characteristic of the parent compounds. These are focused and accelerated through the second quadripole where the charged molecular fragments are separated according to m/z ratio. A detector situated at the outlet of the second quadripole picks up and measures the electrical current generated by the passage of charged molecular fragments.

Quantitative analyses are generally performed by addition of internal standards of specific compounds labeled with deuterium (^{2}H) to the original sample and comparing the signals produced by the natural compounds in the mixture being analyzed with the signals from the labeled standards of known concentration. Analysis characteristically requires sophisticated computer-assisted data analysis and reporting.

Tandem MSMS instruments are modifiable to extend the range of compounds and the sensitivity of analysis. One of the more common modifications is the addition of up-stream high-performance liquid chromatography (HPLC) to produce a preliminary separation of isomeric compounds with the same molecular weight, such as leucine and isoleucine, prior to injection into the first quadripole. The development of the computer software and robotics required for the analysis of hundreds of samples per day has made tandem MSMS a particularly attractive technique for

Table 9.8 Some common causes of secondary abnormalities of porphyrin excretion

ALA	_Coproporphyrin_
Acute and chronic alcohol ingestion	Normal variant
Lead poisoning	Ingestion of brewer's yeast
Acute iron loading	Chronic alcohol ingestion
Hereditary tyrosinemia	Liver disease
Some malignancies	Chronic renal failure
ALA and PBG	Lead poisoning
Some malignancies	Exposure to mercury or arsenic
Uroporphyrin	Some malignancies
Chronic renal failure	_Protoporphyrin_
Some malignancies	Iron deficiency
	Anemia of chronic disease
	Lead poisoning

Abbreviations: ALA, 5-aminolevulinic acid; PBG, porphobilinogen.
Source: Table is adapted from Nuttall (1994).

newborn screening for disorders of organic acid and amino acid metabolism (see Chapter 8).

Tandem MSMS differs from GC-MS in many important respects. Both are capable of sensitive qualitative and quantitative analysis of organic metabolites in physiological fluids, such as plasma, CSF, and urine. However, tandem MSMS is significantly more sensitive, and the time taken for analysis is a fraction of that required for GC-MS. Depending on the type of analysis being performed and the sensitivity required, the analysis of acylcarnitines and amino acids in blood spots obtained during newborn screening typically takes only minutes per specimen. The marked improvement in sensitivity also decreases significantly the number of false positive screening tests occurring in conventional newborn screening programs.

Porphyrins

The investigation of porphyria presents some special challenges. Acquired or secondary disorders of porphyrin metabolism, such as that caused by lead poisoning, exposure to other toxins, chronic alcoholism, chronic liver disease, or some malignancies (Table 9.8), are more common causes of porphyria than primary hereditary disorders of porphyrin metabolism. Secondary acute porphyria, caused by inhibition of 5-aminolevulinic acid dehydratase by succinylacetone, is also a common manifestation of hepatorenal tyrosinemia. Many carriers of autosomal dominant mutations causing acute porphyria never show any clinical manifestations of the diseases, and conversely, between acute attacks, many individuals with acute porphyria show only subtle biochemical evidence of the defect. The relationship between the various enzymes involved in heme biosynthesis and the different porphyrias is shown in Figure 9.2.

The excretion of porphyrins in urine and stool is highly variable, even in patients with severe disorders of porphyrin metabolism, such as acute intermittent porphyria. Severe abnormalities that are easily identifiable during acute attacks, in the case of the acute porphyrias, are often not present when the patient is clinically well, between attacks. In general, porphyrin abnormalities in urine are more evanescent than those commonly observed in feces. Analyses of feces is often, therefore, more productive than urine analyses in asymptomatic patients between acute attacks.

Porphyrins are photosensitive, and special care needs to be taken to avoid degradation in biological samples between the time the sample is collected and it is analyzed. Samples need to be protected from exposure to air, heat, and light, and analyzed as soon as possible after collection. Collection into air-tight tubes with minimum deadspace, wrapped in aluminum foil to protect the sample from light, and storage on dry ice, is necessary for reliable results if any delay is anticipated in testing. Analysis of random urine samples is usually adequate for diagnosis of the acute porphyrias during acute attacks; however, 24-hour urine collections are often necessary for diagnosis between attacks. In addition to the precautions listed above, the pH of urine should be adjusted to pH 8 by addition of sodium carbonate to minimize non-enzymatic degradation of PBG.

In all the acute neurovisceral porphyrias, except 5-aminolevulinic acid (ALA) dehydratase deficiency, the marked increase in urinary porphobilinogen (PBG) excretion occurring during acute attacks causes the urine to turn pink or red on standing. Urinary screening tests for PBG are almost always positive if the urine is tested during an acute attack. In the case of acute intermittent porphyria (AIP), the diagnosis is confirmed by demonstration of deficiency of PBG deaminase in erythrocytes; in rare cases, erythrocyte PBG deaminase activity may not be decreased, and the diagnosis of AIP requires analysis of tissue porphyrins. Analysis of porphyrins in erythrocytes, plasma, urine, bile, and stool is helpful in the diagnosis and classification of porphyria (Table 9.9). Abnormalities in the water-soluble porphyrin precursors, ALA and PBG, are generally most obvious in urine; whereas abnormalities in the more distal, relatively water-insoluble, porphyrins, coproporphyin and protoporphyrin, which are exreted in bile, are best demonstrated by analysis of feces. The collection of bile, by duodenal intubation, obviates the need for collection and analysis of feces, which is sometimes difficult and always unpleasant, and it also greatly decreases confusion caused by the presence in feces of dietary porphyrins and porphyrins produced by gut bacterial action.

Because the biochemical abnormalities occurring in the hereditary porphyrias may not be obvious when the patient is clinically well, or in asymptomatic carriers,

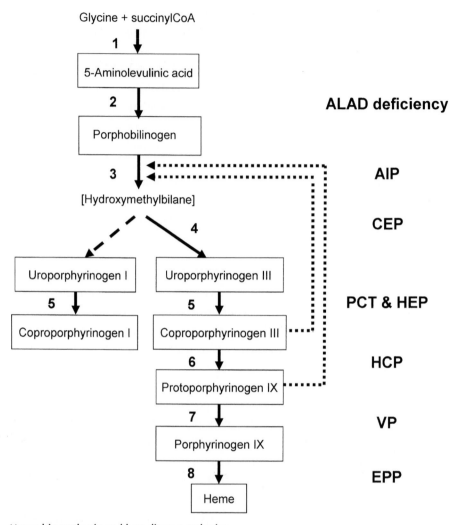

Figure 9.2   Heme biosynthesis and hereditary porphyrias.

Enzymes involved in heme biosynthesis: **1**, 5-aminolevulinic acid synthase; **2**, 5-amino-levulinic acid dehydratase; **3**, porphobilinogen deaminase; **4**, uroporphyrinogen III cosyn-thase; **5**, uroporphyrinogen decarboxylase; **6**, coproporphyrinogen oxidase; **7**, protopor-phyrinogen oxidase; **8**, ferrochetalase. The broken line indicates spontaneous non-enzymatic reactions; the dotted line indicates feedback inhibitory actions.

Abbreviations: ALAD, 5-aminolevulinic acid dehydratase; AIP, acute intermittent porphyria; CEP, congenital erythropoietic porphyria; PCT, porphyria cutanea tarda; HEP, hepatoerythro-poietic porphyria; HCP, hereditary coproporphyria; VP, variegate porphyria; EPP, erythropoi-etic protoporphyria.

Table 9.9 Biochemical abnormalities in the hereditary porphyrias

Disease	Inheritance	Enzyme defect	Urine				Feces	
			ALA	PBG	URO	COPRO	COPRO	PROTO
Acute porphyrias								
Neurovisceral only								
ALA dehydratase deficiency	AR	ALA dehydratase	↑↑↑	±↑	↑	↑	↑	↑
AIP	AD	PBG deaminase	↑↑↑	↑↑↑	↑	↑	±↑	±↑
Neurovisceral ± cutaneous								
HCP	AD	Coproporphyrinogen oxidase	↑↑	↑↑	±↑	↑↑	↑↑	↑
VP	AD	Protoporphyrinogen oxidase	↑↑	↑↑	↑	↑	↑↑	↑↑↑
Non-acute porphyrias								
Cutaneous only								
CEP	AR	Uroporphyrinogen III cosynthase	N	N	↑↑[1]	↑↑[1]	↑↑[1]	↑↑[1]
PCT	AD	Uroporphyrinogen decarboxylase	N	N	↑↑[2]	↑↑[2]	↑[3]	N
HEP	AR	Uroporphyrinogen decarboxylase	N	N	↑↑[2]	↑↑[2]	↑[3]	N
EPP	AD	Ferrochetalase	N	N	N	N	N	±↑[4]

Abbreviations: AR, autosomal recessive; AD, autosomal dominant; ALA, 5-aminolevulinic acid; URO, uroporphyrinogen III; COPRO, coproporphyrinogen III; AIP, acute intermittent porphyria; PBG, porphobilinogen; CEP, congenital erythropoietic porphyria; PCT, porphyria cutanea tarda; HCP, hereditary coproporphyria; HEP, hepatoerythropoietic porphyria; VP, variegate porphyria; EPP, erythropoietic protoporphyria;

[1] The increases in CEP are in uroporphyrin I and coproporphyrin I isomers.

[2] The porphyrins are a mixture of 7- & 8-carboxylated porphyrins as a results of partial decarboxylation of uroporphyrinogens I & III.

[3] Isocoproporphyrin.

[4] Marked increase in protoporphyrin in erythrocytes.

specific enzyme assay or molecular genetic studies to identify disease-causing mutations are particularly valuable in the identification of individuals who are at high risk for life-threatening acute attacks of the disease.

Approaches to the investigation of metabolic disorders

Cellular metabolic screening studies

A number of specialized laboratories now offer metabolic screening studies based on analysis of the metabolism of specific, radiolabeled substrates by intact cells in culture. Although simple in principle, these are generally cumbersome and require fastidious laboratory technique to produce reliable, interpretable results.

Screening for fatty acid oxidation defects by analysis of the release of $^{14}CO_2$ from radiolabeled fatty acid or organic acid substrates incubated with intact cultured skin fibroblasts

The principle here is straightforward; however, the application has proved to be technically demanding and for practical purposes restricted to a handful of research laboratories with special expertise in the area. When cultured fibroblasts are incubated *in situ* with [^{14}C]-labeled fatty acids, oxidation of the substrates results in the production of $^{14}CO_2$ which is trapped by concentrated NaOH or KOH. By the use of labeled fatty acid substrates of differing chain length, the relative efficiency of short-chain, medium-chain, and long-chain fatty acid oxidation can be determined. However, interpretation of the results may be difficult owing to the overlap in substrate specificities of the various enzyme systems involved in fatty acid oxidation. Selective inactivation of specific fatty acyl-CoA dehydrogenases, by precipitation with monospecific antibodies, greatly improves the diagnostic power of the technique. Identification of a presumptive defect generally requires confirmation by specific enzyme analysis or specific mutation analysis.

Complementation analysis

Complementation analysis has been widely used to demonstrate the genetic heterogeneity of conditions that may resemble each other very closely, but are the result of mutation sin different genes with gene products that are mutually complementing. The principles involved are illustrated diagrammatically in Figure 9.3.

Rosenblatt and others have developed elegant techniques for classifying hereditary defects in cobalamin metabolism by complementation analysis. This involves analysis of combinations of fibroblast cell lines from different patients, fused together to produce hybrids in which the enzymic defect in one cell line may be corrected (i.e., complemented) by the presence of normal enzyme in the other. Cross-correction (complementation) only occurs if the defects in the two cell lines are different and either the enzymes involved, or their substrates, are freely diffusible. The analysis in this example involves incubation of various pairs of mutant fibroblast cell lines with radiolabeled propionic acid and determination of the extent of incorporation of label into protein. In the course of its normal metabolism, propionate is converted into methylmalonate, and the carbon skeleton of the methylmalonate becomes incorporated into various nonessential amino acids, which are then incorporated into protein. The metabolism of methylmalonate requires the presence of activated cobalamin (vitamin B_{12}). By complementation analysis, it was

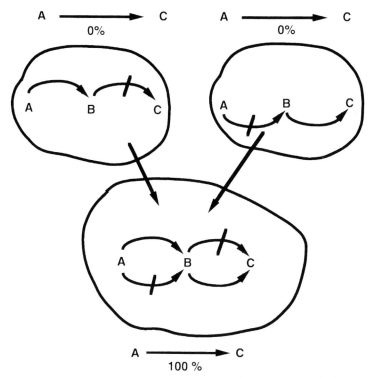

Figure 9.3　Schematic diagram showing principles of complementation analysis.

possible to identify a wide spectrum genetic defects in cobalamin metabolism long before the specific enzymes involved had been identified.

Testing for deficiency of one of the sphingolipid activator proteins, or for pseudodeficiency of lysosomal enzyme activities, by measuring the hydrolysis of radiolabeled, natural substrate by intact cultured skin fibroblasts *in situ*

Most of the lysosomal enzymes involved in the metabolism of sphingolipids require the participation of one of a group of nonenzymic glycoprotein activators for activity towards the natural substrate. When the activities of these enzymes are measured *in vitro*, the detergents used to maintain the substrates in aqueous solution substitutes for the glycoprotein activators: in order to identify defects involving one of the activator proteins, enzyme activity must be measure using the natural substrate, *without* any added detergent. One way to do this is to suspend radiolabeled substrate in buffer as a micellar suspension and layer this on a confluent monolayer of cultured fibroblasts. After several hours of incubation, the distribution of radioactivity between the labeled substrate and product reflects the activator-dependent enzyme activity.

Screening for defects in NADH oxidation by analysis of lactate/pyruvate (L/P) ratios in cultured fibroblasts

This procedure exploits the fact that the intracellular lactate dehydrogenase-catalyzed interconversion of lactate and pyruvate reaches thermodynamic equilibrium so rapidly that the L/P ratio is a direct reflection of the intracellular $NADH/NAD^+$ ratio. Defects causing NADH accumulation are associated with increased L/P ratios, one of the principal characteristics of mitochondrial electron transport chain defects.

Screening for defects in the mitochondrial ETC by culturing fibroblasts in medium containing galactose as the sole source of carbohydrate

As a result of impaired capacity for the production of energy from mitochondrial NADH oxidation, fibroblasts from patients with ETC defects rely heavily on glycolysis to meet their energy needs. When the energy-generating efficiency of glycolysis is decreased by substituting galactose for glucose in the culture medium, the viability of the cells is compromised. Fibroblasts with intact mitochondrial ETC survive – those with ETC defects die. Cells that fail to survive in galactose-containing medium are subjected to more detailed biochemical analysis to identify the specific ETC defect.

Cybrid analysis

The mitochondrial genome codes for the production of 2 ribosomal RNAs (rRNA), 22 transfer RNAs (tRNA), and only 13 of the estimated 69 polypeptides of the ETC; over 50 of the polypeptides of the ETC are encoded by nuclear genes. Cybrid analysis is a type of complementation analysis used to differentiate between mitochondrial ETC defects caused by mutations in nuclear genes from mtDNA mutations. A key element of the technique is the production of cultured cells containing a nucleus, but no mtDNA, by serial passage in medium supplemented with ethidium bromide. These mtDNA-less cells, called $\rho°$ ('rho zero'), are able to survive and grow in medium supplemented with pyruvate and uridine. By fusion of $\rho°$ cells with platelets, which contain mitochondria, but no nuclear DNA, or with cells from which the nucleus has been extracted, and analysis of ETC activity, the relative contributions of nDNA and mtDNA to ETC defects is determined (Figure 9.4).

Blue native polyacrylamide gel electrophoresis (BN-PAGE analysis)

Isolated mitochondria, from cells or tissues, are solubilized with 6-aminocaproic acid. A dye, Serva Blue G (Coomassie Blue G250), is added to introduce a charge shift on each of the complexes, and the five electron transport chain complexes (see Figure 9.12) are separated according to their molecular mass. by electrophoresis on a native polyacrylamide gel gradient. The proteins are transferred to a membrane

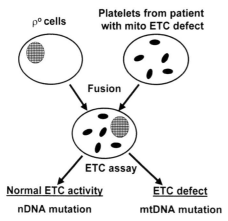

Figure 9.4   Principles of cybrid analysis.

and visualized by treatment with antibodies that recognize the individual native complexes (Figure 9.5).

BN-PAGE analysis requires only small amounts of material (a single flask of skin fibroblasts, or less than 50 mg of tissue), and the total amount of fully assembled enzyme can be measured. BN-PAGE also leaves the protein intact and enzymatically active, permitting semi-quantitative histochemical estimates to be made of the activity of the complexes. Finally, nearly all of the known autosomal recessive oxidative phosphorylation disorders in infants apparently result from a failure in the assembly of one or more of the oxidative phosphorylation enzyme complexes, rather than from mutations affecting the catalytic activity of individual components of the complexes; in most cases, a biochemical diagnosis can be made by investigating the amount of fully assembled complexes.

Provocative testing

Diagnostic tolerance tests are based on the notion that increasing the flux through a metabolic pathway that is impaired as a result of a defect in one of the specific enzymatic steps produces an increase in the concentration of the immediately proximal substrate of the defective reaction without producing an increase in the concentration of the product of the reaction. The ratio of substrate to product is increased, and normally minor metabolites often appear in easily measurable quantities. Tolerance tests are useful for evaluating, by one procedure, the integrity of an entire metabolic pathway in which equilibration between different subcellular compartments is not rate-limiting. Metabolic flux may be increased by:

• exogenous administration of one of the substrates of the pathway under investigation, such as phenylalanine loading for detection of carriers of PKU;

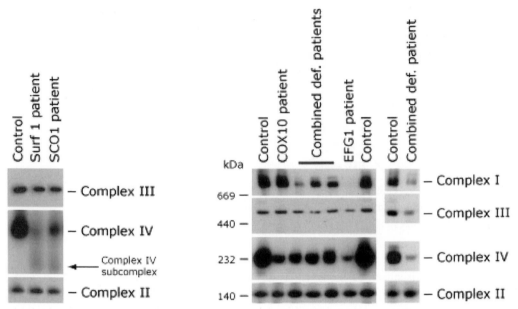

Figure 9.5   Blue native polyacrylamide gel electrophoresis (BN-PAGE) analysis of mitochondrial electron transport chain defects.

The figure shows the results of analysis of Complexes I–IV in cultured skin fibroblasts from patients with isolated cytochrome c oxidase deficiency caused by mutations in the assembly factors *SURF1*, *SCO1* and *COX10*, a patient with a combined deficiency due to a mutation in the translation elongation factor *EFG1*, and patients with combined enzyme deficiencies of known etiology. Patients with isolated cytochrome c oxidase deficiencies have reduced amounts of the fully assembled Complex IV, but normal amounts of the other complexes. Two of them (*SURF1* and *SCO1*) show clear evidence of a partially assembled complex. Patients with a combined deficiency show decreased amounts of more than one enzyme complex. Isolated deficiency of Complex II is very rare, and it is used as a loading control in most instances. (Courtesy of Dr. Eric Shoubridge).

- physiologic manipulation of flux, such as by prolonged fasting, by exercise, etc.;
- exogenous hormone administration, such as administration of glucagon to test the integrity of glycogenolysis or gluconeogenesis.

Loading tests

The number of ways for evaluating the integrity of various metabolic pathways by administering supranormal amounts of one or more of the intermediates is limited only by the imagination of the investigator. However, the reliability of the testing may be limited by problems of absorption, slow equilibration among different subcellular compartments, and potential toxicity of the test metabolite. All loading tests are attended by some risk to the patient, particularly if the symptoms of disease, as is common, are the result of accumulation of the substrate of the defective reaction. In some cases, such as fructose loading for the diagnosis of hereditary fructose intolerance, the risk of morbidity is high. Once commonly used in an effort to localize metabolic defects, metabolic loading tests are now rarely used to screen for genetic defects of intermediary metabolism. This is partly because tolerance tests are dangerous. In most cases, analysis of the specific enzyme presumed to be involved in the defect is available, it is more specific, and it is safer.

Physiologic stress tests

Closely monitored, controlled starvation is one of the most commonly employed stress tests used to assess the physiologic response to fasting. During the transition from the fed to the fasting state, important adjustments in the energy economy of the body occur to ensure an adequate continuing supply of energy to vital organs, like the brain, while minimizing the mobilization of energy substrates from tissues like muscle protein.

A typical test for the evaluation of the efficiency of mitochondrial fatty acid oxidation takes up to 24 hours, depending on the age of the patient and the history of tolerance of fasting (see Chapter 4). Fasting is generally begun in the early evening with occasional biochemical monitoring during the night. On the following morning, a slowly running intravenous infusion of 0.9% NaCl is established to facilitate blood sampling and the rapid administration of glucose should the need arise. After obtaining blood and urine for baseline analysis of glucose, 3-hydroxybutyrate and acetoacetate, free fatty acids, and carnitine (free and total) in plasma, and ketones (by Acetest: Ames), organic acids, carnitine (free and total), acylcarnitines, and acylglycines, in urine, the blood glucose is monitored hourly until the patient develops symptoms of hypoglycemia, or until 20 hours has elapsed, whichever comes first. All urine passed should be tested for ketones. At the termination of the fast, blood and urine are again obtained for the same studies done at baseline. If the patient is symptomatic or hypoglycemic by finger-prick monitoring, the test blood sample should be obtained without delay and the patient given glucose by intravenous infusion until asymptomatic and stable.

The normal response to fasting includes a gradual fall in plasma glucose, rise in plasma ketones (3-hydroxybutyrate and acetoacetate), rise in plasma free fatty acids, and the appearance of ketones and small quantities of medium-chain dicarboxylic acids in the urine. The ratio of free fatty acids to 3-hydroxybutyrate normally does not exceen 3.0. Patients with fatty acid oxidation defects often become hypoglycemic during this procedure, but the ketone levels in plasma do not rise significantly, resulting in a marked elevation of the free fatty acid to 3-hydroxybutyrate ratio. Analysis of urinary organic acids, acylcarnitines, and acylglycines shows the presence of intermediates typical of the underlying defect.

Hormone stimulation tests

Glucagon stimulation is an excellent way to evaluate the integrity of glycogenolysis and gluconeogenesis. However, accurate interpretation of the results requires careful preparation of the patient. For example, the absence of a glycemic response to intramuscular administration of an appropriate dose of the hormone after several hours of fasting may be the result of a defect in glycogen mobilization, such as glycogen debranching enzyme deficiency, or to prior depletion of liver glycogen by prolonged starvation (see Chapter 4).

Enzymology

A strong presumptive diagnosis of a specific inherited metabolic condition is often possible on the basis of the results of analysis of the substrates and products of a particular enzyme reaction, and awareness of the significance of various secondary metabolic abnormalities. This is particularly true of defects in the metabolism of water-soluble metabolites, such as amino acids. However, the definitive diagnosis of many other inherited metabolic diseases is not possible without demonstrating specific deficiency of the enzyme involved. Prenatal diagnosis, in particular, requires access to specific enzyme assay or to DNA analysis in cases in which the diagnosis of the disease under investigation is established and the specific mutations, or appropriate linkage markers, are known.

The practical application of clinical diagnostic enzymology demands attention to a number of variables affecting the results of any particular assay. Although the details of the conditions for measurement of specific enzyme activities vary tremendously from one enzyme to another, the nature of the variables is the same for any diagnostically important enzyme. They include:
- the source of the enzyme to be assayed (tissue specificity). Many enzymes are tissue specific, and diagnostic analysis requires sampling of the relevant tissue.
- the stability of the enzyme during handling and storage.
- the reaction conditions. It goes without saying that the assay conditions used for the analysis of enzyme activities should be optimum for the measurement of the rate of enzyme-catalyzed conversion of substrate to product.
- the substrate specificity of the enzyme.
- the influence of metabolic regulators on activity.
- the phenomenon of 'pseudodeficiency'. A number of situations have been identified in which apparently completely healthy individuals were found to have marked deficiency of the activity of a particular enzyme, as measured *in vitro* under normal assay conditions. This phenomenon of pseudodeficiency is particularly common among the lysosomal hydrolases and has the potential to produce major diagnostic confusion.

Molecular genetic studies

Clinicians are relying increasingly on molecular genetic studies to confirm the diagnosis of genetic disease, including genetic metabolic diseases, and the availability of specific molecular testing is expanding rapidly. In many cases, confirmation of the presumptive diagnosis of a metabolic condition by conventional metabolic laboratory testing is so cumbersome that it has been replaced completely by mutation analysis. Therefore, the clinician needs to be aware of the pitfalls of molecular genetic testing and how they can be avoided.

The techniques currently available for the detection of specific disease-associated mutations are generally well standardized and technically relatively simple, and the results are usually unambiguous: either the mutation is present or it is not. If homozygosity for the mutation is known to cause a particular disease, then the demonstration of two copies of the mutant allele is virtually diagnostic of the condition. However, the power of the approach is diluted by the problem of allelic diversity.

With few exceptions, in all inherited metabolic diseases for which the responsible gene has been isolated and disease-producing mutations characterized, no single mutation accounts for all cases of the disease. Instead, the mutations associated with each disease usually number in the dozens with single specific alleles accounting for no more than a simple majority of the mutant alleles. The problem is particularly acute in the case of X-linked disorders in which each kindred affected with a particular disease, such as Fabry disease or Hunter disease, for example, often has a different disease-causing mutation in the relevant gene. The clinician is often faced with the question: Is the demonstration of a sequence variation *necessary* for confirmation of a diagnosis? And when is the demonstration of a nucleotide sequence variation *sufficient* for confirmation of the diagnosis of a specific disease?

In practice, most inherited metabolic diseases are associated with sequence variations in the exons of the gene or in intron-exon boundaries, which are relatively easy to identify by current diagnostic laboratory techniques. In some cases, such as large deletions, the sequence variation is relatively easy to detect. In others, such as in Pelizaeus-Merzbacher disease, duplications of the gene may be very large, but they are technically difficult at times to demonstrate.

The failure to demonstrate more subtle abnormalities may result from practical limitations on the extent of the molecular genetic analysis, particularly for very large genes with many exons or a very large coding sequence. Many molecular genetic diagnostic laboratories limit analysis to a search for common mutations or sequencing of exons and intron-exon boundaries. Uncommon defects, or defects in non-coding regions, such as within introns or in regulatory sequences flanking the

Table 9.10 Some common mutations causing specific inherited metabolic diseases

Disease	Gene	Mutation*
MCAD deficiency	*MCAD*	K329E
Tay-Sachs disease (Ashkenazi Jews)	*HEXA*	$+TATC_{1278}$[†]
Gaucher disease (Ashkenazi Jews)	*GBA*	N370S
α_1-Antitrypsin deficiency	*PI*Z*	E342K
LCHAD deficiency	*LCHAD (α-subunit)*	E510Q
Galactosemia	*GALT*	Q188R
MPS IH	*IDUA*	W420X
LHON	*ND4*	G11778A[‡]
PKU	*PAH*	R408W

Abbreviations: MCAD, medium-chain acyl-CoA dehydrogenase; LCHAD, long-chain 3-hydroxyacyl-CoA dehydrogenase; MPS IH, Hurler disease; LHON, Lebers hereditary optic neuropathy; PKU, phenylketonuria.
*Mutations are described in general by the amino acid substitution in the gene product polypeptide.
†Nucleotide change in the cDNA.
‡Nucleotide change in the mtDNA.

gene, will be missed. What this means in practical terms is that while the detection of a significant DNA nucleotide sequence variation in tissue from a patient is generally considered strong support for the diagnosis of the related disease, the failure to demonstrate the presence of the mutation does not rule out the diagnosis. The patient may simply have mutant alleles that have not yet been characterized, or they are sufficiently rare that testing for them in a routine diagnostic testing facility is not economically feasible. Nonetheless, in certain cases, and within some specific ethnic groups, the number of different alleles accounting for a high proportion of the cases of a particular disease may be small enough to enable strong diagnostic inferences to be made on the basis of molecular genetic analysis. The absence of specific mutant alleles should always be interpreted with care: the disease in any specific individual may be caused by a mutation that has not previously been identified with the disorder. In such cases, the analysis of the gene product, by measurement of enzyme activity, for example, is a more powerful test of the presence of disease-causing mutations in the relevant gene. Some conditions in which specific mutant alleles occur with sufficient frequency in selected populations to be useful as a primary diagnostic test are shown in Table 9.10.

A number of techniques have been developed to screen for abnormalities anywhere in coding sequences and adjacent intron-exon junctions of specific genes. These have proved to be particularly useful in the identifying mutations in X-linked genes in which each family tends to have a different mutation. Southern blot analysis, though cumbersome, is useful for the detection of significant deletions, insertions, or rearrangements, or for the identification of sequence changes producing new restriction sites or deleting restriction sites present in the normal gene. Many laboratories employ single-strand conformation polymorphism (SSCP) analysis or heteroduplex analysis to screen for sequence abnormalities in general, then follow up with more detailed polymerase chain-reaction (PCR) amplification and sequence analysis of coding regions and adjacent intron-exon boundaries. This process has been simplified by the development of automated techniques for sequence analysis.

Unless a particular mutation has been found in family members affected with the same condition, the failure to identify sequence abnormalities by this approach decreases, but does not eliminate, the possibility that a disease-causing alteration in the expression of the gene exists in the patient. For example, most of the gene screening techniques used for routine detection of mutant alleles do not examine regulatory sequences flanking coding sequences. A mutation in the regulatory region of a gene would, therefore, likely be missed.

The question, is the demonstration of a nucleotide sequence variation *sufficient* for confirmation of the diagnosis of a specific disease? is important because nucleotide sequence variations are, in general, extremely common, and only a fraction of them are associated with disease. The confirmation that a specific sequence abnormality, resulting for example in a single amino acid substitution, is responsible for disease, and is not simply a benign polymorphism, is often time-consuming and cumbersome. Benign polymorphisms are useful for linkage analysis, but are otherwise not diagnostically important in the individual patient. As mentioned previously, the problem of predicting the significance of single nucleotide substitutions is particularly important in the investigation of X-linked disorders, in which new mutations are a major contributor to disease, and every kindred tends to have a different, private mutation.

Some of the properties of disease-causing mutations are:

- Most, though not all, occur in exons or in intron-exon boundaries.
- They segregate with the disease in blood relatives of the affected patient.
- The same defect has been demonstrated in patients with the disease in other families. This is particularly important in situations in which a small number of defects account for the majority of patients with the disease, such as medium-chain acyl-CoA dehydrogenase (MCAD) deficiency in caucasians and Tay-Sachs disease in Ashkenazi Jews.
- They often predict obviously severe alterations in the amino acid sequence of the gene product. For example, insertions and deletions generally produce frameshifts in the reading frame, causing major changes in the downstream amino acid sequence and premature termination of translation.

- They may cause substitutions involving amino acids with profoundly different physico-chemical properties, such as substitution of an asparagine for a serine. Or the substitution involves a change from a codon coding for a specific amino acid to a stop codon, resulting in premature termination of translation.
- The predicted amino acid substitution involves one that is highly conserved, meaning that the same amino acid is present in the same position of the same gene in phylogenetically different organisms.
- The same sequence variation reproduces the predicted metabolic abnormality, usually deficiency of enzyme activity, when it is expressed in appropriate cells in culture. This is actually the gold standard for confirming the pathologic importance of a specific sequence abnormality. However, for obvious reasons, it is well beyond the scope of routine molecular diagnostic testing. Instead, most laboratories providing diagnostic services will report on the presumed significance of previously unreported sequence abnormalities, either with the original report or when asked.

The identification and characterization of specific mutations causing inherited metabolic diseases is occurring at a dizzying pace. Staying abreast of clinically important discoveries and reports is facilitated by the availability of various Internet-accessible databases. The best known is OMIM (Online Mendelian Inheritance in Man), an outgrowth of the massive catalogue first launched some decades ago by Victor McKusick. The website address of the catalogue, which is updated frequently, is http://www3.ncbi.nlm.nih.gov/Omim/.

Investigation of 'organelle disease'

Lysosomal disorders

Lysosomes are single-membrane subcellular organelles that contain a large number of enzymes involved in the hydrolysis of high molecular weight or water-insoluble compounds, like membranes, complex lipids, proteins, and nucleic acids, derived either from the normal turnover of intracellular structures or from similar materials taken up from the extracellular environment by endocytosis/phagocytosis. Lysosomal hydrolases are glycoproteins that become localized in lysosomes by virtue of modification of the oligosaccharide part of the enzyme molecule to contain a mannose-phosphate signal moiety, which is subsequently removed inside the lysosome. Defects in the synthesis of this signal moiety cause I-cell disease, a condition characterized by failure of lysosomal enzymes to become localized within lysosomal vesicles. Some lysosomal enzymes, like most of the sphingolipid hydrolases, require the presence of genetically distinct, non-catalytic, activator proteins for activity against their natural substrates. Disease resulting from mutations affecting activator proteins is clinically indistinguishable from that caused by deficiency of the respective lysosomal enzyme. Other lysosomal enzymes, such as α-neuraminidase and β-galactosidase, require the presence of a protective protein to prevent premature breakdown. Mutations affecting production of the protective protein cause combined deficiency of both enzymes and a disease called galactosialidosis.

Most of this class of enzymes exhibit relatively relaxed substrate specificity. Lysosomal hydrolases, with some important exceptions, are highly specific for the leaving group of the reaction. As a group, the glycosidases are specific for the monosaccharide removed from the substrate glycoconjugate; they are also very specific for the anomeric configuration of the glycosidic linkage, α or β. In contrast, they are not as fastidious with regard to the specific structure of the aglycone, the non-carbohydrate part of the molecule. Accordingly, the lysosomal enzyme, β-galactosidase, which catalyzes the hydrolysis of the galactose residue from the non-reducing end of the oligosaccharide of the sphingolipid, GM1 ganglioside, is very specific for an unsubstituted galactose in β-anomeric glycosidic linkage to the rest of the substrate molecule, the aglycone. However, a large number of compounds can be substituted for the aglycone for the purposes of the measurement of β-galactosidase activity. When the substituting aglycone is a relatively simple, water-soluble, chromogenic or fluorogenic compound, the measurement of enzyme activity becomes easy: the rate of enzyme-catalyzed hydrolysis of the synthetic, 'artificial', substrate is measured by the change in the absorbance of fluorescence at specific wavelengths depending on the nature of the aglycone. Lysosomes have an acid *p*H, and the *p*H optima of all lysosomal hydrolases, regardless of the substrate, is in the acid range (*p*H 4.5–6.0)

The laboratory investigation of diseases caused by hereditary deficiency of lysosomal enzymes involves three sorts of studies of increasing specificity and sophistication:

• morphologic studies;
• identification of the chemical nature of compounds accumulating as a result of the enzyme deficiency; and
• demonstration of a specific enzyme deficiency.

Morphologic studies

Many lysosomal storage diseases are characterized by the presence of morphologic changes identifiable on radiographs of bones (see Chapter 6), or on histologic, histochemical, or electron microscopic studies on tissues obtained by biopsy. One of the simplest tests is microscopic examination of a routine Wright-stained peripheral blood smear for the presence of metachromatic granules (Alder-Reilly bodies) in monocytes and large lymphocytes (Figure 6.3), which is a feature of many, though not all, mucopolysaccharide storage diseases. However, although the test is inexpensive and widely available, the differentiation of Alder-Reilly bodies from other types of inclusions requires some experience, and failure to demonstrate their presence does not eliminate the possibility of an MPS disorder.

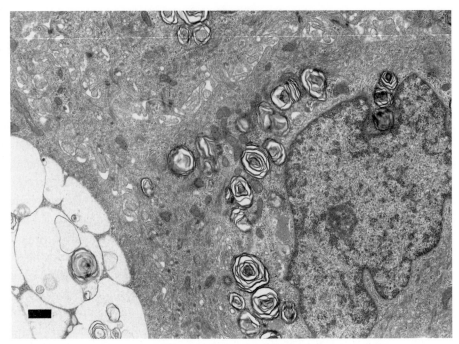

Figure 9.6   Electron micrograph of conjunctival biopsy in mucolipidosis type IV.
Figure shows fibrillogranular flocculent material (lower left) and abundant membranous
lamellar bodies. The bar represents 1 μm. (Courtesy of Dr. Venita Jay.)

Bone marrow is also a readily accessible tissue that often shows diagnostically significant morphologic changes in patients with lysosomal storage diseases. In some cases, like Gaucher disease, the morphology of the storage cell is sufficiently characteristic that a strong presumptive diagnosis can be made on the basis of these findings alone (Figure 6.5).

Conjunctival biopsy is technically simple, and coupled with electron microscopic examination, it provides important, often diagnostic, information in patients with neurodegenerative lysosomal disorders, such as neuronal ceroid lipofuscinosis (Figure 2.3) and mucolipidosis type IV (Figure 9.6). It is generally just as informative and less invasive than rectal or brain biopsy.

Joseph Alroy has shown that electron microscopic examination of skin biopsies is particularly useful in the diagnostic work-up of patients with presumed lysosomal disorders. Diseases in which the pathology is generally considered to be limited to the central nervous system, such as Tay-Sachs disease, are associated with characteristic ultrastructural abnormalities in skin (Figure 9.7). This approach to investigation is inexpensive, and a single test covers a number of lysosomal disorders.

Biopsies of brain or nerve, or of parenchymatous organs, like liver, are rarely required for the diagnosis of lysosomal diseases. On the one hand, the pathologic changes are rarely specific enough to make a diagnosis that could not be made

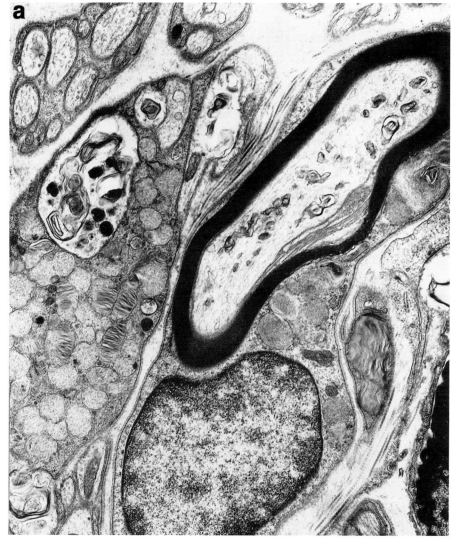

Figure 9.7   Electron micrographs of skin biopsies in some lysosomal storage diseases.
Panels **a**, from a 9-month-old girl with classical Tay-Sachs disease, showing Schwann cells
containing numberous secondary lysosomes packed with lamellar membrane structures, i.e.,
zebra bodies. Magnification × 10,500; **b**, from a 22-month-old Ashkenazi Jewish boy with
mucolipidosis type IV, showing two Schwann cells containing numerous secondary lysosomes packed with lamellar membranous structures called 'fingerprints'. Magnification ×
17,900; **c**, from a 13-year-old boy with acid lipase deficiency, showing a fibroblast containing numerous secondary lysosomes filled with lipid cholesterol clefts and some membrane
structures. Magnification × 16,900; **d**, from a 4 $\frac{1}{2}$-year-old Arab boy with infantile neuronal
ceroid-lipofuscinosis, showing endothelial cells and pericytes. One endothelial cell contains
a large secondary lysosome and a pericyte containing a chain of secondary lysosomes. The
lysosomes are packed with curvilinear bodies which are diagnostic of the disease. Magnification × 25,800. (Courtesy of Dr. Joseph Alroy.)

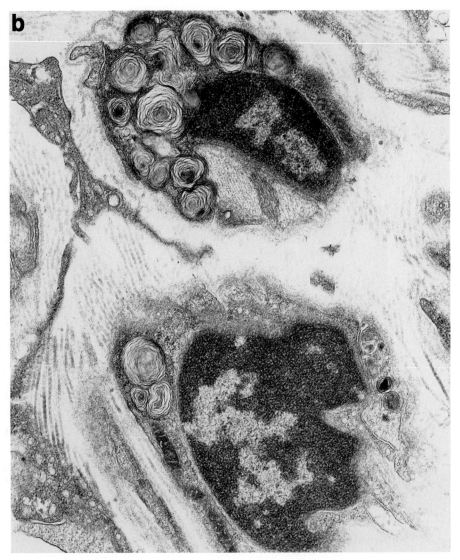

Figure 9.7 (*cont.*)

biochemically or by biopsy of more accessible tissues. On the other hand, if tissue is available, histochemical and ultrastructural studies may provide guidance for further more definitive studies.

Identification of accumulating compounds (storage material)

In general, chemical analyses of stored compounds sufficiently sophisticated to suggest a specific enzyme deficiency are rarely practical in the clinical diagnosis of lysosomal storage disorders. The amount of tissue required is too large to be

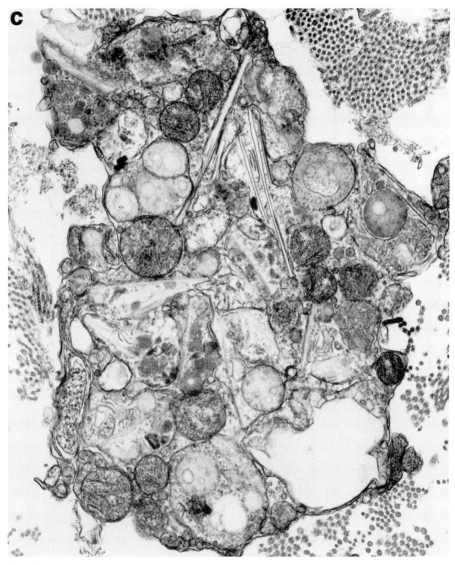

Figure 9.7   (*cont.*)

obtainable before death, and the type of studies required to establish the structure of the stored material are usually available only in research laboratories. However, with some idea of the class of compound involved, derived from morphologic investigation and some relatively unsophisticated biochemical tests, such as the urinary MPS screening test discussed below, the specific enzyme defect can be identified by assaying several enzymes in a suitable tissue, such as leukocytes or fibroblasts.

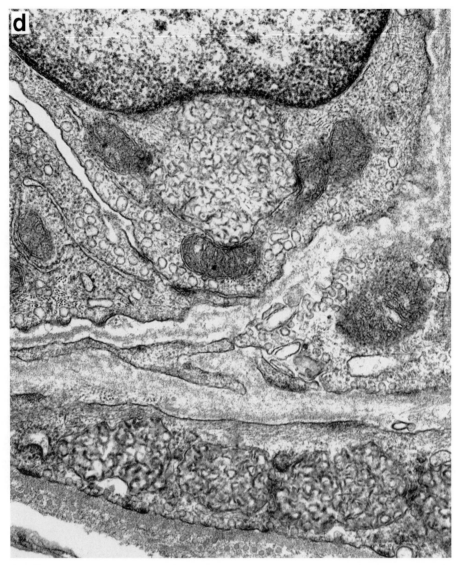

Figure 9.7   (*cont.*)

Urinary mucopolysaccharide (MPS) tests. There are many screening tests for excess acidic mucopolysaccharide in urine; almost all of them are based on tests for the presence of increased amounts of high molecular weight polyanions in urine. This may involve precipitation of the MPS by the addition of a detergent or a change in the color of a metachromatic dye, such as toluidine blue or Alcian blue. Various laboratory test manufacturers have developed methods to simplify testing, such as impregnating a metachromatic dye in paper. Only a few drops of urine are required, and the test takes only seconds to perform. The sensitivity of all MPS screening tests is high. However, false positives are common, particularly in young infants.

Table 9.11 Urinary MPS in the different mucopolysaccharidoses (MPS)

Disease	Dermatan sulfate	Heparan sulfate	Keratan sulfate	Chondroitin sulfate
MPS I	++++	+	−	+
MPS II	+++	+	−	+
MPS III	−	+++	−	+
MPS IV	−	−	++	+
MPS VI	+++	±	−	+
MPS VII	++	±	−	++*
Normal	±	±	±	+

Note: *Reported early in the course of some cases of the disease.

False negatives also occur, particularly in patients with Morquio disease (MPS IV) and less often in Sanfilippo disease (MPS III). The amount of MPS in urine can be estimated by measuring the turbidity of a urine specimen after precipitation with detergent or by quantitating spectrophotometrically the amount of Alcian blue bound by precipitated MPS. Thin-layer chromatographic analysis (TLC) or high-voltage electrophoresis of urinary MPS is more cumbersome, but it provides information important to the classification of the disorder by indicating the relative proportions of specific mucopolysaccharides (Table 9.11).

Urinary oligosaccharide analysis. Oligosaccharides are low molecular weight carbohydrate polymers made up of at least three monosaccharide subunits. The oligosaccharides in urine are derived in part from the incomplete breakdown of the carbohydrate side-chains of complex glycoproteins. The general structure of excreted oligosaccharides and the role that various lysosomal enzymes play in their metabolism is shown in Figure 9.8. TLC of unconcentrated urine is the most widely employed method for screening for the glycoproteinoses. Only a very small aliquot of urine (< 0.5 ml) is needed for the analysis. The amount of urine spotted for TLC is adjusted to correspond to a constant amount of creatinine to obviate the need for 24-hour collections of urine. Urine specimens require no preservative, but they should be stored frozen at −20 °C until analyzed.

Unfortunately, this technically simple and inexpensive screening test for glycoproteinoses is not particularly sensitive, and the specificity is also low. Patients with GM1 gangliosidosis, galactosialidosis, sialidosis, or Schindler disease are rarely missed − the urinary oligosaccharide abnormality is generally obvious. On the other hand, the excretion of oligosaccharides by patients with other glycoproteinoses is variable. Urine of patients with α-mannosidosis, α-fucosidosis, Sandhoff disease, or aspartylglucosaminuria usually shows increased amounts of oligosaccharides, although the abnormalities may be very subtle. Urine specimens from patients with β-mannosidosis, I-cell disease (mucolipidosis II) or pseudo-Hurler

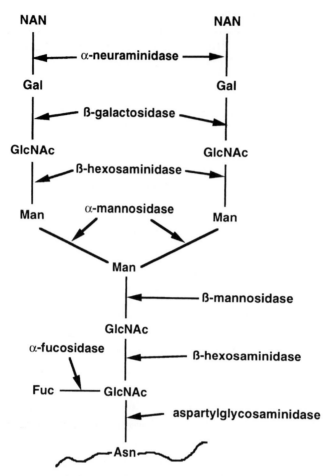

Figure 9.8   Summary of glycoprotein degradation.

polydystrophy (mucolipidosis III) generally do not contain excess amounts of oligosaccharides. Oligosacchariduria is a feature of some glycogen storage diseases, such as Pompe disease (GSD II), and we have seen it in some patients with Gaucher disease. Spurious oligosacchariduria occurs in patients infused with large amounts of complex carbohydrate, such as dextran. Breast-fed neonates also commonly show the presence of oligosaccharide bands that would be interpreted as abnormal in older children. The cost of pursuing false positive oligosacchariduria has been so high that some reputable laboratories have abandoned the test altogether and screen for the glycoproteinoses by testing leukocytes with batteries of several lysosomal enzyme assays. Some representative TLC analyses of urinary oligosaccharides are shown in Figure 9.9. Structural analysis of individual oligosaccharides detected by TLC is beyond the scope of most diagnostic laboratories.

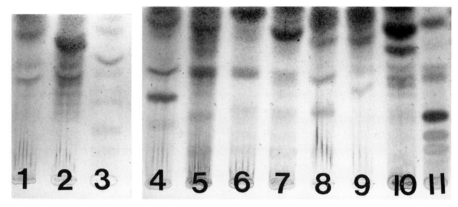

Figure 9.9 Thin-layer chromatographic analysis of urinary oligosaccharides.
The various lanes show analyses of urine from patients with different glycoproteinoses.
Lane **1**, Normal; **2**, α-mannosidosis; **3**, α-fucosidosis; **4**, aspartylglucosaminuria; **5**, Farber
lipogranulomatosis; **6**, MPS IH (Hurler disease); **7**, I-cell disease; **8**, galactosialidosis; **9** glycogen storage disease, type III; **10**, glycogen storage disease, type II (Pompe disease); **11**, GM1
gangliosidosis.

Demonstration of specific enzyme deficiency

Owing to the clinical similarity between various lysosomal disorders, the final
diagnosis in each case rests on the ability to demonstrate a specific enzyme deficiency
to account for the disease. Table 9.12 shows a summary of the enzyme defects in each
of the known lysosomal enzyme deficiency diseases and the most readily accessible
source of enzyme for diagnostic analysis.

Fibroblasts are probably the best material for diagnosis of lysosomal disorders
by enzyme assay. However, obtaining enough cells for reliable analyses often takes
some weeks in culture. The analysis of enzyme activities in leukocytes is equally reliable in some cases. In others, the presence of non-lysosomal isozymes may obscure
deficiency of the lysosomal enzyme when the assay is carried out with leukocytes.
For example, leukocytes contain a neutral, non-lysosomal α-glucosidase. In order
to make the diagnosis of GSD II on the basis of measurements of lysosomal
α-glucosidase in leukocytes, particular care must be taken to account for enzyme
activity attributable to the non-lysosomal enzyme. Enzyme analysis is still the most
common technique used for detection of carriers of lysosomal storage disease mutations. However, in many cases, the overlap between enzyme activities in leukocytes
from carriers and homozygous normal individuals is sufficient to cause misclassi-
fication in 10–15% of carriers. The advent of molecular genetic testing for carrier
detection is a major advance in genetic counselling of family members of individuals
affected with lysosomal enzyme deficiency diseases in which specific disease-causing
mutations have been identified.

Table 9.12 Summary of assays useful in the investigation of lysosomal storage diseases

Disease	Enzyme	Enzyme source
Mucopolysaccharide storage diseases		
Hurler disease and allelic variants (MPS IH, MPS IH/S, MPS IS)	α-L-iduronidase	L, F
Hunter disease (MPS II)	Iduronate 2-sulfatase	S, L, F
Sanfilippo disease, type A (MPS IIIA)	Heparan *N*-sulfatase	L, F
Sanfilippo disease, type B (MPS IIIB)	α-*N*-Acetylglucosaminidase	L, F
Sanfilippo disease, type C (MPS IIIC)	Acetyl-CoA:α-glucosaminide acetyltransferase	F
Sanfilippo disease, type D (MPS IIID)	*N*-Acetylglucosamine 6-sulfatase	L, F
Morquio disease, type A (MPS IVA)	*N*-Acetylgalactosamine 6-sulfatase	L, F
Morquio disease, type B (MPS IVB)	β-Galactosidase	S, L, F
Maroteaux-Lamy disease (MPS VI)	*N*-Acetylgalactosamine 4-sulfatase (arylsulfatase B)	L, F
Sly disease (MPS VII)	β-Glucuronidase	S, L, F
Glycoproteinoses		
Aspartylglucosaminuria	Aspartylglucosaminidase	L, F
GM1 gangliosidosis	β-Galactosidase	S, L, F
α-Mannosidosis	α-Mannosidase	L, F
β-Mannosidosis	β-Mannosidase	L, F
Sialidosis	α-Neuraminidase	F
Galactosialidosis	α-Neuroaminidase + β-Galactosidase	F
α-Fucosidosis	α-Fucosidase	S, L, F
Schindler disease	α-Glucosaminidase (α-galactosidase B)	L, F
Pycnodysostosis	Cathepsin K	F
I-Cell disease or pseudo-Hurler polydystrophy (ML III)	β-Hexosaminidase	S **and** L F **and** culture medium
Sphingolipidoses		
Fabry disease	α-Galactosidase A	S, L, F
Gaucher disease	Glucocerebrosidase (β-glucosidase)	L, F
Niemann-Pick disease, type A or B	Acid sphingomyelinase	L, F
Niemann-Pick disease, type C	Cholesterol esterification (or specific mutation analysis)	F (or DNA)
Metachromatic leukodystrophy	Arylsulfatase A	L, F
Krabbe globoid cell leukodystrophy	Galactocerebrosidase	L, F
Farber lipogranulomatosis	Ceramidase	L, F

Abbreviations: L, peripheral blood leukocytes; F, cultured skin fibroblasts; S, serum.

Disorders of mitochondrial energy metabolism

Muscle is almost always involved to some extent, if not primarily, in inborn errors of mitochondrial energy metabolism (see Chapter 2). Histochemical, electron microscopic, and biochemical studies on the tissue are the principal means be which definitive diagnosis is made in most cases, though studies on cultured fibroblasts are often helpful.

Morphologic studies

Lytic lesions in the basal ganglia and thalamus, sometimes extending into the midbrain, are often seen in CT and MRI scans of the CNS in patients with chronic encephalopathies associated with mitochondrial ETC defects (see Figure 2.5 and 2.6). However, the histochemical and electron microscopic findings in skeletal muscle are perhaps the most characteristic morphologic abnormalities in patients with mutations affecting mitochondrial energy metabolism. Skeletal and cardiac muscle typically shows accumulation of lipid and glycogen. However, the changes produced by proliferation, aggregation, and distortion of mitochondria are particularly instructive, especially in older patients with disease caused by mtDNA mutations. The subsarcolemmal accumulation of mitochondria produces a typical ragged-red fiber appearance when sections of the tissue are stained by the modified Gomori trichrome method. This is illustrated in Figure 2.15 and discussed in Chapter 2 where mitochondrial myopathies are discussed in more detail. Ragged red fibers are uncommon in young infants with Leigh disease caused by autosomal recessive nuclear gene defects affecting mitochondrial ETC. Electron microscopic examination often shows distortion of the mitochondria, with abnormalities of the cristae and matrix, and accumulation of paracrystalline inclusions between the mitochondrial membranes or in the cristae.

Biochemical studies

The ultimate definition of abnormalities arising from mutations affecting mitochondrial energy metabolism rests on biochemical evaluation of mitochondrial function. The assessment of mitochondrial function *in vitro* has been advanced tremendously by:

- the development of techniques for the analysis of ETC function in lymphocytes, fibroblasts, and mitochondria isolated from very small samples of tissue, particularly muscle;
- methods for studying mitochondrial function *in situ* in lymphocytes and cultured skin fibroblasts by permeablization of the cell membrane by treatment with detergents;
- the development of monospecific antibodies for measuring the activities of different enzymes, such as the acyl-CoA dehydrogenases, with overlapping substrate specificities;

• the use of various synthetic chromogenic electron acceptors, along with specific electron transport inhibitors, to evaluate the integrity of the different multiprotein complexes of the mitochondrial ETC;

• the rapidly growing application of molecular genetic techniques to the characterization of the various components of mitochondrial energy metabolism.

Familiarity with some of the theoretical and technical issues involved in the assessment of this very complex system makes the clinical investigation of disorders of mitochondrial energy metabolism easier to follow. Assessment of mitochondrial energy metabolism embraces three types of process, each associated with defects producing disease. Detailed analysis of most of these is available only in laboratories doing active research on disorders of energy metabolism.

Substrate transport. Most of the energy derived from fatty acid oxidation is generated by the process of β-oxidation, which takes place in the mitochondrial matrix. The transport of fatty acids into mitochondria involves the participation of four distinct gene products, two enzymes and two membrane transporters (Figure 9.10).

Fatty acids entering the cytosol are rapidly esterified to form coenzyme A derivatives. Transport into mitochondria requires transesterification with free carnitine to form fatty acylcarnitine in a reaction catalyzed by the enzyme carnitine palmitoyltransferase I located in the outer mitochondrial membrane. Transport of the fatty acylcarnitine through the inner mitochondrial membrane involves carnitine-acylcarnitine translocase, a co-transporter that facilitates transport of acylcarnitine in one direction and free carnitine in the other. Finally, the fatty acylcarnitine inside mitochondria is transesterified to regenerate long-chain fatty acyl-CoA in a reaction catalyzed by carnitine palmitoyltransferase II. The fourth gene product required for the process to work is the carnitine transporter in the cell membrane which, along with carnitine-acylcarnitine translocase, ensures adequate cytosolic concentrations of free carnitine to support production of fatty acylcarnitines.

Substrate utilization. Pyruvate carboxylase (PC) catalyzes the most important of the anaplerotic reactions that function to ensure the supply of tricarboxylic acid (TCA) cycle intermediates is adequate to support the cycle. It is a biotin-dependent enzyme that catalyzes the carboxylation of pyruvate to form oxaloacetate. It is dependent for activity on the presence of acetyl-CoA, an allosteric activator of the enzyme. In addition to its role in fueling the TCA cycle, PC catalyzes a key, early step in gluconeogenesis.

PDH is a huge multicomponent enzyme complex made up of multiple units of 4 enzymes: pyruvate decarboxylase (E_1, 30 units), dihydrolipoyl transacetylase (E_2, 60 units), dihydrolipoamide dehydrogenase (E_3, 6 units), and protein X (6 units). The enzyme catalyzes the oxidative decarboxylation of pyruvate to

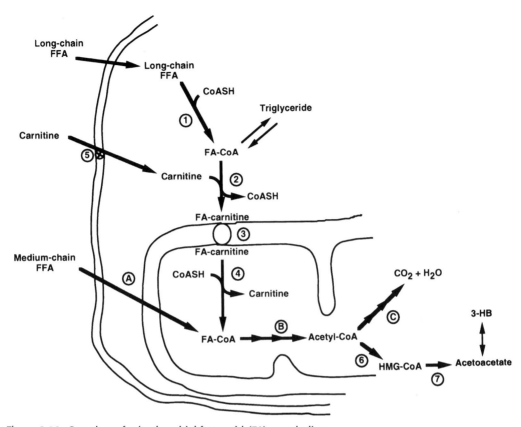

Figure 9.10   Overview of mitochondrial fatty acid (FA) metabolism.

Specific enzymes are shown here as numerals, and processes are represented by letters of the alphabet. The processes shown are: **A**, medium-chain free fatty acid (FFA) uptake and diffusion into mitochondria without activation to coenzyme A (CoA) esters; **B**, fatty acid β-oxidation; **C**, oxidation of acetyl-CoA via the tricarboxylic acid cycle. The enzymes involved in various reactions are: **1**, long-chain fatty acid:CoA ligase; **2**, carnitine palmitoyltransferase I (CPT I); **3**, carnitine-acylcarnitine translocase; **4**, carnitine palmitoyltransferase II (CPT II); **5**, transmembrane carnitine translocase; **6**, 3-hydroxy-3-methylglutaryl-CoA (HMG-CoA) synthetase; **7**, HMG-CoA lyase.

acetyl-CoA. Enzyme activity is regulated by phosphorylation (inactivation)-dephosphorylation (activation) in reactions catalyzed by PDH kinase and PDH phosphatase, respectively. It is customary when measuring PDH activity in tissue extracts to do the assay in the presence and absence of dichloroacetate, an inhibitor of PDH kinase, to determine total PDH activity and the proportion in the active form, respectively.

PC deficiency and PDH deficiency are both associated with persistent, severe, lactic acidosis (see Chapter 3). The majority of cases of PDH deficiency are the

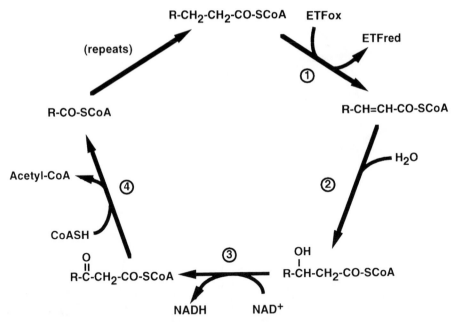

Figure 9.11 Mitochondrial fatty acid β-oxidation.
The enzymes involved in mitochondrial fatty acid β-oxidation are: **1**, fatty acyl-CoA dehydrogenases (short-chain, medium-chain, long-chain, and very long-chain); **2**, 2-enol-CoA hydratase; **3**, L-3-hydroxyacyl-CoA dehydrogenase; **4**, 3-ketoacyl-CoA thiolase.

result of mutations in the X-linked α subunit of E_1. Overall, males and females are equally affected except among patients with the mildest form of the disease, which is characterized by intermittent ataxia and appears only to occur in males (see Chapter 2).

Defects in fatty acid oxidation may arise as a result of mutations affecting any one of several enzymes involved in the process. The fatty acyl-CoA dehydrogenases are FAD-containing enzymes that catalyze the first step in the mitochondrial β-oxidation of fatty acids (Figure 9.11), the introduction of a *trans* double bond, and transfer of electrons from the substrate to electron transfer flavoprotein (ETF). The four genetically distinct mitochondrial fatty acyl-CoA dehydrogenases (SCAD, MCAD, LCAD, and VLCAD) differ in their substrate specificities, though there is considerable overlap between them in this regard. Long-chain 2-enoyl-CoA hydratase, 3-hydroxyacyl-CoA dehydrogenase, and 3-ketoacyl-CoA thiolase activities exist in the mitochondrion as a single trifunctional protein. The corresponding short-chain substrate-specific enzymes appear to exist as separate proteins.

Analytical screening techniques have been developed to assess fatty acid oxidation *in situ* in cultured fibroblasts using [^{14}C]-labeled fatty acids and measuring

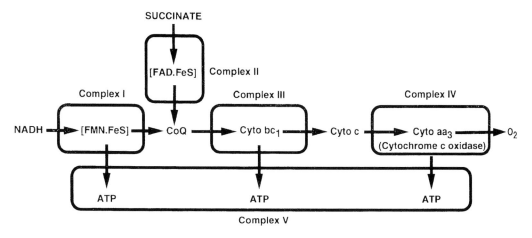

SUCCINATE

Figure 9.12 Complexes of the mitochondrial electron transport chain.

the production of $^{14}CO_2$. This has been coupled with assays to identify defects in specific enzymes involved in fatty acid oxidation. The analysis of steps in fatty acid β-oxidation catalyzed by more than one enzyme with different chain-length specificities, such as the fatty acyl-CoA dehydrogenases, is complicated by overlapping substrate specificities. Measurement of medium-chain acyl-CoA dehydrogenase (MCAD) activity inevitably includes activity contributed by long-chain and short-chain acyl-CoA dehydrogenases (LCAD and SCAD), respectively, unless these enzymes are inactivated. This can be done by specific immunoprecipitation of the dehydrogenases contaminating the measurement of the enzyme activity of interest.

Complementation analysis is another approach to pin-pointing a defect in fatty acid oxidation. Cells with a known defect are fused with cells from the patient, and the effect on [^{14}C]fatty acid oxidation is determined. If the defect in the two cell lines is the same, fusion of the cells will have no effect on $^{14}CO_2$ production from labeled substrate. But, if the defects in the two cell lines are different, they will be mutually corrected when cells from the two lines are fused.

Electron transport chain (ETC). The mitochondrial ETC encompasses an assemblage of polypeptide gene products arranged in the mitochondrial membrane to transfer the energy derived from the oxidation of NADH and succinate to produce ATP. The process is achieved by the consecutive participation of as many as 83 polypeptides, arranged in five multicomponent complexes, Complexes I to V, through which the electrons pass to be accepted finally by O_2 to form H_2O and generate ATP (Figure 9.12). The majority of the polypeptides involved are the products of nuclear genes and cytosolic protein biosynthesis, the rest are coded by mitochondrial genes

Table 9.13 Subunits of mitochondrial electron transport chain

Electron transport complex	Inhibitor	Subunits coded by	
		mtDNA	nDNA
Complex I (NADH:ubiquinone oxidoreductase)	Rotenone	7	39±
Complex II (Succinate:ubiquinone oxidoreductase)		0	4
Complex III (Ubiquinol:ferrocytochrome c oxidoreductase or cytochrome bc_1 complex)	Antimycin	1	10
Complex IV (Ferrocytochrome c:oxygen oxidoreductase or cytochrome c oxidase)	Cyanide	3	10
Complex V (ATP synthase)	Oligomycin	2	14±

and synthesized within the mitochondrion (Table 9.13). Most of the diseases caused by nuclear gene mutations are transmitted as autosomal recessive disorders.

The laboratory investigation of mitochondrial ETC defects is similar, in principle, to the investigation of fatty acid β-oxidation defects. Respiration of intact lymphocytes, fibroblasts, or isolated muscle mitochondria is assessed polarographically (i.e., by measurement of oxygen utilization) using various energy substrates and specific ETC inhibitors. ETC activity of the individual complexes is then measured spectrophotometrically. Cytochrome c oxidase (COX, Complex IV) is measured directly by spectrophotometry. Marked deficiency of the activity of the complex can sometimes be determined histochemically. Complexes I and III are measured together by spectrophotometric analysis of rotenone-sensitive NADH-cytochrome c reductase activity. Complexes II and III are evaluated together by measurement of succinate-cytochrome c reductase activity. Complex I alone is evaluated by measurement of rotenone-sensitive NADH oxidation in the presence of decyl ubiquinone as electron acceptor.

The quality of results of enzyme assays is highly variable due to differences in techniques used in different laboratories, and in the technical difficulty of measuring the activities of some of the complexes. This is particularly true for the measurement of the activity of Complex I, which requires a relatively large number of cells or tissue and which is plagued by the presence of interfering and confounding activities. Estimation of individual ETC complexes by blue native polyacrylamide gel (BN-PAGE) analysis, alone or coupled with enzyme analysis of the isolated complexes, represents a significant breakthrough in this respect (see Figure 9.5).

Molecular genetic studies

The approach to the diagnosis of mitochondrial disorders caused by mtDNA mutations has been revolutionized by the application of molecular genetic mutation detection techniques. The mitochondrial genome is not large, slightly more than 16,000 nucleotides in size. However, the relatively high concentrations of benign sequence variations, particularly in the D-loop, and the phenomenon of hetero-plasmy make interpretation of the results more difficult than similar studies on nuclear gene sequences. Some mutant mtDNA alleles are relatively common among disease-associated sequence abnormalities (Table 9.14), and specific analysis is particularly useful for the diagnosis of disease.

In recent years, considerable progress has been made in the identification of nuclear gene defects causing mitochondrial respiratory chain abnormalities. Table 9.13 shows that the majority of the polypeptides of the various subunits of the electron transport chain are encoded by nuclear genes.

Peroxisomal disorders

Peroxisomes are single-membrane subcellular organelles that contribute both biosynthetic and catabolic functions to tissues throughout the body. Some of the key functions of peroxisomes are shown in Table 9.15.

Morphologic studies

The appearance on electron microscopy of the peroxisomes in liver obtained by biopsy is particularly informative in the investigation of peroxisomal disorders. Abnormalities in shape or number, including total absence of the organelle, are characteristic of the peroxisomal assembly defects, such as classical Zellweger syndrome. However, in many of the diseases caused by single peroxisomal enzyme deficiencies, such as X-linked adrenoleukodystrophy, peroxisomal morphology is normal.

Biochemical studies

The clinical biochemical abnormalities in patients with peroxisomal disorders reflect, to a large extent, the underlying metabolic defects. Defects in peroxisomal biogenesis are, in general, associated with numerous abnormalities, particularly increased levels of very long-chain fatty acids in plasma. Table 9.16 summarizes key laboratory abnormalities in some of the more common peroxisomal disorders.

None of the laboratory investigations shown in Table 9.16 is routine. They are performed primarily in laboratories set up specifically to study peroxisomal disorders.

Plasma very long-chain fatty acids and phytanic acid. The quantitative analysis of very long-chain fatty acids and phytanic acid (a 20-carbon branched-chain fatty acid derived from chlorophyll) requires preliminary extraction and derivatization of complex lipids, followed by preparatory TLC isolation and capillary GC analysis of the fatty acid methyl esters. The analysis is technically challenging, and it is

Table 9.14 Mitochondrial mutations

Disease group	Specific features (see also Chapter 2)	Gene product, mutation
MELAS (Mitochondrial encephalomyopathy, lactic acidosis, stroke-like episodes)	Seizures, dementia, lactic acidosis, strokes, cortical blindness, migraine, recurrent vomiting, failure to thrive, muscle weakness	tRNA^Leu(UUR): **A3243G**, A3251G, A3252G, T3271C, T3291C, T3308C COXIII: T9957C
MERRF (Myoclonus epilepsy with ragged-red fibers)	Myoclonus, seizures, ataxia, myopathy with ragged-red fibers, dementia, short stature, neuropathy, optic atrophy	tRNA^Lys: **A8344G**, T8356C tRNA^Ser(UCN): 7472insC
Leigh disease or NARP (Neurogenic muscle weakness, ataxia, and retinitis pigmentosa	Relapsing acute encephalopathy; progressive cerebral neurodegeneration, lactic acidosis, apnea/tachypnea, hypotonia, seizures (Leigh disease)	ATPase6: **T8993G**, T8993C tRNA^Lys: A8344G, T8356C, G8363A tRNA^Val: G1644T
	Developmental delay, proximal muscle weakness, recurrent acute ataxia, retinitis pigmentosa, ± lactic acidosis (NARP)	
Bilateral striatal necrosis		ATPase6: T8851C, T9176C
Other encephalomyopathies	with diabetes mellitus, CPEO, deafness	tRNA^Leu(UUR): C3256T
	with cerebral calcifications	tRNA^Leu(UUR): 3271delT
	with diabetes mellitus	tRNA^Glu: T14709C
MM (Mitochondrial myopathy)		tRNA^Leu(UUR): T3250C, T3251G, A3302G, C3303T
		tRNA^Ile: A4269G
		tRNA^Pro: G15990A
	Fatal infantile variant	tRNA^Thr: A15923G*
	MM + progressive external ophthalmoplegia, and chronic intestinal pseudo-obstruction	tRNA^Gly: A10006G
		tRNA^Ser(GCU): C12246A
		tRNA^Asn: T5692G, G5703A
CPEO (Chronic progressive external ophthalmoplegia)		tRNA^Ile: T4285C
		mtDNA deletions ± rearrangements

(cont.)

Disease	Clinical features	Mutations
Deafness	Nonsyndromic sensorineural or aminoglycoside-induced	12S rRNA: A1555G tRNA$^{Ser(UCN)}$: A7445G
LHON (Leber hereditary optic neuropathy)		ND1: G3460A ND4: **G11778A** ND6: T14484C ATPase6: T9101C
	LHON + dystonia	ND6: G14459A ND4: G11696 + ND6: T14596A
Cardiomyopathies	Fatal infantile hypertrophic	tRNA^{Ile}: A4317G, C4320T
	Infantile/childhood onset hypertrophic	tRNA$^{Leu(UUR)}$: C3303T
	Childhood onset hypertrophic + hearing loss + encephalopathy	tRNA^{Gly}: T9997C
	Adult onset	tRNA^{Ile}: A4269G tRNA^{Lys}: G8363A
	Adult onset + myopathy	tRNA^{Ile}: A4300G tRNA$^{Leu(UUR)}$: A3260G
KSS (Kearns-Sayre syndrome)	Ophthalmoplegia, myopathy, hearing loss, cardiomyopathy, cardiac conduction defects, neuropathy, ataxia, failure to thrive	mtDNA deletions ± rearrangements
Pearson marrow pancreas syndrome	Severe macrocytic, sideroblastic anemia ± neutropenia and thrombocytopenia, pancreatic insufficiency, failure to thrive, lactic acidosis, myopathy, progressive neurodegeneration	mtDNA deletions ± rearrangements

Note: Mutations shown in bold type are particularly common causes of disease.

Source: Modified in part from Suomalainen (1997).

Table 9.15 Some key functions of peroxisomes

Biosynthetic processes	Catabolic processes
Synthesis of plasmalogens, a special class of membrane phospholipids	Elimination, by the action of catalase, of H_2O_2 generated by the activity of some peroxisomal oxidases
Synthesis of cholesterol and other isoprenoid derivatives, such as dolichol, a complex lipid with an important role in glycoprotein biosynthesis	β-Oxidation of fatty acids, long-chain dicarboxylic acids, the side-chain of cholesterol, and other compounds
Synthesis of bile acids	Oxidation of pipecolic acid, a normally minor intermediate in lysine metabolism
Transamination of glyoxylate to glycine (by the action of alanine:glyoxylate aminotransferase)	Spermine and spermidine oxidation

Table 9.16 Laboratory abnormalities in some of the peroxisomal disorders

Laboratory test	Zellweger syndrome	Ketoacyl-CoA thiolase deficiency	NALD or IRS	XL-ALD	Adult Refsum disease	RCDP
Increased plasma VLCFA	+++	+++	+++	++	−	−
Increased urinary pipecolic acid	+++	+++	++	−	−	−
Decreased red cell plasmalogens	+++	−	++	−	−	+++
Increased plasma phytanic acid	+	−	+ − ++	−	+++	++
Increased plasma bile acid metabolites	+++	+++	+++	−	−	−

Abbreviations: NALD, neonatal adrenoleukodystrophy; IRS, infantile Refsum syndrome; XL-ALD, X-linked adrenoleukodystrophy; RCDP, rhizomelic chondrodysplasia punctata; VLCFA, very long-chain fatty acids.

offered by only a small number of specialized laboratories specifically interested in the diagnosis of inborn errors of peroxisomal metabolism.

Plasma and urinary pipecolic acid. L-Pipecolic acid is an intermediate in lysine metabolism. Accumulation of the compound is a characteristic of inherited defects of peroxisome biogenesis. Levels in plasma and urine are normally extremely low. Even in patients with peroxisomal disorders, in whom plasma and urine concentrations may be 100 times normal, the levels are relatively low compared with other diagnostically important biological compounds. After extraction and derivatization, pipecolic acid is usually measured by HPLC, GC, or GC-MS. The sensitivity and accuracy of quantitation are increased by using an isotope-dilution approach to analysis of the compound. Plasma levels may be spuriously elevated in children with hepatocellular disease or by ingestion of vegetables rich in pipecolate.

Red cell plasmalogens. Plasmalogens are major components of the phospholipids of myelin and other membranes, including red cells. Deficiency of plasmalogen biosynthesis in peroxisomal disorders results in decreased concentrations in red cell membranes. Plasmalogens are measured by extraction of membrane lipids and measurement of lipid phosphorus after saponification to remove phosphoglycerides.

SUGGESTED READING

Applegarth, D. A., Dimmick, J. E. & Hall, J. G. (eds). (1997). *Organelle Diseases: Clinical Features, Diagnosis, Pathogenesis and Management.* London: Chapman & Hall Medical.

Bauer, M. F., Gempel, K., Hofmann, S., Jaksch, M., Philbrook, C. & Gerbitz, K. D. (1999). Mitochondrial disorders. A diagnostic challenge in clinical chemisty. *Clinical Chemistry and Laboratory Medicine,* **37**, 855–76.

Bernier, F. P., Boneh, A., Dennett, X., Chow, C. W., Cleary, M. A. & Thorburn, D. R. (2002). Diagnostic criteria for respiratory chain disorders in adults and children. *Neurology,* **59**, 1406–11.

Blau, N., Duran, M., Blaskovics, M. E. & Gibson, K. M. (eds) (2003). *Physician's Guide to the Laboratory Diagnosis of Metabolic Diseases,* 2nd ed, Heidelberg: Springer-Verlag.

Ceuterick-de Groote C. & Martin, J. J. (1998). Extracerebral biopsy in lysosomal and peroxisomal disorders. Ultrastructural findings. *Brain Pathology,* **8**, 121–32.

Chamoles, N. A., Blanco, M. B., Gaggioli, D. & Casentini, C. (2001). Hurler-like phenotype: enzymatic diagnosis in dried blood spots on filter paper. *Clinical Chemistry,* **47**, 2098–102.

DiMauro, S. (2004). Mitochondrial diseases. *Biochimica Biophysica Acta,* **1658**, 80–8.

DiMauro, S. & Schon, E. A. (2003). Mitochondrial respiratory-chain diseases. *New England Journal of Medicine,* **348**, 2656–68.

Goebel, H. H. (1999). Extracerebral biopsies in neurodegenerative diseases of childhood. *Brain and Development,* **21**, 435–43.

Hanson B. J., Capaldi R. A., Marusich M. F., Sherwood S. W. (2002). An immunocytochemical approach to detection of mitochondrial disorders. *Journal of Histochemistry and Cytochemistry,* **50**, 1281–8.

Hyland, K. (2003). The lumbar puncture for diagnosis of pediatric neurotransmitter diseases. *Annals of Neurology,* **54** (suppl 6), S13–S17.

Nuttall, K. L. (1994). Porphyrins and disorders of porphyrin metabolism. In: Burtis, C. A. & Ashwood, E. R. (eds). *Tietz Textbook of Clinical Chemistry,* 2nd ed, Philadelphia: W. B. Saunders, pp. 2073–106.

Prasad, A., Kaye, E. M. & Alroy, J. (1996). Electron microscopic examination of skin biopsy as a cost-effective tool in the diagnosis of lysosomal storage diseases. *Journal of Child Neurology,* **11**, 301–308.

Roe, C. R. & Roe, D. S. (1999). Recent developments in the investigation of inherited metabolic disorders using cultured human cells. *Molecular Genetics and Metabolism*, **68**, 243–57.

Schagger, H. & von Jagow, G. (1991). Blue native electrophoresis for isolation of membrane complexes in enzymatically active form. *Analytical Biochemistry*, **199**, 223–31.

Shoffner, J. M. (1999). Oxidative phosphorylation disease diagnosis. *Seminars in Neurology*, **19**, 341–51.

Shoubridge, E. A. (2001). Nuclear gene defects in respiratory chain disorders. *Seminars in Neurology*, **21**, 261–7.

Steiner, R. D. & Cederbaum, S. D. (2001). Laboratory evaluation of urea cycle disorders. *Journal of Pediatrics*, **138** (1 Suppl), S21–9.

Suomalainen, A. (1997). Mitochondrial DNA and disease. *Annals of Medicine*, **29**, 235–46.

Wong, L. J. (2004). Comprehensive molecular diagnosis of mitochondrial disorders: qualitative and quantitative approach. *Annals of the New York Academy of Sciemces.* **1011**, 246–58.

Zaider, E. & Bickers, D. R. (1998). Clinical laboratory methods for diagnosis of the porphyrias. *Clinics in Dermatology*, **16**, 277–93.

Zerbetto, E., Vergani, L. & Dabbeni-Sala, F. (1997). Quantification of muscle mitochondrial oxidative phosphorylation enzymes via histochemical staining of blue native polyacrylamide gels. *Electrophoresis*, **18**, 2059–64.

10

Treatment

The purpose of this chapter is to present some general principles of the management of inherited metabolic diseases using specific examples to illustrate various points. It is not meant to be a detailed guide to the specific treatment of any particular disease. Instead, it is intended to provide a conceptual scaffold to aid in understanding the strategy behind the management of various inborn errors of metabolism, particularly strategies involving environmental manipulation.

A logical approach to treatment would be to determine how various point defects in metabolism cause disease, and to reverse or neutralize them, either by dietary, pharmacologic, or some other form of metabolic manipulation. However, in many cases, our understanding of how a particular point defect in metabolism produces disease is still incomplete. Often the abnormality is metabolically or physically inaccessible to environmental manipulation. In the discussion to follow, examples are provided of how rational approaches to treatment grew out of an understanding of the primary and secondary consequences of inborn errors of metabolism. The emphasis is on instances in which treatment is at least partially successful.

Control of accumulation of substrate

When disease is caused by accumulation of the substrate of a reaction that is impaired as a result of deficiency of an enzyme or transport protein, a reasonable approach to treatment would be to try to control levels of the toxic metabolite, either by decreasing its accumulation or accelerating its removal by alternative reactions.

Restricted dietary intake

Phenylketonuria

The treatment of PKU by dietary phenylalanine restriction is successful largely because the most obvious clinical abnormalities of the disease are due to accumulation of phenylalanine, and ultimately all the phenylalanine in the body is derived from dietary protein. It is not synthesized endogenously. Moreover, it is water soluble, and it equilibrates rapidly among various compartments in the body, including the circulation. In theory, regulation of phenylalanine levels in the body would appear to be relatively easy. However, the practical management of the disease turns out to be somewhat more complicated. Phenylalanine is an essential amino acid. Failure to provide amounts in the diet adequate to support normal protein biosynthesis will result in malnutrition. In some of the original infants with PKU treated by dietary phenylalanine restriction, this was severe enough to cause death. Most of the phenylalanine in the body by far exists as protein. As such, it is not neurotoxic. However, even subtle shifts in the balance between endogenous protein synthesis and breakdown, such as occur during intercurrent illnesses, can have profound effects on levels of the free amino acid. Marked increases in plasma phenylalanine levels are routinely seen in children with PKU during relatively trivial intercurrent illnesses. The same can be said, by the way, about branched-chain amino acids in MSUD. The levels of toxic branched-chain amino acids, especially leucine, in plasma are the net result of the balance between protein biosynthesis and protein breakdown. Marked increases in plasma branched-chain amino acids occur often in children with MSUD during intercurrent illnesses.

When the conversion of phenylalanine to tyrosine is impaired, as it is in PKU, tyrosine becomes an essential amino acid. PKU diets have generally been considered to contain enough tyrosine to meet the needs for protein, neurotransmitter, and hormone biosynthesis. However, a number of observations on children with PKU suggest that this may not be the case. Some of the suboptimal results of dietary treatment of the disease may be the result of tyrosine deficiency. This is still being examined by some investigators.

In order to avoid inadvertent phenylalanine deficiency, the diets of children with PKU are designed to maintain blood levels of the amino acid two to five times above normal, levels that appear not to be neurotoxic. Although malnutrition and the direct and immediate neurotoxicity of phenylalanine may be avoided in this manner, the increased concentrations of the amino acid interfere with the transport of other amino acids, such as leucine, sharing the same cellular transport systems. The long-term effects of this are unknown.

Despite the theoretical and practical imperfections of the treatment of PKU by dietary phenylalanine restriction, it is the model on which the management of other inborn errors of metabolism is based (Table 10.1).

Galactosemia

Propelled in part by the success experienced with the dietary treatment of PKU, investigators developed a similar strategy for the management of galactosemia. Disease is caused by accumulation of galactose-1-phosphate and, to a lesser extent,

Table 10.1 Some examples of inborn errors of metabolism treatable by dietary manipulation

Disease	Defect	Clinical aspects	Treatment
Disorders of amino acid metabolism			
PKU	Phenylalanine hydroxylase	Progressive mental retardation	Phenylalanine-restricted diet
MSUD	Branched-chain 2-ketoacid decarboxylase	Acute encephalopathy, metabolic acidosis, mental retardation	Dietary restriction of leucine, isoleucine, and valine
Homocystinuria	Cystathionine β-synthase	Tall stature, dislocated ocular lens, intravascular thrombosis, mental retardation	Methionine-restricted diet, supplemented with vitamin B_6 and betaine
Hepatorenal tyrosinemia	Fumarylacetoacetase	Acute liver failure, cirrhosis	Dietary phenylalanine and tyrosine restriction
LPI	Dibasic amino acid transport defect	Hyperammonemic encephalopathy	Dietary protein restriction supplemented with citrulline
UCED	Any of several enzymes involved in urea biosynthesis	Hyperammonemic encephalopathy, mental retardation	Dietary protein restriction supplemented with sodium benzoate, sodium phenylbutyrate, arginine, citrulline
Disorders of organic acid metabolism			
Methylmalonic acidemia	Methylmalonyl-CoA mutase	Metabolic acidosis, hyperammonemia	Dietary isoleucine, valine, methionine, and threonine restriction supplemented with carnitine
Propionic acidemia	Propionyl-CoA carboxylase	Metabolic acidosis, hyperammonemia	Dietary isoleucine, valine, methionine, and threonine restriction supplemented with carnitine

(*cont.*)

Table 10.1 (*cont.*)

Disease	Defect	Clinical aspects	Treatment
Isovaleric acidemia	Isovaleryl-CoA dehydrogenase	Metabolic acidosis, hyperammonemia	Dietary protein restriction supplemented with carnitine and glycine
Glutaric aciduria, type I	Glutaryl-CoA dehydrogenase	Metabolic acidosis, dystonia, seizures	Dietary tryptophan and lysine restriction
Disorders of carbohydrate metabolism			
Galactosemia	GALT	Hepatocellular dysfunction, hemolytic anemia, cataracts	Dietary galactose and lactose restriction
HFI	Fructose-1-phosphate aldolase	Hypoglycemia, lactic acidosis	Dietary fructose and sucrose restriction
GSD, type I	Glucose-6-phosphatase	Hypoglycemia, lactic acidosis, hypertriglyceridemia	Frequent feeds of glucose or glucose polymer; dietary fructose and galactose restriction
Intestinal disaccharidase deficiencies	Any of several enzymes involved in the digestion of various dietary disaccharides	Chronic diarrhea, failure to thrive	Dietary avoidance of relevant disaccharide
Congenital disorders of glycosylation			
CDG Ib	Phosphomannose isomerase	Protein-losing enteropathy, coagulopathy, hypoglycemia, hepatic dysfunction, recurrent vomiting and diarrhea	Dietary D-mannose supplementation

Abbreviations: MSUD, maple syrup urine disease; GALT, galactose-1-phosphate uridyltransferase; HFI, hereditary fructose intolerance; GSD, glycogen storage disease; LPI, lysinuric protein intolerance; UCED, urea cycle enzyme defects; PKU, phenylketonuria; CDG, congenital disorder of glycosylation.

galactitol. On the surface, controlling galactose-1-phosphate levels by dietary galactose restriction might appear to be easier than the management of PKU by phenylalanine restriction. It is a significant component of only a limited number of foods, and it is not essential for adequate nutrition. However, it is synthesized endogenously for use in the synthesis of galactose-containing compounds, such as the myelin lipid, galactocerebroside. The inability to control endogenous biosynthesis limits the extent to which galactose accumulation can be controlled by diet alone. This may be why the outcome of the dietary treatment of the disease is not generally as good as the treatment of PKU.

Many inborn errors of metabolism in which disease is caused by accumulation of a water-soluble metabolite resemble the galactosemia model. In order to be successful, therapeutic strategies must be developed to take into consideration the need to control endogenous production, as well as dietary intake of the toxic metabolite. In some cases, this has been achieved by pharmacologic inhibition of endogenous production of the metabolite.

Propionic acidemia

Propionic acidemia, caused by deficiency of the biotin-containing enzyme, propionyl-CoA carboxylase, is characterized by persistent metabolic acidosis as a result of propionic acid accumulation. Treatment is based on controlling propionic acid production by limiting dietary intake of propionic acid precursors: isoleucine, valine, threonine, methionine, thymine, uracil, cholesterol side-chain, and odd-chain fatty acids. The accumulation of the essential amino acids, isoleucine, valine, and threonine, is controllable to some extent by diet. The contribution of dietary and endogenously produced thymine and uracil to propionate accumulation is unknown, but it is probably small. The contribution of the side-chain of cholesterol may be important, and the cholesterol content of therapeutic diets for children with propionic acidemia should be decreased to a minimum.

What sets propionic acidemia and related organic acidopathies (methylmalonic acidemia and isovaleric acidemia) apart from other inborn errors of metabolism is the important contribution of intestinal flora to the accumulation of toxic metabolites. The normal diet contains very small amounts of odd-chain fatty acids, and they are not synthesized endogenously. However, they are produced by intestinal bacteria, which also produce large amounts of propionic acid itself in the gut. These compounds formed in the gut are rapidly absorbed and added to the total body propionic acid pool. Intermittent oral administration of non-absorbable antimicrobials, such as metronidazole, routinely causes a decrease in plasma levels of organic acid.

Control of endogenous production of substrate

Controlling the endogenous production of potentially toxic substrates is a basic aspect of the management of many inherited metabolic diseases. During intercurrent illnesses, patients with amino acidopathies or urea cycle enzyme defects are routinely treated with high-calorie, nonprotein feeds, taken either orally or intravenously, in an effort to minimize breakdown of body protein. During recovery, amino acids or protein are reintroduced into the diet in a fashion calculated to optimize reparative protein biosynthesis and avoiding starvation-induced catabolism. In the event of acute metabolic decompensation, high-calorie intakes are sometimes combined with infusions of insulin and glucose to further decrease protein breakdown and to promote protein biosynthesis during recovery.

Most of the morbidity associated with inherited fatty acid oxidation defects is preventable by avoiding high fat dietary loads or situations in which the body is required to draw on fat to meet its energy needs. This is achievable by careful adherence to a high-carbohydrate, low-fat diet and sedulous avoidance of fasting. Intervention during intercurrent illnesses should include measures to ensure adequate, uninterrupted delivery of simple carbohydrates, especially glucose, along with fluids and electrolytes. This often requires early consideration of intravenous therapy if the patient is vomiting or otherwise unable to take in adequate amounts of carbohydrate by mouth.

NTBC treatment of hepatorenal tyrosinemia

Disease in hepatorenal tyrosinemia is caused by accumulation of fumarylacetoacetate and maleylacetoacetate, intermediates in the oxidative metabolism of tyrosine. Marked improvement in infants with the disease is often achievable by carefully managed restriction of dietary phenylalanine and tyrosine intakes. However, dietary treatment has generally not arrested some of the more serious complications of the disease, such as recurrent attacks of acute porphyria and the development of cirrhosis and hepatocarcinoma. A major advance in the management of the disease was the introduction of treatment with a drug, 2-(2-nitro-4-trifluoromethylbenzoyl)-1,3-cyclohexanedione (NTBC), which blocks the production of the toxic tyrosine intermediates by inhibiting the enzyme, p-hydroxyphenylpyruvate dioxygenase (Figure 10.1).

While it is too early to determine what the overall long-term effects of treatment with NTBC will be, the short-term results have been dramatic in many infants with the disease.

Substrate reduction therapy of glycosphingolipid storage diseases

In patients with lysosomal disorders of glycosphingolipid metabolism, who have low levels of residual activity of the deficient enzyme, accumulation of the substrate is theoretically controllable by decreasing substrate production. The drug, miglustat (N-butyldeoxynojirimycin), originally developed for the treatment of HIV infection, suppresses glycosphingolipid synthesis by inhibiting the synthesis of

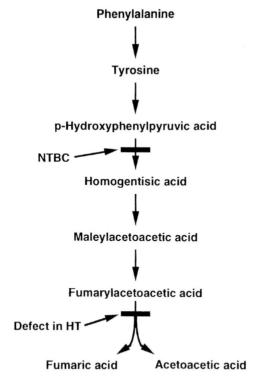

Figure 10.1 Effects of NTBC (2-(2-nitro-4-trifluoromethylbenzoyl)-1,3-cyclohexane-dione) on tyrosine metabolism.

glucosylceramide. Studies in patients with Gaucher disease have shown that short-term treatment with the drug results in decreases in the sizes of the spleen and liver, as well as improvement in hemoglobin and platelet concentrations. Clinical trials are currently underway to evaluate this approach to treatment in Fabry disease, late-onset GM2 gangliosidosis, and Niemann-Pick disease type C. Treatment with miglustat is associated with unpleasant side-effects, particularly diarrhea and weight-loss, and the safety of this approach to treatment in children has not been established. At present, it is approved in Europe and America only for the treatment of patients with Gaucher disease who are unable for some reason to tolerate enzyme replacement therapy.

Acceleration of removal of substrate

Dialysis (including peritoneal dialysis, hemodialysis, and continuous venous-venous hemofiltration)

One of the most effective methods for the rapid removal of water-soluble toxic substrates is some form of dialysis. Peritoneal dialysis is technically the least demanding.

However, it is also the slowest way to remove amino acids, organic acids, or ammonium. Hemodialysis is more rapid, but it is technically difficult to perform, particularly in neonates, because of the difficulty achieving adequate vascular access. In this respect continuous venous-venous hemofiltration (CVVH) is often preferred because it is generally easier to establish. Exchange transfusion is only effective for short periods of time. As a rule, any patient with an inherited metabolic disease who is considered a candidate for exchange transfusion, as treatment of acute metabolic decompensation, should be dialyzed.

Dialysate volumes and cycling time are probably more important variables in clearing water-soluble metabolites than the pH and composition of the fluid. Nonetheless, an alkaline pH is generally preferred for the optimum clearance of ammonium, and bicarbonate is a better anion than lactate for the treatment of severe metabolic acidosis.

Treatment of UCED with sodium benzoate and sodium phenylbutyrate

Sodium benzoate is a nontoxic food preservative, which is absorbed extremely well from the gut and condenses with glycine to form hippuric acid, which is cleared very efficiently from the circulation by the kidney. Each molecule of hippuric acid formed results in the removal of one atom of waste nitrogen. Sodium 4-phenylbutyrate is oxidized *in vivo* to phenylacetate, which is theoretically even more efficient because it condenses rapidly with glutamine to form 4-phenylacetylglutamine. Phenylacetylglutamine is excreted taking with it two waste nitrogen atoms per molecule of the drug. These medications are particularly useful for the interval control of ammonium levels in patients with UCED, and for the anticipatory management of newborn infants who are at high risk, on the basis of the family history, for having UCED.

Treatment of homocystinuria with betaine

Homocystinuria is a characteristic of a group of disorders caused by inborn errors of the biosynthesis of cystathionine by condensation of the amino acids, homocysteine and serine, and inherited defects in the methylation of the amino acid to form methionine. Cystathionine biosynthesis is catalyzed by the pyridoxine-requiring enzyme, cystathionine β-synthase (CBS) (see Figure 6.14). Initial efforts to treat CBS deficiency focused on limiting endogenous production of the amino acid through dietary methionine restriction. However, the modifications to diet necessary to maintain plasma methionine and homocysteine concentrations at normal levels are difficult, and compliance beyond early childhood is generally poor.

In patients who have homocystinuria as a result of CBS deficiency that is not responsive to pharmacologic doses of pyridoxine, homocysteine accumulation has been treated by administration of betaine (*N, N, N*-trimethylglycine). Betaine promotes methylation of the amino acid to methionine with the production of N, N-dimethylglycine (DMG) in a reaction catalyzed by the enzyme, betaine-homocysteine methyltransferase (Figure 6.14). Treatment causes increased concentrations of methionine, above the already elevated levels occurring in untreated patients with CBS deficiency. This has been a matter of some concern because methionine is toxic to the liver, at least in experimental animals. Nevertheless, betaine treatment is widely used in an effort to control the complications of homocysteine accumulation in patients with homocystinuria who are not responsive to pyridoxine therapy.

In very young infants with homocystinuria caused by defects in the methylation of homocysteine to methionine, such as severe methylenetetrahydrofolate reductase (MTHFR) deficiency, treatment with betaine has rapid and dramatic clinical effects on activity, attention, muscle tone, and feeding. The brisk response of these diseases to treatment is probably the result of restoration of tissue methionine levels to concentrations required to support the methylation reactions involved in the biosynthesis of a wide range of compounds important in the metabolism of the central nervous system.

Treatment of organic acidopathies with carnitine or glycine

In many of the inborn errors of metabolism, the substrate of the reaction affected is the coenzyme A ester of one or more low molecular weight organic acids, such as propionic acid or methylmalonic acid. Accumulation of the compounds sequesters coenzyme A making it unavailable for other important processes and reactions in which it plays a central role. These include a critical role in fatty acid oxidation (see Chapter 4), fatty acid biosynthesis, pyruvate oxidation (see Chapter 3), and a vast assortment of biological acetylations. One of the latter is acetylation of glutamate, a reaction catalyzed by N-acetylglutamate synthetase, which is required for the activation of carbamoylphosphate synthase I, the first reaction in urea biosynthesis. One of the important secondary metabolic consequences of organic acid accumulation is hyperammonemia, which appears to be caused by impaired ureagenesis resulting from insufficiency of N-acetylglutamate.

Transesterification of organic acyl-CoA ester, with the release of free coenzyme A, appears to be one of the important roles of carnitine. The formation of organic acylcarnitines not only restores free coenzyme A levels, it facilitates excretion of the organic acids because the renal clearance of acylcarnitines is greater than that of the free acids. This is the reason why accumulation of organic acids, including many drugs, ultimately causes carnitine depletion. It is also why analysis of urinary or plasma acylcarnitines by gas chromatography-mass spectrometry (see Chapter 9) is helpful in the diagnosis of inborn errors of organic acid metabolism. Treatment of organic acidopathies with carnitine is an important adjunct to the dietary management of the diseases. It restores tissue carnitine concentrations for use in processes like the transport of fatty acids into mitochondria (see Chapter 4). Carnitine treatment also contributes to ensuring adequate supplies of free coenzyme A, and it facilitates removal of toxic organic acid metabolites.

Some organic acids condense readily with glycine to form acylglycine esters. In the case of isovaleric acidemia, most of the isovaleric acid recovered in urine occurs as isovalerylglycine. The alacrity with which this occurs is exploited to enhance excretion of accumulated organic acid in the urine by treating affected patients with large oral doses of glycine.

Replacement of product

Replacement of the reaction product is the most logical approach to the management of inherited metabolic diseases in which the symptoms of disease are due to deficiency of the product. For example, this would apply to all the disorders of hormone biosynthesis. However, it also applies to metabolic situations in which intermediary metabolites become sequestrated as a result of defects in membrane transport.

Reaction product replacement

Thyroid treatment of congenital goitrous hypothyroidism

The treatment of inborn errors of thyroid hormone biosynthesis is not fundamentally different from the treatment of athyrotic hypothyroidism. Administration of thyroid hormone is all that is needed to control symptoms arising as a result of thyroid hormone deficiency. The same is true of other inherited disorders of hormone biosynthesis, such as congenital adrenal hyperplasia due to 21-hydroxylase deficiency, rickets in 25-hydroxycholecalciferol-1α-hydroxylase deficiency, megaloblastic anemia in disorders of cobalamin metabolism, and others.

Treatment of hyperammonemia-hyperornithinemia-homocitrullinemia (HHH) syndrome with ornithine

Most of the symptoms and disability associated with HHH syndrome are the result of chronic and acute-on-chronic hyperammonemia due to intramitochondrial ornithine deficiency arising from an inborn error of mitochondrial ornithine transport. Plasma ornithine concentrations in affected patients are elevated. However, a low-protein diet supplemented with pharmacologic amounts of L-ornithine greatly enhances urea biosynthesis by forcing ornithine into mitochondria where it is needed to condense with carbamoylphosphate to form citrulline, an early step in the elimination of ammonium (see Figure 2.12). This approach to management of the disease is not without some risk: excess intramitochondrial ornithine is probably what causes the ocular damage in patients with gyrate atrophy, a disease caused by intramitochondrial ornithine accumulation arising from deficiency of ornithine aminotransferase (OAT).

Treatment of argininosuccinic aciduria (ASAuria) with arginine

The hyperammonemia in patients with ASAuria is caused by intramitochondrial ornithine deficiency resulting from deficiency of arginine from which ornithine is formed by enzymic elimination of urea. Argininosuccinate lyase (ASAL) deficiency blocks the formation of arginine by ASAL-catalyzed elimination of fumaric acid in the urea cycle (see Figure 2.12). Treatment of the acute hyperammonemia in patients with ASAuria by administration of arginine, either as the hydrochloride or the free base, produces a dramatic resolution of the hyperammonemia. It is because the response to administration of arginine is so dramatic that patients with newly recognized, symptomatic hyperammonemia should be treated early with intravenous arginine hydrochloride, which is generally easily available, immediately the possibility of a UCED is considered. It may be life saving and often obviates the need for treatment with dialysis in patients with the disease.

Gene product replacement

In many inherited metabolic diseases, disease-producing accumulation of substrate is not affected by dietary manipulation or conventional pharmacologic interventions. This is the case, for example, with all the lysosomal storage disorders. The lysosomal breakdown of complex carbohydrates and lipids is a constitutive degradative process that is not significantly influenced by practical environmental manipulations. However, the relatively indiscriminant uptake of 'foreign' proteins into secondary lysosomes by the process of endocytosis has been exploited in the development of enzyme replacement strategies for the management of at least some of these diseases.

Lysosomal enzymes are synthesized in the rough endoplasmic reticulum like other proteins. In the course of biosynthesis, they are glycosylated by a complex co-translational process, followed by specific modifications of the oligosaccharide in the Golgi apparatus, which produces a recognition signal for targeting the nascent enzyme glycoprotein to primary lysosomes. This involves the production of mannose-6-phosphate residues, which bind specific receptors in lysosomal membranes. Inside primary lysosomes, further proteolytic modification of the pro-enzyme polypeptide occurs, and the mannose phosphate residues are removed. Similar systems of receptor-mediated binding and uptake of lysosomal enzymes exist at the cell surface. As a result, lysosomal enzyme infused into the circulation tend to be taken up by cells of various types and to become localized in lysosomes, precisely where they would normally become localized for the metabolism of complex, water-insoluble compounds, such as glycosphingolipids.

Early attempts to treat various lysosomal storage diseases by enzyme replacement were limited by shortages of suitably purified enzymes, adverse allergic reactions, and the inaccessibility of the target tissue, especially the brain, to infused enzyme. The development of methods to produce human enzyme on an industrial scale by recombinant DNA technology has drastically changed this situation. ERT is now generally accepted to be the treatment of choice of Gaucher disease, Fabry disease, and attenuated variants of MPS I, and clinical trials are currently in progress to evaluate the effectiveness this approach to the treatment of MPS II (Hunter disease), Pompe disease, and MPS VI (Maroteaux-Lamy disease).

Enzyme replacement therapy of Gaucher disease

The successful treatment of Gaucher disease by infusions of 'engineered' human glucocerebrosidase represents a major milestone in the management of inherited metabolic diseases. Glucocerebrosidase, originally extracted and purified from pooled human placenta, but now produced by recombinant DNA technology, is enzymically modified to remove the terminal sialic acid, galactose, and N-acetylglucosamine residues from the glycoprotein oligosaccharide. This modification of the enzyme had been shown to greatly enhance uptake by tissue macrophages by exposing mannose residues involved in receptor-mediated uptake of the enzyme. Intravenous infusion of adequate doses of suitably modified enzyme, called imiglucerase, as infrequently as every two to four weeks produces a dramatic decrease in spleen and liver sizes and improvements of hemoglobin concentrations and platelet counts in patients with Gaucher disease within a few months. The bone lesions of the disease are slower to respond to treatment. Treatment may delay, but does not prevent, the onset of neurologic symptoms in patients with acute neuronopathic Gaucher disease (type II). In patients with subacute disease (type III), the visceral manifestations of the disease respond well to enzyme replacement therapy; the effect on neurologic symptoms is still unclear.

Adverse reactions to imiglucerase treatment are rare and almost always mild. Unfortunately, expansion of the use of enzyme replacement therapy for severe non-neuronopathic Gaucher disease has been limited, not by concerns about its efficacy or safety, but by its enormous cost. The cost of the first year of treatment of an average adult with the disease could easily exceed $250,000 US.

The success of enzyme replacement of Gaucher disease has spawned numerous efforts to develop similar treatments for a wide range of lysosomal storage diseases. One of the most advanced initiatives is the treatment of Fabry disease by infusion of human lysosomal α-galactosidase, which has been shown to have dramatic effects on glycosphingolipid accumulation and symptoms of the disease.

Enzyme replacement therapy has also been approved for clinical use in the treatment of MPS I, though the role of the treatment in the most severe form of the disease, Hurler disease, has still to be established. One of the most vexing problems of enzyme replacement therapy is the apparent inability of enzyme administered intravenously to penetrate the blood-brain barrier to gain access to the brain. This severely limits the application of this approach to the management of lysosomal diseases involving the central nervous system. Clinical studies of the treatment of MPS I and Hunter disease (MPS II) have tended to focus on patients with milder variants of the diseases in which primary CNS involvement is minimal. Although studies are in progress to develop methods to circumvent the blood-brain barrier, none has so far shown significant clinical practicability.

Gene product stabilization

Over the past several years, studies on the properties of mutant proteins, including enzymes, have shown that one of the most common effects of mutations producing single amino acid substitutions is abnormal folding of the primary transcript, resulting in aggregation and rapid degradation of the polypeptide by an intracellular 'quality control' process. The details of the process are incompletely understood. What is of potentially major clinical significance is the demonstration that mutant enzymes are often catalytically active, and that treatment of mutant cells with relatively simple 'chemical chaperones' stabilizes the mutant polypeptides enough to produce marked increases in enzyme activity. At least one patient with cardiomyopathy due to Fabry disease improved clinically on treatment with intravenous galactose, which was shown to produce a signficant increase in α-galactosidase A activity in leukocytes. However, the full potential of this approach to therapy has not yet been established. One aspect of the treatment that has excited a great deal of attention is the common observation that most potential chemical chaperones do cross the blood-brain barrier readily, increasing enormously the potential for the effective treatment of lysosomal diseases affecting the CNS.

Cofactor replacement therapy

The catalytic properties of many enzymes depend on the participation of non-protein prosthetic groups, such as vitamins or minerals, as obligatory cofactors. In fact, the nutritional value of vitamins stems largely from their role as catalytically important prosthetic groups of specific enzymes (Table 10.2).

Nutritional vitamin deficiency affects most or all enzymatic reactions in which the particular vitamin plays a role as a prosthetic group. The clinical effects of nutritional vitamin deficiency cannot always be traced to the effect of the deficiency on one specific enzyme. Treatment of diseases caused by nutritional vitamin deficiencies

Table 10.2 Various cofactors involved in intermediary metabolism and implicated in some cofactor-responsive inborn errors of metabolism

Cofactor	Function	Cofactor responsive disorders
Thiamine (Vitamin B_1)	Reactions involving transfers of acetate groups (e.g., transaldolase, transketolase)	Some cases of lactic acidosis due to PDH deficiency Thiamine-responsive megaloblastic anemia–diabetes mellitus-deafness Rare cases of MSUD
Riboflavine (Vitamin B_2)	Oxidation and reduction reactions	Some cases of multiple acyl-CoA dehydrogenase deficiency (glutaric aciduria, type II)
Pyridoxine (Vitamin B_6)	Transaminations, decarboxylations, rearrangements of many amino acids	About 50% of cases of homocystinuria due to cystathionine β-synthase deficiency Pyridoxine-responsive seizures of infancy Cystathioninuria Xanthurenic aciduria Hyperornithinemia with gyrate atrophy
Cobalamin (Vitamin B_{12})	Methyl group ($-CH_3$) transfer reactions	Methylmalonic acidemia (*cblA*, *cblB*) Homocystinuria and methylmalonic acidemia (*cblC*, *cblD*, *cblF*)
Folic acid	One-carbon metabolism, particularly in nucleic acid synthesis	Some cases of homocystinuria
Ascorbic acid (Vitamin C)	Hydroxylation of proline and lysine in collagen synthesis; enzymic conversion of *p*-hydroxyphenylpyruvic acid to homogentisic acid	Some disorders of mitochondrial electron transport chain (unproven)
Biotin	Reactions involving chemical transfers of CO_2 (e.g., pyruvate carboxylase)	Biotinidase deficiency Holocarboxylase synthetase deficiency
Vitamin K	Carboxylation of glutamate residues of proteins of the blood clotting system	Some disorders of mitochondrial electron transport chain (unproven)
Cholecalciferol (Vitamin D)	Calcium absorption and mineralization of bone	Vitamin D-dependent rickets
Pantothenic acid	Functions as acyl group carrier in fatty acid and organic acid metabolism (as part of coenzyme A)	Metabolic acidosis, dystonia, seizures
Nicotinamide	Oxidation and reduction reactions throughout metabolism	Hartnup disease
Coenzyme Q_{10}	Mitochondrial electron transport	Some disorders of mitochondrial electron transport chain (unproven) Coenzyme Q_{10} deficiency
Lipoic acid	Oxidation, reduction and acyl transfer reactions (e.g., pyruvate dehydrogenase)	Some cases of PDH deficiency

Abbreviations: MSUD, maple syrup urine disease; PDH, pyruvate dehydrogenase.

by administration of amounts of the relevant vitamin only five to ten times higher than the amounts required to prevent deficiency in the first place generally results in rapid resolution of the symptoms of deficiency, though the effects of secondary tissue damage may persist.

Defects in the absorption of specific vitamins or mineral cofactors may have widespread metabolic effects similar to those produced by dietary deficiency. In some cases, the cause of the malabsorption can be traced to a genetic defect in intestinal or renal uptake caused by mutations affecting a specific receptor required for transport of the cofactor across the intestinal or renal epithelium. Whether the vitamin or cofactor deficiency is due to malabsorption resulting from acquired disease, or to a mutation affecting receptor function, the effect and the response to therapy is the same. The symptoms of deficiency are generally indistinguishable from those caused by dietary deficiency of the specific vitamin. Moreover, treatment with relatively small amounts of the vitamin, administered by injection, to circumvent the barrier of the intestinal mucosa, generally results in rapid resolution of the symptoms of deficiency. An example of this type of problem is anemia due to defects in the intestinal absorption of vitamin B_{12}. Treatment with injections of as little as 1 mg of vitamin B_{12} per month is generally sufficient to prevent the development of symptoms of deficiency.

Disease may also arise as a result of mutations affecting the normal metabolic processing of a vitamin or cofactor. For example, one form of vitamin D-dependent rickets is caused by deficiency of the enzyme that converts the relatively inactive vitamin precursor, 25-hydroxycholecalciferol, to fully active 1α, 25-dihydroxycholecalciferol. The clinical effects are indistinguishable from severe nutritional vitamin D deficiency. Treatment with very large doses of vitamin precursor or physiologic doses of the active vitamin produces rapid resolution of the symptoms of disease.

Disease may also occur as a result of mutations in the enzyme protein affecting the utilization or binding of the vitamin or mineral cofactor. In these cases, the effect of the defect is specific and limited to the reaction catalyzed by the mutant enzyme protein. In cases like this, the outcome is often clinically indistinguishable from the effects of mutations involving any other site in the enzyme protein affecting its catalytic properties. Treatment of disease caused by this class of mutations with amounts of the cofactor several hundred times the dosages generally required to prevent the development of symptoms of nutritional deficiency often results in correction of the metabolic defect and reversal of the signs of disease. These conditions have been called vitamin or cofactor *dependencies* to distinguish them from the more generalized metabolic effects of nutritional *deficiencies*, which are, moreover, correctable by low doses of the relevant vitamin or cofactor. Table 10.2 shows several examples of vitamin responsive inborn errors of metabolism.

Pyridoxine-responsive homocystinuria

CBS requires pyridoxine as a prosthetic group for catalytic activity. In about half the patients with CBS-deficiency homocystinuria, methionine and homocysteine levels in plasma are markedly decreased, and thromboembolic complications of the disease are prevented, by administration of vitamin B_6 (pyridoxine) in dosages (250 to 500 mg per day) far in excess of those necessary to prevent clinical pyridoxine deficiency in otherwise healthy humans. The catalytically active form of vitamin B_6 is pyridoxal phosphate, derived from the metabolism of dietary pyridoxal, pyridoxine, and pyridoxamine. In the course of the CBS-catalyzed reaction of serine with homocysteine, a covalently bound pyridoxal-homocysteine intermediate is formed followed by rapid condensation with serine and release of the pyridoxal aldehyde group. Pyridoxal phosphate is tightly bound by noncovalent interactions with amino acids at the active site of the apoenzyme protein. The specificity and affinity of binding are determined by the amino acid sequence of the active site, which is determined by the nucleotide sequence of the CBS gene. Pyridoxine responsiveness in some patients with homocystinuria has been shown to be caused by a decrease in the affinity of pyridoxal phosphate binding by the mutant apoenzyme with the result that the production of active holoenzyme is insufficient to control accumulation of the amino acid.

Vitamin B_{12}-responsive methylmalonic acidemia

Methylmalonic acidemia is caused by deficiency of the mitochondrial cobalamin-dependent enzyme, methylmalonyl-CoA mutase. The resulting accumulation of methylmalonic acid in tissues often causes severe metabolic acidosis (see Chapter 3). Deficiency of methylmalonyl-CoA mutase may occur as a result of mutations in the apoenzyme, or as a consequence of defects in the biosynthesis or binding of the obligatory cofactor, adenosylcobalamin. By the application of genetic complementation analysis using cultured skin fibroblasts, a number of genetically distinct defects in cobalamin metabolism have been identified in patients with methylmalonic acidemia (see Figure 3.5). *CblA* and *cblB* mutations are both characterized by specific defects in adenosylcobalamin biosynthesis, and the resulting diseases are clinically indistinguishable at presentation. However, patients with *cblA* defects respond, at least initially, to treatment with large doses of vitamin B_{12}; the response of patients with *cblB* disease is generally poor.

Biotin-responsive multiple carboxylase deficiency

Biotin participates as an obligatory cofactor in four carboxylase-catalyzed reactions: acetyl-CoA carboxylase, propionyl-CoA carboxylase, pyruvate carboxylase, and 3-methylcrotonyl-CoA carboxylase. In each case, the cofactor is bound covalently to the apoenzyme in a reaction catalyzed by the enzyme, holocarboxylase synthetase. Biotin is salvaged during the course of normal enzyme protein degradation by a reaction catalyzed by another enzyme, biotinidase. Deficiency of either holocarboxylase synthetase or biotinidase causes combined deficiency of all four carboxylases. In the first case, deficiency of holocarboxylase synthetase results in failure to form the required active holoenzymes. In the second, failure to hydrolyze the biotin from the degraded enzyme proteins ultimately results in loss of the cofactor by excretion as a protein breakdown product, producing systemic biotin deficiency. In both conditions, the response to treatment with relatively low doses (10–20 mg per day) of oral biotin is often dramatic.

Mitochondrial electron transport defects

Mitochondrial electron transport involves the participation of a number of low molecular weight, nonprotein cofactors, such as flavins, nicotinamide, ubiquinone, iron-sulfur clusters, and heme. Moreover, many compounds not normally involved in mitochondrial electron transport may function as electron transporters under special circumstances. Experience with other systems in which nonprotein cofactors are involved has stimulated attempts to treat mitochondrial electron transport chain (ETC) defects with pharmacological dosages of the various prosthetic groups normally implicated in the transport process, or by administration of other electron acceptors, such as ascorbate or various vitamin K derivatives (e.g., menadione phylloquinone).

Another approach currently being explored is to decrease reliance on electron transport via Complex I by enhancing complex II activity. This is done by treating the patient with large doses of succinate. The rationale might be better understood by reference to Figure 9.12. As a result of studies that have shown accumulation of free radical moieties in the tissues of patients with electron defects, other therapeutic efforts have focused on administration of free radical scavengers, such as dimethylglycine, in an effort to decrease tissue damage resulting from accumulation of these compounds. Dichloroacetate has been used with some success in the treatment of lactic acidosis of various sorts, including that associated with some inherited metabolic diseases. It acts by inhibiting pyruvate dehydrogenase (PDH) kinase and thereby preventing phosphorylation-mediated inactivation of PDH. What place it has in the treatment of mitochondrial ETC defects has yet to be determined.

With some notable exceptions, efforts to treat the various mitochondrial ETC defects by dietary manipulation, vitamin supplements, drugs, or physical therapy have been disappointing. Studies on the effectiveness of treatment of mitochondrial ETC defects have been seriously compromised by the rarity of the conditions, the multisystem involvement, marked clinical heterogeneity, variability of the course of the diseases in individual patients, and relative lack of sensitive means for assessment of the outcome of therapy which have made the evaluation of various treatments difficult. Although anecdotal accounts have appeared of "improvement" in patients with mitochondrial myopathies treated with various combinations of vitamins, drugs, and chemicals, few have withstood critical evaluation or efforts to duplicate the experience under rigorous clinical trial conditions.

In contrast to the situation with mitochondrial ETC defects, some other primary defects in energy metabolism, such as coenzyme Q_{10} deficiency, have been shown to respond, dramatically in some cases, to oral administration of large doses of the cofactor. Similarly, some patients with cerebral creatine deficiency resulting from defects in creatine biosynthesis have been reported to improve significantly on treatment with dietary creatine supplementation in the case of arginine:glycine amidinotransferase (AGAT) deficiency, or creatine supplementation, together with dietary arginine restriction and ornithine supplementation, in the case of guanidinoacetate methyltransferase (GAMT) deficiency.

Gene transfer therapy

The ultimate treatment of single gene disorders would be to replace the disease-producing mutant gene with a normal gene in a fashion that would ensure long-term, normally regulated expression in the tissues and organs affected by the disease. Although this might be theoretically possible by germ cell gene transfer, the risks associated with this form of treatment are generally considered to be unacceptable. Most attention on gene transfer therapies in humans has focused on treatment of somatic cells. The goal of therapy is to achieve the incorporation and expression of sufficient amounts of normal genetic material in appropriate tissues to achieve long-term correction of the genetic defect. This has been approached in two quite different ways.

Organ transplantation

Many primary genetic diseases have been 'cured' by replacement of the entire organ in which expression of the mutant gene causes disease. This is a rather indiscriminant form of gene transfer therapy, for not only is the disease-producing mutant gene replaced, but every other gene in the tissue is replaced as well. In some cases, the organ to be transplanted is so damaged that transplantation is the only way to restore normal function, and the procedure is curative because the root cause of the original organ damage is corrected and the effects of the disease on other systems or organs are either trivial or secondary to the primary organ disease (Table 10.3). In other situations, the primary enzyme defect is generalized, but the effect is primarily on one transplantable organ, at least in the first instance. These are difficult groups of patients and disorders to manage. The ultimate prognosis often

Table 10.3 Some examples of inborn errors of metabolism treatable by solid organ transplantation

Disease	Defect	Organ transplanted	Other systems involved
Disease essentially limited to transplantable organ			
Hepatorenal tyrosinemia	Fumarylacetoacetase	Liver	Renal tubular dysfunction
GSD, type I	Glucose-6-phosphatase	Liver	Renal tubular dysfunction
GSD type IV	Glycogen brancher enzyme	Liver	Skeletal myopathy, cardiomyopathy
Disease affecting primarily one transplantable organ but with significant involvement of other organ systems			
Fabry disease	Lysosomal α-galactosidase A	Kidney	Cerebrovascular disease, cardiomyopathy
Mitochondrial ETC defects	Various	Liver	Chronic and acute encephalopathy, skeletal myopathy, cardiomyopathy
		Heart	
Wilson disease		Liver	Encephalopathy
Disease primarily affecting other organ systems correctable by transplantation of otherwise healthy organ			
Crigler-Najjar, type I		Liver	Kernicterus
Primary hyperoxaluria type I		Liver or combined liver-kidney	Progressive renal impairment due to renal interstitial oxalate accumulation
FH	LDL receptor	Liver	Atherosclerosis
Organic acidopathies	Various	Liver	Recurrent metabolic acidosis with encephalopathy
UCED	Various	Liver	Recurrent hyperammonemic encephalopathy
MSUD	Branched-chain 2-ketoacid decarboxylase	Liver	Chronic and recurrent acute encephalopathy

Abbreviations: GSD, glycogen storage disease; ETC, electron transport chain; UCED, urea cycle enzyme defects; FH, familial hypercholesterolemia; LDL, low-density lipoprotein; MSUD, maple syrup urine disease.

depends on complications of the disease that only emerge after the defect in the primary organ of involvement is corrected by transplantation. In a third group of disorders, the effects of the primary enzyme defect are not on the transplantable organ, but replacement of the organ, such as the liver, corrects the metabolic abnormality causing disease as a result of damage to other non-transplantable organs or tissues. In each case, the donor liver essentially represents a 'factory' provided for the metabolism of some circulating metabolite responsible for the symptoms of disease.

In some diseases, the role of organ transplantation is clear. For example, in Crigler-Najjar syndrome, type I, liver transplantation is the only way to prevent kernicterus. It is also indicated in patients with hepatorenal tyrosinemia who are incompletely responsive to NTBC or who have already evidence of malignancy or advanced cirrhosis. Liver transplantation is the treatment of choice of primary hyperoxaluria type I, before the development of end-stage renal disease, when combined liver-kidney transplantation becomes necessary. Kidney transplantation alone is not indicated – the kidney disease invariably recurs unless the enzyme defect in liver is corrected. Kidney transplantation corrects the end-stage renal disease in Fabry disease, but it has no effect on the non-renal manifestations of the disease, which appear, however, to respond to enzyme replacement therapy.

The role of transplantation in the treatment of many inherited metabolic diseases is not as clear. Patients with glycogen storage diseases associated with cirrhosis or an increased risk of malignancy benefit, at least in the short term; the longer term risks of renal disease, advancing skeletal myopathy or cardiomyopathy appear to vary from patient to patient. Similarly, transplantation of patients with severe hepatocellular dysfunction as a result of mitochondrial electron transport chain defects generally produces salutary short-term benefits; however, the non-hepatic complications of the diseases, such as progressive encephalopathy or cardiomyopathy, invariably seriously compromise long-term outcomes.

The role of liver transplantation in the treatment of the organic acidopathies, urea cycle enzyme defects, and maple syrup urine disease is evolving. These conditions are generally manageable by dietary or mixed dietary-pharmacological treatment, though the rigors of the treatment make management particularly difficult in some patients. Pressure for transplantation usually derives from problems with compliance with dietary management as much as from the danger of metabolic decompensation. Patients generally find it easier to comply with post-transplantation monitoring and drug treatment, required to prevent and treat rejection, than the level of dietary control often required to achieve optimum results. The ultimate place of transplantation in the treatment of these diseases, particularly in older patients, remains to be established, though a rapidly growing number of patients, especially with citrullinemia or argininosuccinic aciduria, are being transplanted with apparently good results.

Bone marrow transplantation (BMT) is another form of gene transfer therapy achieved by organ transplantation. This approach to gene transfer therapy has been used with success in the management of inherited metabolic disorders of hematopoietic tissues, such as severe combined immunodeficiency (SCID) caused by adenosine deaminase (ADA) deficiency. The principle is the same as that applying in the treatment of hepatorenal tyrosinemia by liver transplantation.

In another group of diseases that do not significantly affect hematopoietic tissues, BMT is being employed as a vehicle for delivering gene product to other tissues in the body. This approach has been widely studied in the treatment of lysosomal storage diseases, especially in the mucopolysaccharidoses. It is now regarded as the treatment of choice of MPS IH (Hurler disease), as long as it can be done before age 18–24 months or before the developmental quotient of the patient falls below 70. The effectiveness of the treatment in arresting the effect of the disease on the CNS has generally been thought to be the result of re-population of macrophage-derived microglial cells with donor cells in the brain. However, the situation is almost certainly more complex. For example, while early treatment of Hurler disease (MPS IH) by BMT has a decidedly beneficial effect on the course of the disease, the same treatment has no discernable effect in children with Hunter disease or Sanfilippo disease, two other MPS disorders with prominent CNS involvement. Experience with successful BMT has shown that the non-neurological complications of Hurler disease, especially the effects on the axial skeleton and large joints, are not significantly improved by the procedure, prompting speculation that there may be a role for ERT in this group of patients post-BMT.

BMT is also indicated in the treatment of minimally symptomatic X-linked adrenoleukodystrophy. Experience with other primary metabolic neurodegenerative diseases has been mixed or insufficient to make generalizations or to produce generally accepted guidelines for treatment. Metachromatic leukodystrophy, Krabbe globoid cell leukodystrophy, Gaucher disease (type 3), and Niemann-Pick disease (type A) are a few examples of conditions in which BMT has been tried, with patchy results.

Single gene transfer therapy

Single gene transfer therapy of inherited metabolic diseases is still regarded as experimental. The approach that seems to offer the most promise at present is *ex vivo*, retrovirus-mediated gene transfer into hematopoietic stem cells for the management of diseases primarily affecting blood cells or blood cell derivatives. Clinical protocols have been approved for the evaluation of this approach to the treatment of ADA deficiency and of Gaucher disease. Protocols have also been approved for the evaluation of a similar *ex vivo* retrovirus-mediated gene transfer approach to the treatment of homozygous familial hypercholesterolemia. In this condition, liver is obtained from the patient by open biopsy, and cultured hepatocytes are transduced *ex vivo* with normal LDL receptor cDNA and infused back into the portal vein, anticipating they will become engrafted and the transgene expressed in the host liver.

Supportive measures

To say that a disease is 'untreatable' is not only untrue for even the most devastating inherited metabolic disorders, it fuels the profound sense of despair, abandonment, and loneliness the parents and relatives of a child already feel towards a situation that is both strange and forbidding. Something can almost always be done to ameliorate the child's condition. Supportive treatment may not extend the life of the stricken child, but it has the potential to add significantly to the quality of whatever weeks, months, or years of life the child is given. Measures to control discomfort, to ensure adequate nutrition, to control seizures and relieve spasticity, to facilitate feeding, to control diarrhea or prevent constipation, to prevent skin sores, to diminish the risk of aspiration, and to enhance mobility all contribute to the quality of life of the patient and indirectly to the quality of life of the parents and any unaffected siblings.

Special considerations for adults with inherited metabolic diseases

The identification of inherited metabolic diseases in adults is growing at a rapid rate. This is in part the result of advances in the management of diseases presenting in childhood, with an increasing proportion surviving and even thriving into adulthood. It is also the result of technological advances that have increased the recognition of adult variants of conditions formerly thought to be found only in children, and also the result of the identification of new diseases, specific to adults.

The management of inherited metabolic diseases in adults presents some problems that are not encountered in the treatment of children. In many respects they reflect the difference between internal medicine and pediatrics. In general terms, the management of any disorder in adults is characterized by:

- increased autonomy,
- increased expectation of independence,
- late-onset, previously unrecognized, complications of childhood diseases,
- the higher likelihood of the presence of co-morbidities, and
- problems arising from the possibility of pregnancy

The increased autonomy adults generally take for granted places increased pressure on managing physicians to ensure that the patient themselves understand the nature of their disease and the rationale for treatment. Many programs formerly focusing predominantly on children have developed transition programs to facilitate the assumption of autonomy young adults expect as they 'graduate' into adulthood. This is done through intensive and individualized education directed at ensuring that monitoring and treatment of their disease is maintained at a level appropriate for the prevention of late complications. Failure to engage this problem and to provide adequate social and dietary support services for patients at this stage inevitably results in a breakdown in therapy, sometimes with tragic consequences.

Our relative inexperience with long-term survivors of early-onset disorders increases the pressure on treating physicians to be alert for complications that might only emerge after several years. The majority of women with classical galactosemia suffer from hypergonadotrophic hypogonadism calling for anticipatory counselling, especially with respect to reproduction, and estrogen replacement therapy. The renal disease seen as a late complication of methylmalonic acidemia is another example of this type of problem. The severe late-onset skeletal complications and valvular heart disease of some of the lysosomal storage diseases are another. Patients on restrictive therapeutic diets for several years are at increased risk for the cumulative effects of subtle nutritional deficiencies, such as the hematologic and neurologic complications of vitamin B_{12} deficiency, iron deficiency anemia, and osteoporosis resulting from inadequate calcium or vitamin D intake.

The increased expectation of independence, on the part of parents and society, as well as the patients themselves, requires closer attention to the assessment of those skills specifically required for independent living. In our clinics we employ a standard questionnaire designed to assess independence with respect to activities of daily living, such as dressing, feeding and personal hygiene, as well as more complex skills, such as the ability to tell time, to handle money, the ability to use public transportation, and simple meal preparation. This type of needs assessment is mandatory for the formulation of long-term plans for the care of patients who might be intellectually challenged, but not severely mentally handicapped by their disease.

Many patients with adult-onset variants of diseases causing severe and obvious brain damage in children exhibit only relatively subtle evidence of cognitive dysfunction, in comparison with motor difficulties, for example. The continuing monitoring and management of these patients, and counselling of their families, is enhanced by the routine administration of a mini-mental status examination, suitable for use in adults, recognizing, however, that some domains are poorly sampled in some of the instruments in use. For example, the assessment of executive functioning is not covered well in some of the mini-mental status screening examinations, yet this is a sphere of mental functioning that seems to be prominently affected in some adults with inherited metabolic diseases.

The presence of co-morbidities, often attributable to self-abusive life-styles, to common adult-onset diseases, or simply to aging, is much more frequent in adults than in children. The contribution of problems like hypertension, eating disorders, diabetes, smoking, alcoholism, drug-abuse, emotional stress, and other common, acquired conditions affecting health in general, to the management of inherited metabolic diseases is a medically daunting challenge requiring patience and inge-nuity. Adults with inherited metabolic diseases are, therefore, more likely than children with similar disorders to be on treatment with a variety of prescription drugs, as well as more likely to be taking over-the-counter medications for the treatment of chronic or intercurrent problems. The potential for drug interactions is accordingly increased. Physicians trained as pediatricians may not be as familiar as internists with the management of multiple co-morbidities and the drugs used to treat them.

Pregnancy in women with inherited metabolic diseases poses some special and often challenging problems. The management of pregnancy requires attention to three questions:

What is the effect of the pregnancy on the metabolic disease? For example, pregnancy and parturition are associated with an increased risk of metabolic decompensation in women with OTC deficiency, sometimes with catastrophic effects.

What is the effect of the metabolic disease on the pregnancy? Most inherited metabolic diseases are not associated with significantly increased risks of pregnancy complica-tions. An outstanding exception are the fatty acid oxidation defects. Women who are carriers of conditions like long-chain hydroxyacyl-CoA dehydrogenase (LCHAD) deficiency, and related disorders, are at increased risk of hemolysis, elevated liver enzymes, low platelets (HELLP) syndrome and acute fatty liver of pregnancy when the fetus they are carrying is affected with the disease (see Chapter 4). Women with lysosomal storage diseases associated with dysostosis multiplex are at increased risk of requiring caesarean section for delivery of their infant.

What is the effect of the metabolic disease on the fetus? The probability that the fetus would be affected with the same disease affecting the mother is part of routine genetic counselling. The risk is generally easy to determine if the genetic diagnosis in the mother is correct and the mode of transmission is known.

The risk to the fetus resulting from the adverse intrauterine environment caused by inherited metabolic disease in the mother is generally considered to be low, with one very important and well-known exception. The risk of severe mental retardation, microcephaly, intrauterine growth retardation, and congenital heart disease is very high for the off-spring of women with poorly controlled PKU during pregnancy. The embryopathy is preventable by carefully controlled dietary phenylalanine restriction, begun before conception. However, achieving this requires a high level of commitment from the woman and strong and consistent support from the family and healthcare providers.

Physicians managing inherited metabolic diseases need to be aware that the treatment of the diseases may adversely affect the pregnancy or fetus. The nutritional protein requirements of women increase during pregnancy, something that needs to be taken into consideration in prescribing and monitoring the diets of women with aminoacidopathies or urea cycle enzyme defects who are on protein restricted diets. Little is known about the potential teratologic effects of most of the medications used to treatment metabolic diseases. None of the drugs in common use, such as vitamin B_6, vitamin B_{12}, or folic acid, appears to be obviously teratogenic, but experience is limited.

SUGGESTED READING

Baldellou, A., Andria, G., Campbell, P. E., *et al.* (2004). Paediatric non-neuronopathic Gaucher disease: recommendations for treatment and monitoring. *European Journal of Pediatrics*, **163**, 67–75.

Bosch, A. M., Grootenhuis, M. A., Bakker, H. D., Heijmans, H. S., Wijburg, F. A., Last, B. F. (2004). Living with classical galactosemia: health-related quality of life consequences. *Pediatrics*, **113**, e423–8.

Brown, A. S., Fernhoff, P. M., Waisbren, S. E., *et al.* (2002). Barriers to successful dietary control among pregnant women with phenylketonuria. *Genetics in Medicine*, **4**, 84–9.

Burdelski, M. & Ullrich, K. (1999). Liver transplantation in metabolic disorders: summary of the general discussion. *European Journal of Pediatrics*, **158** (Suppl 2), S95–S96.

Cabrera-Salazar, M. A., Novelli, E. & Barranger, J. A. 2002. Gene therapy for the lysosomal storage disorders. *Current Opinions in Molecular Therapeutics*, **4**, 349–58.

Charrow, J., Andersson, H. C., Kaplan, P., *et al.* (2004). Enzyme replacement therapy and monitoring for children with type 1 Gaucher disease: consensus recommendations. *Journal of Pediatrics*, **144**, 112–20.

Clarke, J. T. R. (2003). The maternal phenylketonuria project: a summary of progress and challenges for the future. *Pediatrics*, **112**, 1584–7.

Cox, T. M., Aerts, F. G., Andria, G., *et al.* (2003). The role of the iminosugar N-butyldeoxynojirimycin (miglustat) in the management of type I (non-neuronopathic) Gaucher disease: a position statement. *Journal of Inherited Metabolic Diseases*, **26**, 513–526.

Desnick, R. J. (2004). Enzyme replacement and enhancement therapies for lysosomal diseases. *Journal of Inherited Metabolic Diseases*, **27**, 385–410.

DiMauro, S., Mancuso, M. & Naini, A. (2004). Mitochondrial encephalomyopathies: therapeutic approach. *Annals of the New York Academy of Sciences*, **1011**, 232–45.

Enns, G. M. & Packman, W. (2002). The adolescent with an inborn error of metabolism: medical issues and transition to adulthood. *Adolescent Medicine*, **13**, 315–29.

Frustaci, A., Chimenti, C., Ricci, R., *et al.* (2001). Improvement in cardiac function in the cardiac variant of Fabry's disease with galactose-infusion therapy. *New England Journal of Medicine*, **345**, 25–32.

Grabowski, G. A. & Hopkin, R. J. (2003). Enzyme therapy for lysosomal storage disease: principles, practice, and prospects. *Annual Review of Genomics and Human Genetics*, **4**, 403–36.

Grompe, M. (2001). The pathophysiology and treatment of hereditary tyrosinemia type 1. *Seminars in Liver Disease*, **21**, 563–71.

Hanley, W. B. (2004). Adult phenylketonuria. *American Journal of Medicine*, **117**, 590–5.

Ioannou, Y. A., Enriquez, A. & Benjamin, C. (2003). Gene therapy for lysosomal storage disorders. *Expert Opinion on Biological Therapeutics*, **3**, 789–801.

Koch, R., Hanley, W., Levy, H., *et al.* (2003). The Maternal Phenylketonuria International Study: 1984–2002. *Pediatrics*, **112**, 1523–9.

Krivit, W., Peters, C. & Shapiro, E. G. (1999). Bone marrow transplantation as effective treatment of central nervous system disease in globoid cell leukodystrophy, metachromatic leukodystrophy, adrenoleukodystrophy, mannosidosis, fucosidosis, aspartylglucosaminuria, Hurler, Maroteaux-Lamy, and Sly syndromes, and Gaucher disease type III. *Current Opinions in Neurology*, **12**, 167–76.

Lee, P. J. (2002). Growing older: the adult metabolic clinic. *Journal of Inherited Metabolic Diseases*, **25**, 252–60.

MacDonald, A. (2000). Diet and compliance in phenylketonuria. *European Journal of Pediatrics*, **159** (Suppl 2), S136–41.

Pastores, G. M. & Barnett, N. L. 2003. Substrate reduction therapy: miglustat as a remedy for symptomatic patients with Gaucher disease type 1. *Expert Opinion on Investigational Drugs*, **12**, 273–81.

Pastores, G. M. & Thadhani, R. (2002). Advances in the management of Anderson-Fabry disease: enzyme replacement therapy. *Expert Opinion on Biological Therapeutics*, **2**, 325–33.

Pastores, G. M., Weinreb, N. J., Aerts, H., *et al.* (2004). Therapeutic goals in the treatment of Gaucher disease. *Seminars in Hematology*, **41** (Suppl 5), 4–14.

Peters, C., Steward, C. G.; National Marrow Donor Program; International Bone Marrow Transplant Registry; Working Party on Inborn Errors, European Bone Marrow Transplant Group. (2003). Hematopoietic cell transplantation for inherited metabolic diseases: an overview of outcomes and practice guidelines *Bone Marrow Transplantation*, **31**, 229–39.

Peters, C., Charnas, L. R., Tan, Y., *et al.* (2004). Cerebral X-linked adrenoleukodystrophy: the international hematopoietic cell transplantation experience from 1982 to 1999. *Blood*, **104**, 881–8.

Platt, F. M., Jeyakumar, M., Andersson, U., *et al.* (2001). Inhibition of substrate synthesis as a strategy for glycolipid lysosomal storage disease therapy. *Journal of Inherited Metabolic Diseases*, **24**, 275–90.

Platt, L. D., Koch, R., Hanley, W. B., *et al.* (2000). The international study of pregnancy outcome in women with maternal phenylketonuria: report of a 12-year study. *American Journal of Obstetrics and Gynecology*, **182**, 326–33.

Rouse, B. & Azen, C. (2004). Effect of high maternal blood phenylalanine on offspring congenital anomalies and developmental outcome at ages 4 and 6 years: the importance of strict dietary control preconception and throughout pregnancy. *Journal of Pediatrics*, **144**, 235–9.

Russo, P. A., Mitchell, G. A. & Tanguay, R. M. (2001). Tyrosinemia: a review. *Pediatric and Developmental Pathology*, **4**, 212–21.

Schwahn, B. C., Hafner, D., Hohlfeld, T., Balkenhol, N., Laryea, M. D. & Wendel, U. (2003). Pharmacokinetics of oral betaine in healthy subjects and patients with homocystinuria. *British Journal of Clinical Pharmacology*, **55**, 6–13.

Schiffmann, R. & Brady, R. O. (2002). New prospects for the treatment of lysosomal storage diseases. *Drugs*, **62**, 733–42.

Schon, E. A. & DiMauro, S. (2003). Medicinal and genetic approaches to the treatment of mitochondrial disease. *Current Medicinal Chemistry*, **10**, 2523–33.

Scriver, C. R. & Lee, P. J. (2004). The last day of the past is the first day of the future: transitional care for genetic patients. *American Journal of Medicine*, **117**, 615–7.

Singh, R. H., Kruger, W. D., Wang, L., Pasquali, M. & Elsas, L. J., II. (2004). Cystathionine beta-synthase deficiency: effects of betaine supplementation after methionine restriction in B6-nonresponsive homocystinuria. *Genetics in Medicine*, **6**, 90–5.

Van den Hout, J. M., Kamphoven, J. H., Winkel, L. P., *et al.* (2004). Long-term intravenous treatment of Pompe disease with recombinant human alpha-glucosidase from milk. *Pediatrics*, **113**, e448–57.

Walter, J. H., Collins, J. E. & Leonard, J. V. (1999). Recommendations for the management of galactosaemia. *Archives of Disease in Childhood*, **80**, 93–6.

Weinreb, N. J., Aggio, M. C., Andersson, H. C., *et al.* (2004). Gaucher disease type 1: revised recommendations on evaluations and monitoring for adult patients. *Seminars in Hematology*, **41** (Suppl 5), 15–22.

Weinreb, N. J., Charrow, J., Andersson, H. C., *et al.* (2002). Effectiveness of enzyme replacement therapy in 1028 patients with type 1 Gaucher disease after 2 to 5 years of treatment: a report from the Gaucher Registry. *American Journal of Medicine*, **113**, 112–9.

Widaman, K. F. & Azen, C. (2003). Relation of prenatal phenylalanine exposure to infant and childhood cognitive outcomes: results from the International Maternal PKU Collaborative Study. *Pediatrics*, **112**, 1537–43.

Wraith, J. E., Clarke, L. A., Beck, M., *et al.* (2004). Enzyme replacement therapy for mucopolysaccharidosis I: a randomized, double-blinded, placebo-controlled, multinational study of recombinant human alpha-L-iduronidase (laronidase). *Journal of Pediatrics*, **144**, 581–8.

Zimran, A. & Elstein, D. (2003). Gaucher disease and the clinical experience with substrate reduction therapy. *Philosophical Transactions of the Royal Society London B: Biological Sciences*, **358**, 961–6.

Index